A Professional Guide to Management
and Nutrition Education Resources

Diabetes Medical Nutrition Therapy

Harold J. Holler, RD
Joyce Green Pastors, MS, RD

THE AMERICAN DIETETIC ASSOCIATION/AMERICAN DIABETES ASSOCIATION

ISBN: 0-88091-146-8

©1997, The American Dietetic Association. All rights reserved. No part of this publication may be reproduced, stored in a retrieval system, or transmitted in any form or by any means, without the prior written consent of the publisher. Printed in the United States of America.

The views expressed in this publication are those of the authors and do not necessarily reflect policies and/or official positions of The American Dietetic Association. Mention of product names in this publication does not constitute endorsement by the authors or The American Dietetic Association. The American Dietetic Association disclaims responsibility for the application of the information contained herein.

10 9 8 7 6 5 4 3 2 1

Contributors

Harold J. Holler, RD
Governance Team, Association Management Group
The American Dietetic Association
Chicago, Illinois

Joyce Green Pastors, MS, RD
Diabetes Nutrition Specialist
University of Virginia Diabetes Center
Charlottesville, Virginia

Co-authors/ Editors

Sections from Chapters 1, 2, 4, 5, 6, 8, and 9 were adapted with permission from *Maximizing the Role of Nutrition in Diabetes Management*, published by the American Diabetes Association in 1994. The following authors contributed to that publication.

Marion Franz, MS, RD
International Diabetes Center
Minneapolis, Minnesota

Karmeen Kulkarni, MS, RD
Diabetes Treatment Center, St Mark's Hospital
Salt Lake City, Utah

Carolyn Leontos, MS, RD
Nevada Cooperative Extension
Las Vegas, Nevada

Melinda Maryniuk, MEd, RD, FADA
Joslin Diabetes Center
Boston, Massachusetts

Sue McLaughlin, RD
Consultant in Private Practice
Omaha, Nebraska

Margaret A. Powers, MS, RD
Powers and Associates
St. Paul, Minnesota

Contributing Authors
(Chapters 1, 2, 4, 5, 6, 8, and 9)

Contributing Authors
(Other Chapters)

Robert Anderson, EdD
Michigan Diabetes Research and Training Center
Ann Arbor, Michigan

Marilynn S. Arnold, MS, RD
Michigan Diabetes Research and Training Center
Ann Arbor, Michigan

David S. Bell, MD
University of Alabama Medical School
Birmingham, Alabama

Brenda A. Broussard, MPH, MBA, RD
Indian Health Service Diabetes Program
Albuquerque, New Mexico

Anne Daly, MS, RD
Springfield Diabetes and Endocrine Center
Springfield, Illinois

Marion Franz, MS, RD
International Diabetes Center
Minneapolis, Minnesota

Sandy Gillespie, MMSc, RD, FADA
Atlanta Diabetes Associates
Atlanta, Georgia

Lea Ann Holzmeister, RD
Phoenix Children's Hospital
Phoenix, Arizona

Karmeen Kulkarni, MS, RD
Diabetes Treatment Center, St Mark's Hospital
Salt Lake City, Utah

Melinda Maryniuk, MEd, RD, FADA
Joslin Diabetes Center
Boston, Massachusetts

Mary Lou Perry, MS, RD
University of Virginia Health Sciences Center
Department of Nutrition Services
Charlottesville, Virginia

Margaret A. Powers, MS, RD
Powers and Associates
St. Paul, Minnesota

Rebecca S. Reeves, DrPH, RD, FADA
Baylor College of Medicine
Houston, Texas

Reviewers

Hope Warshaw, MMSc, RD
Hope Warshaw Associates
Alexandria, Virginia

Madelyn L. Wheeler, MS, RD, FADA
Diabetes Research & Training Center
Indiana University Medical Center
Indianapolis, Indiana

Phyllis Barrier, MS, RD
American Diabetes Association
Alexandria, Virginia

Mary Carey, PhD, RD
MGH Institute of Health Professions
Boston, Massachusetts

Melinda Maryniuk, MEd, RD, FADA
Joslin Diabetes Center
Boston, Massachusetts

Rebecca Schafer, MS, RD
VA Medical Center
Bay Pines, Florida

Madelyn L. Wheeler, MS, RD, FADA
Diabetes Research & Training Center
Indiana University Medical Center
Indianapolis, Indiana

Editorial Coordinator

Gill Robertson, MS, RD
Nutrition Writer/Editor
Sun Prairie, Wisconsin

Contents

Foreword xi
Preface xiii

**Part I
Diabetes Management**

Chapter 1. Introduction to Diabetes Medical Nutrition Therapy 3
The Diabetes Control and Complications Trial 4
The American Diabetes Association 1994
  Nutrition Recommendations 4
Scope of Practice for Qualified Dietetics Professionals 5
Nutrition Practice Guidelines 7
Summary 7

Chapter 2. Classification, Pathophysiology, and Diagnosis of Diabetes 9
Impact of Diabetes 9
Classification of Diabetes 9
Pathophysiology of Diabetes 10
Diagnosis 13
Summary 14

Chapter 3. Management of Diabetes: Medical Nutrition Therapy 15
Diabetes Control and Complications Trial (DCCT) 15
The 1994 American Diabetes Association
  Nutrition Recommendations 17
Goals of Medical Nutrition Therapy for Type I Diabetes 18
Goals of Medical Nutrition Therapy for Type II Diabetes 18
Nutrient Recommendations 19
Nutrition Practice Guidelines 26
Summary 27

Chapter 4. Management of Diabetes: Exercise 29
Metabolic Effects of Exercise 29
Benefits of Exercise 30
Risks of Exercise 31
Exercise Recommendations 32
Exercise Guidelines 32
Summary 33

vii

Chapter 5.	**Management of Diabetes: Medications**	35
	David S. Bell	
	Oral Glucose-Lowering Medications	35
	Insulin	37
	Insulin Regimens	39
	Insulin Pumps	41
	Summary	42
Chapter 6.	**Management of Diabetes: Self-Monitoring of Blood Glucose**	43
	Frequency of Monitoring	43
	Reviewing Blood Glucose Monitoring Records	45
	Summary	49
Chapter 7.	**Management of Diabetes: Intensive Insulin Therapy**	51
	Sandy Gillespie	
	Selecting Insulin Regimens	51
	Glucose Monitoring	53
	Insulin Adjustment	53
	Candidates for IIT	56
	Clinical Setting	58
	Length of Time to Teach	58
	Advantages/Disadvantages	58
	Summary	59
Chapter 8.	**Management of Diabetes: Different Life Stages**	61
	Children and Adolescents	61
	Pregnancy	64
	Older Adults	68
Chapter 9.	**Management of Diabetes: Complications**	75
	David S. Bell	
	Acute Complications	75
	Chronic Complications	78
	Summary	82
Chapter 10.	**Special Topics in Meal Planning**	83
	Alcohol	83
	Delay of Meals	86
	Eating Out	86
	Snacking	87
	Hypoglycemia	88
	Sick-Day Management	91

Part II
Diabetes Nutrition Education

Chapter 11. From Philosophy to Practice — 95
Robert Anderson and Marilynn S. Arnold

Chapter 12. Process of Diabetes Medical Nutrition Therapy — 99
- Nutrition Assessment — 99
- Goal Setting — 105
- Intervention — 106
- Evaluation — 107
- Summary — 110
- Case Study — 111

Part III
Basic Nutrition Intervention

Chapter 13. Introduction to Basic Nutrition Intervention — 127
- Time Frame — 128
- Other Issues That Should Be Addressed — 128
- Educational Resources — 129

Chapter 14. Basic Nutrition Guidelines — 131
- *Dietary Guidelines for Americans* — 131
- *Guide to Good Eating* — 132
- *Food Guide Pyramid* — 134

Chapter 15. Diabetes Nutrition Guidelines — 137
Madelyn Wheeler, Brenda Broussard, Margaret Powers, and Marion Franz
- The First Step in Diabetes Meal Planning — 137
- *Healthy Food Choices* (Guideline Section) — 139
- *Healthy Eating* — 142

Chapter 16. *Single-Topic Diabetes Resources* — 147
Lea Ann Holzmeister and Hope Warshaw
- Definition — 147
- Historical Background — 148
- Method of Use — 148
- Intended Population — 150
- Clinical Setting — 151
- Length of Time to Teach — 151
- Advantages/Disadvantages — 151

Part IV
In-depth Nutrition Intervention

Chapter 17. Introduction to In-depth Nutrition Intervention — 155
- Advancing to the In-depth Stage of Nutrition Intervention — 155
- In-depth Nutrition Educational Resources — 156

Chapter 18. Menus — 157
Melinda Maryniuk and Anne Daly
- Individualized Menus — 157
- *Month of Meals* — 161
- Summary — 165

ix

Chapter 19.	**Exchanges**	167
	Exchange Lists for Meal Planning	167
	Healthy Food Choices (Poster Section)	175
Chapter 20.	**Carbohydrate Counting**	179
	Sandy Gillespie, Anne Daly, and Karmeen Kulkarni	
	Definition	179
	Historical Background	180
	Method of Use	180
	Intended Population for Use	188
	Clinical Setting	189
	Length of Time to Teach	189
	Advantages/Disadvantages	189
	Summary	190
Chapter 21.	**Calorie and Fat Counting**	193
	Mary Lou Perry and Rebecca S. Reeves	
	Calorie Counting	193
	Fat Counting	195

Part V
Case Studies and Conclusion

Chapter 22.	**Case Studies of Clinical Application**	201
	Case Study 1	201
	Case Study 2	206
	Case Study 3	215
	Case Study 4	217
	Case Study 5	223
	Case Study 6	228
	Case Study 7	231
Chapter 23.	**Conclusion**	245
	Diabetes Medical Nutrition Therapy	245
	Diabetes Nutrition Education Resources	245

Appendixes

Appendix 1. Laboratory Values for Diabetes Mellitus	251
Appendix 2. Clinical Data	252
Appendix 3. Nutrition History	256
Appendix 4. Diabetes Knowledge Checklist	259
Appendix 5. Goal Setting	260
Appendix 6. Sample Completed *Single-Topic Diabetes Resources* Handouts	261
Appendix 7. Database for the *Exchange Lists for Meal Planning*	265
Index	285

Foreword

People with diabetes mellitus have to coordinate foods, exercise, and possibly medication (oral glucose-lowering agents or insulin) to normalize their blood glucose and other metabolic parameters. They must learn to self-manage by monitoring, recognizing patterns, and changing behavior (eating and physical activity) and perhaps medications as well. None of the over 16 million people in the United States who have diabetes can accomplish this monumental task by themselves. All of these people need the expertise and counseling skills of a number of health professionals on a continuing basis. One of the major players in this team approach is the dietitian, with the skills and expertise he or she has to offer via diabetes medical nutrition therapy.

But what does this abstract term *diabetes medical nutrition therapy* mean? How can we integrate the many aspects of diabetes medical nutrition therapy, such as practice guidelines, outcomes evaluation, nutrition assessment, goal setting, behavior change, and interventions, into a global "picture"? *Diabetes Medical Nutrition Therapy* helps us do just that! It provides concrete, applicable information and a framework within which we can help all people with diabetes to reach their goals.

This book follows a number of significant recent events, including:

▶ The Diabetes Control and Complications Trial (DCCT), which proved that dietitians could make a difference in diabetes outcomes. These techniques used in the DCCT intervention (for example, carbohydrate counting) needed to be shared on a nationwide level.
▶ Updated diabetes nutrition recommendations, based on current scientific evidence. Not only do these recommendations need to be disseminated and implemented in clinical practice, but also up-to-date nutrition resources to reflect them.

This book also pulls together a number of resources:

▶ The expertise of the Clinical Education Program Developed by the American Diabetes Association and The American Dietetic Association's Diabetes Care and Education Practice Group, exemplified in *Maximizing the Role of Nutrition in Diabetes Management,*
▶ The ever-changing arena of meal-planning methods, based on the first and second editions of *Meal Planning Approaches for Diabetes Management,*

➤ The mandate of The American Dietetic Association's and the American Diabetes Association's Diabetes Nutrition Education Resources Steering Committee that methods for use of products newly developed or updated must be disseminated to dietitians and other interested health practitioners.

Joyce Green Pastors and Harold Holler have done a superb job of merging this diverse but relevant and necessary information into one integrated resource. The book's framework is the cyclic, four-step process of assessment, goal setting, intervention, and evaluation, and diabetes practice guidelines provide the key components. This is not an abstract textbook. It is filled with practical information, sample forms to use, and case studies which illustrate the use of meal-planning resources. Educators will find this book appropriate for use as a text for undergraduate students majoring in nutrition and dietetics, as well as for dietetic interns. It is a must for all dietitians who encounter clients with diabetes. And other health professionals will welcome this book as it provides the nutrition perspective for the team approach to treatment of diabetes.

Madelyn L. Wheeler, MS, RD, FADA

Coordinator, Research Dietetics
Diabetes Research and Training Center
Indiana University School of Medicine

Chairman, The American Dietetic Association's and
American Diabetes Association's Diabetes Nutrition Education
Resources Steering Committee, 1993–1995

Preface

Diabetes medical nutrition therapy is an extremely important aspect of diabetes self-management training. This publication is intended to provide guidance during the various stages of diabetes medical nutrition therapy. The role of the registered dietitian is to provide leadership and expertise in the area of diabetes medical nutrition therapy. The nurse educator's role, as well as that of other members of the diabetes care team, is to support the nutrition-related goals and intervention provided by the registered dietitian. However, in some instances the nurse educator may initiate intervention if a dietitian is not available. When a client's needs extend beyond one's resources or skills in nutrition assessment and intervention, he or she should be referred to a dietitian with expertise in diabetes medical nutrition therapy.

In fact, all health professionals caring for people with diabetes should have a clear understanding of the process of diabetes medical nutrition therapy. This process requires a considerable amount of time and should be viewed as a critical component of diabetes care.

This professional guide incorporates components of two previously published resources: *Maximizing the Role of Nutrition in Diabetes Management*[1] and *Meal Planning Approaches for Diabetes Management*.[2] In addition, the publication includes discussions related to the newly developed/revised nutrition education resources created by The American Dietetic Association and American Diabetes Association Diabetes Nutrition Education Resources Steering Committee:

➤ *The First Step in Diabetes Meal Planning* (Chapter 15)
➤ *Exchange Lists for Meal Planning*, 1995 edition (Chapter 19)
➤ *Carbohydrate Counting*, Levels 1, 2, and 3 (Chapter 20)
➤ *Facilitating Lifestyle Change: A Resource Manual* (Chapter 12)
➤ *Single-Topic Diabetes Resources* (Chapter 16)

This guide emphasizes the need to individualize meal plans through the process of medical nutrition therapy. It is divided into five sections:

Part I — Diabetes Management
Part II — Diabetes Nutrition Education
Part III — Basic Nutrition Intervention
Part IV — In-Depth Nutrition Intervention
Part V — Case Studies and Conclusion

In addition, the appendixes provide the reader with laboratory values, tables for collection of nutrition assessment data, and the Exchange/Carbohydrate Counting Database. The database contains the nutrient composition that was used to develop the 1995 *Exchange Lists for Meal Planning* and the *Carbohydrate Counting* food lists. It will serve as a valuable resource for professionals and clients.[3]

This professional guide reviews knowledge that should be integrated into medical nutrition therapy so that improved blood glucose control can be achieved. It is the integration of medical, nutritional, and behavioral sciences that enables registered dietitians to make a significant difference in the lives of people with diabetes. Patients need more than just a meal plan—they need the integrated care that a diabetes care team can provide. This guide emphasizes the need to individualize meal plans through the process of diabetes medical nutrition therapy. We hope it will challenge you to broaden your nutrition intervention approach and implement some of the information into your current practice.

Harold J. Holler, RD
Joyce Green Pastors, MS, RD

1. *Maximizing the Role of Nutrition in Diabetes Management.* Alexandria, Va: American Diabetes Association; 1994.
2. Diabetes Care and Education Dietetic Practice Group of The American Dietetic Association. *Meal Planning Approaches for Diabetes Management.* 2nd ed. Chicago, Ill: The American Dietetic Association; 1994.
3. Wheeler ML, Franz M, Barrier P, Holler H, Cronmiller N, Delahanty LM. Macronutrient and energy database for the 1995 Exchange Lists for Meal Planning: A rationale for clinical practice decisions. *J Am Diet Assoc.* 96(11):1167–1171.

Part 1
Diabetes Management

Introduction to Diabetes Medical Nutrition Therapy

The term *medical nutrition therapy* was introduced in 1994 by The American Dietetic Association primarily because of legislative efforts to promote reimbursement. It is defined as the use of specific nutrition services to treat an illness, injury, or condition and involves two phases: 1) assessment of the nutritional status of the client and 2) treatment, which includes diet therapy, counseling, and the use of specialized nutrition supplements.[1]

Nutrition services are vital in the treatment of diabetes, and reimbursement of these services is of paramount importance in the current evolutionary period of health care. Thus, the term *diabetes medical nutrition therapy* is more commonly used today than either *diabetes nutrition management* or *diabetes nutrition education*. However, because of the chronic nature of diabetes, the definition of diabetes medical nutrition therapy has been expanded to include not only assessment and treatment, but also goal setting and evaluation. Therefore, diabetes medical nutrition therapy stresses a four-pronged approach that includes:

➤ assessment of the client's metabolic, nutrition, and lifestyle parameters;
➤ identification and negotiation of nutrition goals;
➤ intervention designed to achieve the individualized goals;
➤ evaluation of the outcomes.[2]

In this approach an individually developed nutrition prescription based on metabolic, nutrition, and lifestyle requirements replaces a simple calculated caloric prescription. As with insulin regimens and exercise programs, no one nutrition prescription will work for all people with diabetes. For most people, this means modifying—not abandoning—their usual eating habits.

Diabetes medical nutrition therapy is integral to total care and management of diabetes. It can be successfully implemented by evaluating self-monitoring of blood glucose (SMBG) records, by recommending medication adjustments, and by teaching about hypoglycemia and the interactions of diabetes medication, food, and activity. In this approach, *evaluation of changes* expands upon the typical nutrition review of lipids, blood pressure, and body weight, and includes HbA_{1c} and SMBG results. Diabetes medical nutrition therapy is critical for achieving and maintaining optimal glycemic control.

Several recent milestone events, which will be discussed in depth, have influenced and altered the status of diabetes medical nutrition therapy. These include the following:

- the Diabetes Control and Complications Trial (DCCT) results, which highlighted the successful use of diverse meal-planning approaches and innovative teaching techniques;[3]
- the American Diabetes Association's 1994 Diabetes Nutrition Recommendations, which emphasized the need for individualizing diabetes medical nutrition therapy;[4,5]
- the Diabetes Care and Education dietetic practice group's Scope of Practice for Qualified Professionals in Diabetes Care and Education,[6] which assists dietetics professionals in understanding their roles and responsibilities and promoting effective communication with other members of the diabetes care team; and
- practice guidelines for diabetes medical nutrition therapy, which provide a systemic approach to increasing the quality and consistency of therapy.[7,8]

The Diabetes Control and Complications Trial

Recent results from the DCCT corroborate findings of studies published as early as the 1960s, and have laid to rest the long-standing debate over whether improving glycemic control is worthwhile.[9] Blood glucose control does indeed make a difference in the onset and progression of diabetes complications. Diabetes medical nutrition therapy, integrated with blood glucose monitoring, is essential in establishing and maintaining improved control of blood glucose levels.

The DCCT was a multicenter, prospective, randomized clinical trial designed to compare the effects of intensive insulin therapy, aimed at achieving blood glucose levels as close to normoglycemia as possible, with the effects of conventional therapy on early microvascular complications of type I diabetes.[9] The results of the DCCT have provided valuable information about the role of nutrition intervention in intensive diabetes therapy, especially in demonstrating that many nutritional intervention strategies can be used to achieve consistency in eating and promotion of a more healthful eating pattern. The DCCT demonstrated that the registered dietitian is an integral members of the diabetes care team, and that individualized diabetes medical nutrition therapy and self-management training are vital aspects of diabetes management.[3] The DCCT is examined in more detail in Chapter 3.

The American Diabetes Association 1994 Nutrition Recommendations

The revised "Nutrition recommendations and principles for people with diabetes mellitus" were issued by the American Diabetes Association[4] and endorsed by The American Dietetic Association in 1994.[10] The revised nutrition recommendations mandate:

- a comprehensive approach to diabetes medical nutrition therapy;
- an individualized nutrition prescription based on assessment and treatment goals.

This approach demands more resources than traditional methods and eliminates the universal "diabetic" or "ADA" diet. However, this approach to diabetes medical nutrition therapy can be more effective in assisting an individual with management of his or her diabetes. Detailed information about overall and specific nutritional goals for all people with diabetes is presented in Chapter 12.

Scope of Practice for Qualified Dietetics Professionals

The scope of practice for qualified dietetics professionals in diabetes care and education has expanded beyond simply providing nutrition care.[6] As a diabetes educator, the dietetics professional is now responsible for promoting self-management of diabetes. Communication and effective participation with other members of the diabetes care team are essential to providing proper support to clients with diabetes.

Various health care professionals function as diabetes educators, including registered dietitians (RDs), registered nurses, physicians, pharmacists, social workers, podiatrists, mental health professionals, and exercise specialists. Recognized diabetes education programs now require a dietitian to be a member of the program staff and the diabetes education advisory committee.[11] Education, experience, and credentials determine the level at which dietetics professionals provide and implement diabetes medical nutrition therapy. The three providers of diabetes medical nutrition therapy are:

➤ the dietetic technician, registered (DTR);
➤ the registered dietitian (RD); and
➤ the RD/certified diabetes educator (CDE).

Dietitians who are certified as diabetes educators are uniquely qualified to provide diabetes self-management training, and have expanded their involvement in content areas outside nutrition, such as program management. The appropriate roles for the DTR, RD, and RD/CDE are summarized in *Table 1.1*.

The benefits of a team approach to diabetes management are well documented.[12,13] A diabetes care team consists, at minimum, of a physician, a dietitian (in some practice settings the team may include a dietetic technician), and a nurse *(Figure 1.1)*. More comprehensive teams may include a social worker, pharmacist, podiatrist, mental health professional, or exercise specialist with expertise and special interest in diabetes. However, the client with diabetes should be the central focus, and it should be remembered that he or she is a key member of the diabetes care team. Regardless of the composition of the diabetes care team, communication among its members is critical for integrated and comprehensive care. All members of the team must understand the recommendations of diabetes medical nutrition therapy and agree with the goals in order to provide support to the client with diabetes.

The dietitian should lead the nutritional aspect of self-management and coordinate team efforts to assist the client with diabetes in achieving success.

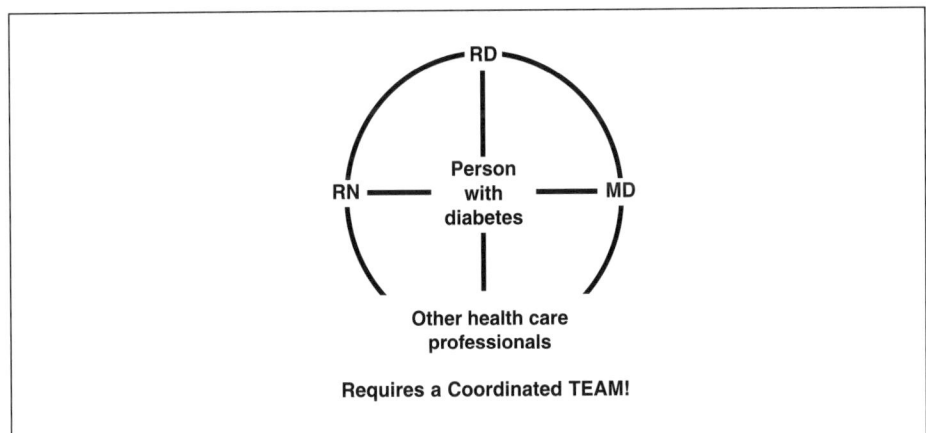

Figure 1.1
Achieving Nutrition Goals

Adapted with permission from *Maximizing Nutrition in Diabetes Management* (Alexandria, Va: American Diabetes Association; 1994).

Table 1.1 Roles and Responsibilities

DTR Roles

- Complete nutrition screening.
- Provide basic diabetes nutrition information.
- Explain restaurant dining and alcohol use guidelines.
- Provide label-reading guidelines.
- Recommend use of modified foods, as appropriate.
- Collaborate and communicate with health care professionals (eg, physician, nurse, RD).

RD Roles

The RD may perform all of the duties mentioned for the DTR, plus the following.

- Complete nutrition assessments.
- Negotiate nutrition goals with the client.
- Provide and individualize an eating plan. (This constitutes more than just an exchange list. An RD may use other types of meal-planning approaches.)
- Recommend and implement modifications to the eating plan to address complications of diabetes.
- Recommend behavior modification, as appropriate.
- Evaluate and adjust a client's plan and goals based on blood glucose levels.
- Explain management of hypoglycemia and hyperglycemia.
- Provide sick-day guidelines for food intake.
- Develop/maintain educational resources appropriate to practice needs.
- Monitor outcomes of diabetes medical nutrition therapy, and revise therapy as needed.
- Monitor and collect data on referral patterns and reimbursement practices.
- Advocate for legislation to improve diabetes care.
- Participate as a member of the multidisciplinary diabetes care team.
- Use a variety of nutrition intervention and lifestyle change strategies.
- Coordinate exercise and diabetes medical nutrition therapy strategies.

RD/CDE Roles

The RD/CDE may perform all of the duties described for the DTR and the RD, plus the following.

- Provide in-depth information on the pathophysiology of diabetes and an overview of diabetes management.
- Provide sick-day management guidelines, beyond those relating to food intake.
- Teach the use of blood glucose meters, depending on the practice setting.
- Interpret blood glucose results and discuss adjustments in food, insulin, or medication.
- Interpret appropriate laboratory results and recommend changes in therapy.
- Review the effect of insulin or oral glucose-lowering medications on blood glucose levels.
- Teach insulin preparation and injection skills/techniques, depending on the practice setting.
- Guide clients to establish problem-solving skills.
- Help select clients as candidates for intensive insulin therapy.
- Recommend protocols to ensure quality diabetes care.
- Refer clients to other team members, as appropriate.
- Provide professional expertise to other members of the diabetes care team and the community.
- Develop, coordinate, and manage diabetes education programs.
- Market diabetes management services to primary care, family practice, and specialty physicians.

Source: Scope of practice for qualified professionals in diabetes care and education, *J Am Diet Assoc*, 1995; 95:607–608.

As members of the diabetes care team, dietitians are in a unique position to explain the relationship of eating variables to blood glucose results, insulin dosage, and episodes of hypoglycemia and hyperglycemia. Effective team management requires dietitians to be knowledgeable about overall diabetes management to effectively integrate nutrition into the medical care and education of clients with diabetes.

Nutrition Practice Guidelines

To assist dietetics professionals in applying the revised nutrition recommendations for diabetes management, nutrition practice guidelines for type I[7] and type II[8] diabetes have been developed to define care that is medically necessary and appropriate in the identification, treatment, or management of specific conditions. Practice guidelines should define care that consistently leads to desired outcomes. More information about nutrition practice guidelines for diabetes is presented in Chapter 3.

Summary

Diabetes medical nutrition therapy is complex, and proper implementation requires changes in practice patterns and in systems for providing diabetes medical nutrition therapy. Health care professionals can no longer depend on preprinted diet sheets, formulated meal patterns, or even computer-individualized meal plans to provide nutrition care to clients with diabetes. They must carefully consider their own approach to education and counseling and how this impacts their effectiveness in counseling clients with diabetes.

This publication has been designed for dietetics professionals and other members of the diabetes care team. It will help them to understand the current management of diabetes and how to effectively empower clients to take responsibility for their diabetes self-care management.

References

1. ADA's definition for nutrition screening and nutrition assessment. *J Am Diet Assoc.* 1994;94(8):838–839.
2. Tinker LF, Heins JM, Holler HJ. Commentary and translation: 1994 nutrition recommendations for diabetes. *J Am Diet Assoc.* 1994;94(5):507–511.
3. Diabetes Control and Complications Trial Research Group. Expanded role of the dietitian in the Diabetes Control and Complications Trial: implications for clinical practice. *J Am Diet Assoc.* 1993;93(7):758–767.
4. Nutrition recommendations and principles for people with diabetes mellitus (position statement). *Diabetes Care.* 1994;17(5):519–522.
5. Franz MJ, Horton ES, Bantle JP, Brunzell JD, Coulston AM, Henry RR, Hoogwerf BJ, Stacpoole PW. Nutrition principles for the management of diabetes and related complications (technical review). *Diabetes Care.* 1994;17(5):490–518.
6. Scope of practice for qualified professionals in diabetes care and education. *J Am Diet Assoc.* 1995;95(5):607–608.
7. Leontos C, Splett PL. Nutrition practice guidelines for Type I diabetes mellitus: development and field testing. *Diabetes Spectrum.* 1996;9(2):128–130.
8. Monk A, Barry B, McClain K, Weaver T, Cooper N, Franz MJ. Practice guidelines for medical nutrition therapy provided by dietitians for persons with non-insulin-dependent diabetes mellitus. *J Am Diet Assoc.* 1995;95(9):999–1006.

9. Diabetes Control and Complications Trial Research Group. The effect of intensive treatment of diabetes on the development and progression of long-term complications in insulin-dependent diabetes mellitus. *N Engl J Med.* 1993; 329(14):977–986.
10. Nutrition recommendations and principles for people with diabetes mellitus. *J Am Diet Assoc.* 1994;94(5):504–506.
11. National standards for diabetes self-care management education programs and American Diabetes Association review criteria. *Diabetes Care.* 1995;18(5):737–741.
12. American Diabetes Association. Standards of medical care for patients with diabetes mellitus. *Diabetes Care.* 1996;19(1):S8–S15.
13. Etzwiler DD. Primary-care teams and a systems approach to diabetes management. *Clinical Diabetes.* 1994;12(3):50, 52.

Classification, Pathophysiology, and Diagnosis of Diabetes

Impact of Diabetes

Diabetes mellitus (types I and II) is a chronic disease that affects almost 16 million Americans—approximately 6% of the population. Nearly 11% of the US population aged 65 to 74 years has diabetes.[1] It results in a considerable increase in morbidity and mortality and is the fourth leading cause of death by disease. Although early diagnosis and treatment can reduce the morbidity and mortality, 8 million Americans, which is 50% of the total population of clients with diabetes, are undiagnosed.[2]

Classification of Diabetes

Diabetes mellitus is a clinically and genetically heterogeneous disorder characterized by elevated blood glucose levels. It occurs because insulin, produced by the beta cells of the pancreas, is either absent, insufficient, or not used properly by target tissues. As a result, the body is unable to normally metabolize macronutrients (carbohydrate, protein, and fat) in foods. When insulin is absent or ineffective, the body cannot convert glucose into energy, and the level of glucose in the blood increases. Elevated blood glucose levels can lead to both short-term and long-term health-related complications.[1] There are several types of diabetes: type I diabetes, type II diabetes, impaired glucose tolerance (IGT), and gestational diabetes mellitus (GDM).

Type I Diabetes

Five to 10 percent of known cases of diabetes are type I diabetes. The onset of type I primarily occurs before the age of 30 years. Clients with type I diabetes produce little or no insulin, indicating insulin deficiency. To survive, they must depend on daily injections of insulin. They are prone to the development of ketoacidosis, a serious condition marked by extremely high blood glucose and ketone levels. Left untreated, ketoacidosis can progress to unconsciousness and death.[1]

Type II Diabetes

A far greater percentage of people with diabetes—90% to 95%—have type II diabetes. Type II diabetes primarily appears after the age of 40 years. In people with type II diabetes, insulin levels may be normal, depressed, or elevated. Typically, high insulin levels, indicating insulin resistance (decreased tissue sensitivity or responsiveness to insulin), are present. Low insulin levels often develop as the disease progresses. People with type II diabetes are not prone to ketoacidosis during normal circumstances, unless they are under physical stress, such as during illness.[1] Type II diabetes is managed by nutrition and lifestyle changes, although oral glucose-lowering medication and/or supplemental insulin may be necessary. Type II diabetes was once considered mild and easy to treat, but it is now known to result in extensive morbidity and mortality. Approximately 40% of clients with type II diabetes require insulin injections to achieve glycemic control.

Impaired Glucose Tolerance (IGT)

Impaired glucose tolerance describes plasma glucose levels that are higher than normal but lower than those considered diagnostic for diabetes mellitus. Twenty-five percent of clients with IGT eventually develop diabetes mellitus.[3] Many clients with IGT are obese; with weight loss, glucose tolerance reverts to normal. Although clients with IGT do not appear to have increased risk for the microvascular (small-vessel) complications of diabetes mellitus, in some populations it has been shown that clients with IGT have a greater-than-normal risk for atherosclerotic disease.[3] Therefore, the treatment goals for IGT depend on the degree of fatness, blood pressure, and evidence of hyperlipidemia. Management of IGT is based on nutrition and lifestyle changes, rather than the administration of medication to lower blood glucose.[3]

Gestational Diabetes Mellitus (GDM)

Gestational diabetes mellitus describes glucose intolerance that is first detected during pregnancy. GDM occurs during pregnancy in about 2% to 5% of all pregnant women, or in approximately 90,000 American women each year, usually during the second or third trimester.[1] This makes it the most common medical disorder affecting pregnancy. It appears to occur only rarely in women younger than 20 years of age. The frequency is greater in women who are older, obese, or who have a family history of diabetes. Although glucose tolerance returns to normal after delivery in the vast majority of these women, 30% to 40% of them eventually develop type II diabetes 10 to 20 years postpartum.[1] Those who maintain a reasonable body weight and exercise on a regular basis have been shown to have a decreased incidence of type II diabetes.

Pathophysiology of Diabetes

The etiology of diabetes is genetically influenced; diabetes often occurs in people with a family history of the disease, although the pattern of inheritance is unknown. Heredity is believed to be a stronger factor in type II than in type I diabetes; other risk factors for type II diabetes are obesity and aging. Ethnic and geographic factors also seem to play a role in the incidence of diabetes. Americans of Puerto Rican, African, Mexican, and Cuban descent are 1.5 to 3.0 times more likely than white Americans to develop type II diabetes.[2] The highest rate of diabetes in the United States, as well as in the world, is found in the Pima Indians of Arizona, where approximately 50% of the population has type II diabetes. It is also widespread and increasing in other Native American groups.[1] Also, the incidence of type I diabetes is lower in Asia and higher in northern Europe.

Type I Diabetes

Type I diabetes is in part an inherited disorder. Geneticists have discovered that certain genetic markers, histocompatibility locus antigens (HLAs), are often found in children who develop diabetes. HLAs are glycoproteins present on all human cell membranes, including the pancreatic beta cells. The exact function of these antigens is unknown, although they are believed to be involved in the detection and destruction of foreign substances in the body, such as viruses and bacteria. Research has shown that certain gene combinations seem to make some people more prone to diabetes. But genes do not cause diabetes on their own. Other events have to occur to make diabetes emerge.[4]

Current theory holds that most people who are susceptible to the development of type I diabetes, because of their genetic predisposition, develop the disease when an environmental stress factor triggers a series of events that result in damage to, or destruction of, the pancreatic beta cells. Viruses may be one such stress factor. The onset of type I diabetes often coincides with or follows infections with mumps, rubella, measles, encephalitis, polio, Epstein-Barr, and Coxsackie viruses.[4] Although viruses seem to be involved in at least some cases of type I diabetes, and although some families have more than one person with diabetes, it is not contagious. The best explanation of why diabetes occurs in some families is that the family members share genes that make them prone to diabetes.

That type I diabetes is an autoimmune disorder is based on the observation that the majority of clients at diagnosis have circulating antibodies to islet cells, to endogenous insulin, and/or to other antigens that are constituents of islet cells. Unlike type II diabetes, it is rarely associated with excess body fat.[4]

Type II Diabetes

Certain predisposing factors make some clients more likely to develop type II diabetes. These risk factors include family history, sedentary lifestyle, obesity, and aging. Type II diabetes is characterized by two primary defects: 1) insulin resistance (diminished tissue sensitivity to insulin) and 2) impaired beta-cell function (delayed or inadequate insulin release). Nearly all clients with type II diabetes exhibit a delayed or sluggish glucose-stimulated insulin response, and most clients have a diminished response. This defective insulin-secretion response of the beta cells of the pancreas results in slow and ineffective suppression of glucose production from the liver and decreased glucose uptake by the peripheral tissues. Hyperglycemia results and provides constant stimulation for insulin secretion.

The resultant chronic hyperinsulinemia causes insulin resistance in the peripheral tissues in two ways. First, since insulin receptors are regulated by ambient insulin levels, high circulating levels of insulin cause "down-regulation" of insulin receptors, referred to as the *binding defect*. Second, chronic hyperinsulinemia can lead to postbinding defects in the metabolism of glucose. This occurs in the peripheral tissues, where uptake of glucose by muscle tissue is decreased, and in the liver, where insulin fails to decrease hepatic glucose production *(Figure 2.1)*. These defects result in elevated glucose levels despite apparently normal or higher than normal insulin levels. The resultant chronic hyperglycemia may further impair insulin secretion and function.

Although defects in insulin secretion and insulin action are clearly present once type II diabetes is established, it is often unclear which defect is the primary or initiating event. Regardless of which defect arises first, the resulting hyperglycemia is thought to play a role in sustaining these defects, a role sometimes referred to as *glucose toxicity (Figure 2.2)*.

Figure 2.1
Pathophysiology of Type II Diabetes

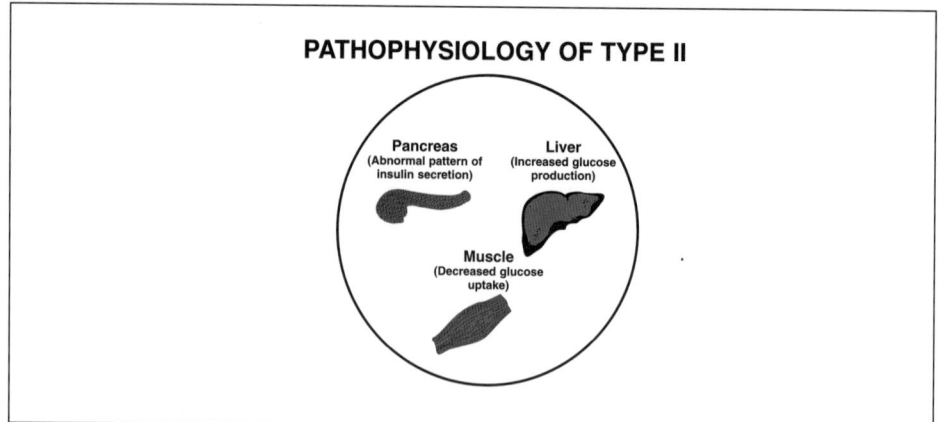

Reprinted with permission from R De Fronzo et al, *Diabetes*, 1988, 37: 667–687.

Figure 2.2
Glucose Toxicity

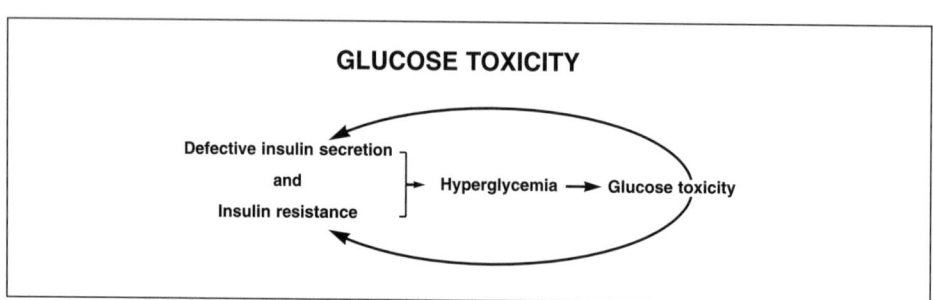

Reprinted with permission from *Maximizing Nutrition in Diabetes Management* (Alexandria, Va: American Diabetes Association; 1994).

Glucose toxicity helps explain the role of chronic hyperglycemia and the resulting vicious cycle. Defective insulin secretion and/or insulin resistance contributes to hyperglycemia.

Impaired Glucose Tolerance

The pathophysiology of IGT is similar to that of type II diabetes; it is just not yet exaggerated enough to cause levels of blood glucose in the range considered diagnostic for type II diabetes.

Gestational Diabetes Mellitus

From the 24th to the 28th week of pregnancy, the body's need for insulin increases dramatically. Two to three times as much insulin is needed during pregnancy to maintain glucose homeostasis. This insulin resistance is a result of the hormones produced for pregnancy (estrogen and progesterone). Another hormone, human placental lactogen (HPL), is a potent insulin antagonist. HPL enhances fat mobilization and reduces maternal glucose utilization and protein degradation so the fetus has a plentiful supply of glucose and amino acids.[5] Insulinase, produced by the placenta, degrades insulin, reducing its supply even further.

Risks for GDM include a history of GDM during an earlier pregnancy, delivery of a previous macrosomic infant (birth weight >9 pounds), a family history of diabetes, maternal obesity (>120% ideal body weight), and older age.

Diagnosis

Diagnosis should be made on the basis of plasma glucose levels. The choice of diagnostic tests and their interpretation are different for nonpregnant adults, children, and pregnant women. Specifically, the criteria for diagnosis in children are more conservative. The following are the criteria for diagnosis of diabetes in various groups.[3,4,6]

Diabetes in Nonpregnant Adults

Criteria for diagnosing diabetes mellitus in nonpregnant adults should be restricted to those who have *at least one* of the following:

- random plasma glucose level higher than 200 mg/dL, plus classic signs and symptoms of diabetes mellitus, including polydipsia, polyuria, polyphagia, and weight loss;
- fasting plasma glucose higher than 140 mg/dL on at least two occasions;
- fasting plasma glucose lower than 140 mg/dL plus sustained elevated plasma glucose levels during at least two oral glucose tolerance tests. The 2-hour sample and at least one other between 0 and 2 hours after a 75-g glucose dose should be higher than 200 mg/dL.

IGT in Nonpregnant Adults

Diagnosis of impaired glucose tolerance in nonpregnant adults should be restricted to those who have *all* of the following:

- fasting plasma glucose less than 140 mg/dL;
- 2-hour tolerance test: plasma glucose between 140 and 200 mg/dL;
- intervening oral glucose tolerance test: plasma glucose greater than 200 mg/dL.

Gestational Diabetes

After a 100-g oral glucose load, diagnosis of gestational diabetes may be made if *two* plasma glucose values equal or exceed the following:

- fasting: 105 mg/dL;
- 1 hour: 190 mg/dL;
- 2 hours: 165 mg/dL;
- 3 hours: 145 mg/dL.

Diabetes in Children

Diagnosis of diabetes mellitus in children should be restricted to those who have *at least one* of the following:

- random plasma glucose higher than 200 mg/dL plus classic signs and symptoms, including polyuria, polydipsia, ketonuria, and rapid weight loss;
- fasting plasma glucose higher than 140 mg/dL on at least two occasions and sustained elevated plasma glucose levels during at least two oral glucose tolerance tests;
- both the 2-hour plasma glucose and at least one other between 0 and 2 hours should be higher than 200 mg/dL after the glucose dose is administered (1.75 g/kg ideal body weight up to 75 g).

Summary

The various forms of glucose intolerance have a tremendous impact on the health status and health care costs of millions of Americans. Although these disorders differ in etiology and pathology, all manifest in abnormal glucose tolerance. If not appropriately managed, the resulting hyperglycemia can cause serious acute and long-term complications.

References

1. American Diabetes Association. *Diabetes 1996: Vital Statistics*. Alexandria, Va: American Diabetes Association; 1996: 3, 7, 8, 13, 14.
2. National Institutes of Health, National Institute of Diabetes and Digestive and Kidney Diseases. *Diabetes in America*. 2nd ed. NIH Publication No. 95-1468, 1995: 1, 52.
3. American Diabetes Association. *Medical Management of Non-Insulin-Dependent Diabetes Mellitus*. 3rd ed. Alexandria, Va: American Diabetes Association; 1994: 6, 9.
4. American Diabetes Association. *Medical Management of Insulin-Dependent Diabetes Mellitus*. 2nd ed. Alexandria, Va: American Diabetes Association; 1994: 11–12.
5. Metzger BE. Pregnancy and diabetes. In: Powers MA, ed. *Handbook of Diabetes Medical Nutrition Therapy*. Gaithersburg, Md: Aspen Publishers, Inc; 1996: 504–506.
6. American Diabetes Association. Office guide to diagnosis and classification of diabetes mellitus and other categories of glucose intolerance. *Diabetes Care*. 1996;19(1):S4.

Management of Diabetes: Medical Nutrition Therapy

3

Diabetes medical nutrition therapy should be accomplished using a four-pronged approach. The first step is a comprehensive nutrition assessment that includes metabolic, nutrition, and lifestyle parameters. The second step is setting goals with the client; these goals must be practical, achievable, and acceptable for the client with diabetes. The third step, nutrition intervention, must incorporate a variety of meal-planning and nutrition education resources that clients with diabetes can easily understand and use. The fourth step is evaluation, which reassesses how the goals have been accomplished and indicates areas for future self-management education.

This chapter presents information that will assist implementation of the four-pronged approach to diabetes medical nutrition therapy. The chapter reviews the results of the Diabetes Control and Complications Trial (DCCT), describes current nutrition recommendations from the American Diabetes Association, differentiates goals of diabetes medical nutrition therapy for type I and type II diabetes, and discusses nutrition practice guidelines for type I and type II diabetes.

Diabetes Control and Complications Trial (DCCT)

The DCCT was a 10-year clinical trial involving 1,441 participants between the ages of 13 and 39 years.[1] They were randomized into two therapy groups, receiving either conventional or intensive therapy. Within the two groups, subgroups of those with no sign of retinopathy at entry into the study were compared to those with mild retinopathy. There were 726 with no retinopathy (primary prevention) at baseline and 715 with mild retinopathy (secondary prevention).

Conventional therapy consisted of one or two daily insulin injections, self-monitoring of blood glucose, routine contact with a physician and the case manager (dietitian or nurse) four times a year, and nutrition education as requested by the participant. Changes in overall management were made if the participant was symptomatic (ie, had polyuria at nighttime or frequent hypoglycemia) or if the glycosolated hemoglobin (HbA_{1c}) value was above an upper limit.

Intensive therapy consisted of three or more daily insulin injections, with the premeal dose of regular insulin adjusted according to blood glucose monitoring results, planned food intake, and anticipated exercise. Each participant in this group was in weekly (at times daily) contact with his or her DCCT case manager and had with monthly visits with the DCCT staff.

Table 3.1
DCCT Results

Reprinted with permission from *Maximizing the Role of Nutrition in Diabetes Management* (Alexandria, Va: American Diabetes Association, 1994).

Intensive management/blood glucose control made a difference.

- 76% reduction in retinopathy
- 60% reduction in neuropathy
- 54% reduction in albuminuria
- 39% reduction in microalbuminuria

Implication: Improved blood glucose control also applies to persons with type II diabetes.

Dietitians had the flexibility to tailor the nutrition intervention approach to each volunteer's lifestyle and capability.[2] The ability to match the meal-planning approach to the participant's needs and individualize the frequency of follow-up as needed promoted better adherence and attainment of treatment of goals. Participants receiving intensive treatment had the same clinical goals as those receiving conventional treatment. They also had specific blood glucose targets (70 to 120 mg/dL preprandially, less than 180 mg/dL postprandially, and HgbA$_{1c}$ values less than 6.05%).

The results demonstrated definitively that blood glucose control, as achieved in the intensive therapy group, effectively delays the onset and slows the progression of long-term complications of type I diabetes: retinopathy, neuropathy, and nephropathy[3] *(Table 3.1)*.

The results were significant for both subgroups in the intensive therapy group. For example, neuropathy was reduced by 60% in the intensive therapy group. The development of microalbuminuria was decreased by 39% in people with no signs of renal disease at entry into the study, and the progression of more severe kidney damage (albuminuria) was slowed by more than 54%. Also, risk for developing retinopathy was reduced by 76% for those in the primary prevention group and its progression was slowed by 54% in the secondary prevention group compared to the conventional therapy groups.

The pathogenesis and natural history of the complications of diabetes are similar in both type I and type II diabetes. Therefore, it is assumed that blood glucose control as near to normal as possible is just as important for clients with type II diabetes as for those with type I diabetes. Any intensification in management that results in an improvement in glycemic control contributes to reduced risk for complications.

Promoting changes in personal eating habits is among the most challenging aspects of diabetes care for the client with diabetes and the diabetes care team.[4] The DCCT affirmed the importance of meal planning in achieving and maintaining desired blood glucose levels *(Figure 3.1)*.

Adopting the nutrition recommendations encourages clients with diabetes to make challenging lifestyle changes, including learning about nutrition and modifying eating habits. Yet emphasis on nutrition education, lifestyle change, and follow-up is often lacking.

The DCCT[2] provided valuable information about the role of nutrition intervention in intensive diabetes therapy, including the following:

- Certain individual profiles and eating habits predict a client's ability to adhere to intensive diabetes treatment.

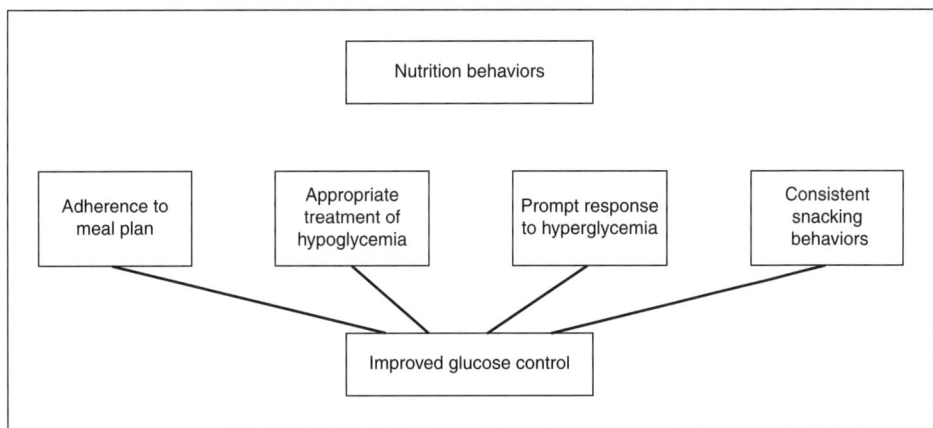

Figure 3.1
Nutrition Behaviors

Reprinted with permission from LM Delahanty and BN Halford, *Diabetes Care*, 1993;16(11):1453–1458.

➤ There are many nutrition intervention strategies that can be used to achieve consistency in eating and promotion of a more healthful eating pattern. The dietitian is the best-qualified health care professional to match appropriate meal-planning approaches to the client's needs and goals.

➤ Careful attention to the relationship between food and insulin is necessary to achieve $HgbA_{1c}$ goals without undue hypoglycemia and weight gain.

➤ Variations in food intake, such as overconsumption of food to treat hypoglycemia and eating extra nighttime snacks, often explain erratic blood glucose results, which are associated with higher $HgbA_{1c}$ levels. As members of the diabetes care team, dietitians are in a unique position to explain the relationship of variability in food consumption to blood glucose results, insulin dosage, and episodes of hypoglycemia and hyperglycemia.

The 1994 American Diabetes Association Nutrition Recommendations

The 1994 nutrition recommendations from the American Diabetes Association[5] strongly state that a dietitian should individualize the diabetes medical nutrition therapy for each client with diabetes. This includes self-management education to promote optimal glycemic control. The goals of diabetes medical nutrition therapy for all people with diabetes are as follows:

➤ achieve blood glucose goals;
➤ achieve optimal blood lipid levels;
➤ provide appropriate calories for reasonable weight, normal growth and development, and pregnancy and lactation;
➤ prevent, delay, or treat nutrition-related complications; and
➤ improve health through optimal nutrition.

These goals can be achieved when the diabetes care team is knowledgeable about diabetes medical nutrition therapy. The team must be able to assess each client's status and individual needs, and should be committed to educating and encouraging each client to participate fully in his or her own diabetes medical nutrition therapy.

Figure 3.2

Nutrition Therapy for Type I Diabetes

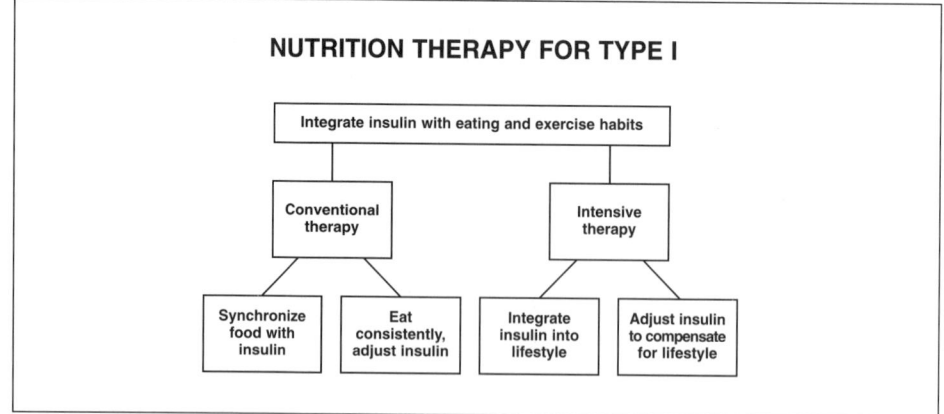

Reprinted with permission from *Maximizing the Role of Nutrition in Diabetes Management* (Alexandria, Va: American Diabetes Association, 1994).

Goals of Medical Nutrition Therapy for Type I Diabetes

For clients with type I diabetes, medical nutrition therapy should emphasize the interrelationships among food, exercise, and insulin. Those receiving conventional insulin therapy must maintain consistency in the timing and amount of their food intake. Ideally, the insulin plan should be designed to match the client's preferred eating pattern. The 1976 nutrition recommendations were for total calories and carbohydrate to be "fractionated" between meals and snacks based on the insulin regimen (eg, 2⁴/₁₀ for meals and ¹/₁₀ for snacks in a split-mixed dosage).[6] This is no longer recommended because it does not promote individualization. However, the timing of food intake should be synchronized with the administration of insulin. Because of the limitations of a conventional insulin regimen (ie, 1 to 2 insulin injections per day), clients on such a regimen may need to alter their usual eating habits by incorporating consistency with timing and amounts of food[5,7] *(Figure 3.2)*.

Clients receiving intensive insulin therapy, ie, multiple daily injections or pump infusion, have considerable flexibility in when and what to eat. Nevertheless, they too need to integrate their insulin regimen with their lifestyle and adjust the insulin dose when they deviate from their usual eating and exercise patterns. These clients can adjust their premeal insulin dose to compensate for departures from their meal plan and exercise program. Even with the increase in flexibility, the more consistent they are with their eating and physical activity, the easier overall management is.[8,9]

Goals of Medical Nutrition Therapy for Type II Diabetes

Blood glucose and lipid goals join weight loss to a reasonable weight (as defined in Chapter 12) as the focus of therapy for overweight clients with diabetes. This recognizes the fact that modification of fat intake, spacing and size of meals, exercise, and reasonable weight loss can be effective in achieving blood glucose and lipid goals in clients with type II diabetes.[5,7]

The primary goal for clients with type II diabetes should be to achieve and maintain near normal blood glucose levels. Making healthy food choices, especially modifying calorie intake, can be beneficial. A moderate caloric modification (250–500 calories less than the average daily intake) and increase in physical activity may lead to improved weight control.

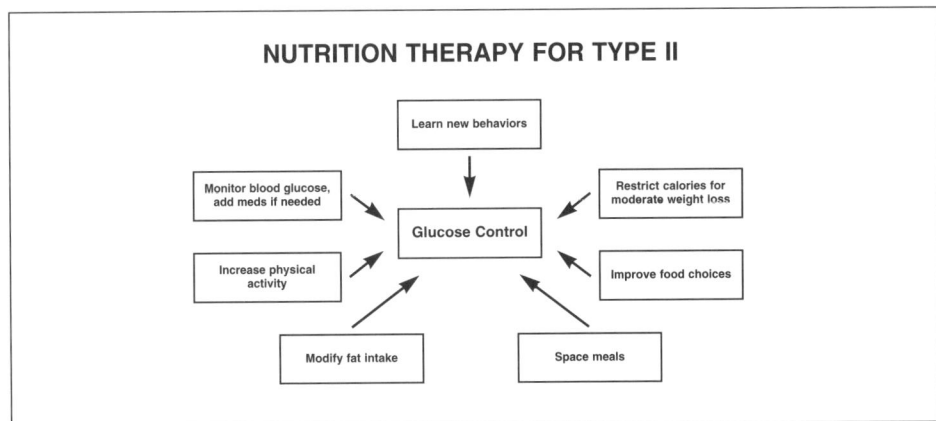

Figure 3.3

Nutrition Therapy for Type II Diabetes

Reprinted with permission from *Maximizing the Role of Nutrition in Diabetes Management* (Alexandria, Va: American Diabetes Association, 1994).

In addition, modifying fat intake may be associated with a reduction in energy intake and weight loss. A nutritionally adequate meal plan with a modification in fat, especially saturated fat, should be implemented. Research has shown that even a weight loss of 5% to 10% is sufficient for improving glycemic control.[5] Weight loss appears to increase insulin sensitivity and normalize hepatic glucose production.

The research on the efficacy of very-low-calorie diets (VLCDs) is inconclusive.[10] Both VLCDs and low-calorie meal plans lead to weight loss and weight regain. VLCDs may be slightly beneficial to clients with type II diabetes because caloric restriction has been shown to improve insulin resistance and blood glucose response. It is unclear, however, if this makes a difference over an extended period of time. More studies need to be conducted investigating other creative alternatives to VLCDs, such as intermittent fasting, which may achieve improved insulin resistance without the yo-yo effect of weight loss and regain.

Due to the impaired insulin secretion in clients with type II diabetes, smaller meals and snacks spaced more frequently throughout the day may prevent exaggerated postmeal hyperglycemia.[10] Also, regular exercise can promote improved metabolic control and weight management.[5] In addition, learning new behaviors and attitudes can promote long-term lifestyle changes. The strategies that have been discussed to promote improved metabolic control for clients with type II diabetes are highlighted in *Figure 3.3*.

Monitoring blood glucose, glycosolated hemoglobin, lipids, and blood pressure is essential to evaluate nutrition-related strategies. If metabolic parameters do not improve, oral glucose-lowering medication, insulin, or lipid-lowering or antihypertensive drugs may be required.[5]

Nutrient Recommendations

One important aspect of diabetes management is optimal nutrition, achieved by the consumption of the proper types and amounts of protein, fat, and carbohydrate. Guidelines for their consumption and that of other nutrition components are provided in the American Diabetes Association recommendations.[5,10] A historic perspective of the distribution of total calories from past American Diabetes Association recommendations is summarized in *Table 3.2*.[7]

Table 3.2
Historic Perspective

Year	Distribution of Calories		
	CHO (%)	Protein (%)	Fat (%)
Before 1921	Starvation diets		
1921	20	10	70
1950	40	20	40
1971	45	20	35
1986	50–60	12–20	30
1994	A	10–20	A, B

A: Based on nutrition assessment.
B: < 10% saturated fat.

Reprinted with permission from *Maximizing the Role of Nutrition in Diabetes Management* (Alexandria, Va: American Diabetes Association, 1994).

Protein

Since current scientific evidence does not support either higher or lower intakes of protein by clients with diabetes, the recommendation for intake is similar to that for the general population: 10% to 20% of total calories.

In clients with type I diabetes and overt diabetic nephropathy, restriction of dietary protein has been shown to retard the progression to renal failure.[11] There is some evidence that this may also be true for people with type II diabetes. Therefore, a protein intake of approximately the adult Recommended Dietary Allowance (RDA), 0.8 g/kg body weight per day (generally equivalent to 10% of daily total calories), is recommended for clients with evidence of macroalbuminuria.[11] However, it has been suggested that once the glomular filtration rate (GFR) begins to fall, further restriction to 0.6 g/kg/day may prove useful in showing the decline of GFR in selected clients. On the other hand, nutrition deficiency may result in some individuals and may be associated with muscle weakness. Nutrition recommendations for clients with renal insufficiency require an individualized approach. In clients with type I and type II diabetes and microalbuminuria, there is inconclusive evidence that a low-protein diet slows the progression of nephropathy.[11]

There is some evidence that the protein source, whether animal or vegetable in origin, may be important in affecting the progression of renal disease.[11] However, the studies are preliminary. If beneficial renal effects of vegetable proteins are confirmed, less drastic dietary protein restriction may be required in the treatment of diabetic nephropathy. Additional research is needed in this area.[12]

Fat

Total fat intake is not specified in the 1994 recommendations. However, guidelines for reducing cardiovascular risk are emphasized. If dietary protein contributes 10% to 20% of total calories, 80% to 90% remains to be distributed between dietary carbohydrate and fat.[5] Less than 10% of caloric intake should be from saturated fats, and daily cholesterol intake should be limited to 300 mg or less. Up to 10% of calories can be from polyunsaturated fats (PUFAs). This leaves 60% to 70% of the calories from monounsaturated fats (MUFAs) and carbohydrates.[5]

The recommended calories from fat depend on desired blood glucose and lipid levels and weight outcomes. The general recommendation for the US population is to limit total dietary fat to 30% or less of total calories, with emphasis on reduction in saturated fat to decrease the risk for developing heart disease. This recommendation continues to apply to people with diabetes who have normal lipid levels and a reasonable body weight. However, if obesity and weight loss are the primary issues, a reduction in dietary fat to reduce caloric intake and weight, combined with increased physical activity, should be considered.

If elevated low-density lipoprotein (LDL) cholesterol is the primary problem, the National Cholesterol Education Program (NCEP) Step II dietary guidelines (7% of total calories from saturated fat, 30% of calories from total fat, and 200 mg/day of dietary cholesterol) should be implemented.[5,13]

If elevated triglycerides and very-low-density lipoprotein (VLDL) cholesterol are the primary concerns, a moderate increase in monounsaturated fat intake, with less than 10% of calories from saturated fats and a more moderate intake of carbohydrate, may be implemented. Clinical studies have shown that a diet with increased monounsaturated fats can lower plasma triglycerides, glucose, and insulin levels more than a high-carbohydrate diet in some individuals.[14,15]

Carbohydrate

The 1994 nutrition recommendations do not specify an amount of carbohydrate. This should be individualized according to current eating habits, treatment goals, metabolic control, and the presence of other medical conditions.[5]

Although various carbohydrates produce different glycemic responses, from a clinical perspective the total amount of carbohydrate consumed is more important than the source of the carbohydrate.[16] The daily total and distribution should be individualized and based on each client's eating habits and blood glucose and lipid goals.

Sucrose

Scientific evidence does not justify the longtime belief that sucrose must be restricted in the meal plans of people with diabetes, based on the assumption that sucrose is more rapidly digested and absorbed than starches and thereby aggravates hyperglycemia. At least 12 studies[10] in which sucrose was substituted for starches found no adverse effect on glycemia. Thus, sucrose can be substituted for other carbohydrates, gram for gram in the context of a healthy meal plan.

Nevertheless, it is still good advice to suggest that clients with diabetes be cautious about consuming foods that contain sucrose. Foods containing sucrose contain minor amounts of vitamins and minerals and tend to be high in fat. Even though these foods do not affect blood glucose levels as previously thought, they do not make a significant contribution to a client's nutrient intake.

When used, sucrose and sucrose-containing foods must be substituted for other carbohydrates and not simply added to the meal plan. Results of two studies[17,18] in which sucrose was substituted for starch in the diets of persons with diabetes are representative of reported research.

In the first study[17] *(Figure 3.4)*, 12 subjects with type II diabetes substituted 19% of calories from sucrose for starch in otherwise comparable diets for 28 days. Since the average reported US intake of sucrose is appropriately 14% of caloric intake, the 19% of calories from sucrose in the study was slightly higher than average intake. No significant differences occurred in average blood glucose levels; fasting and total high-density lipoprotein (HDL) cholesterol, LDL cholesterol, and triglyceride levels; or peak postprandial triglyceride levels when 19% of calories came from sucrose or when less than 3% of calories came from sucrose.

Figure 3.4

Sucrose and Blood Glucose Values (Type II)

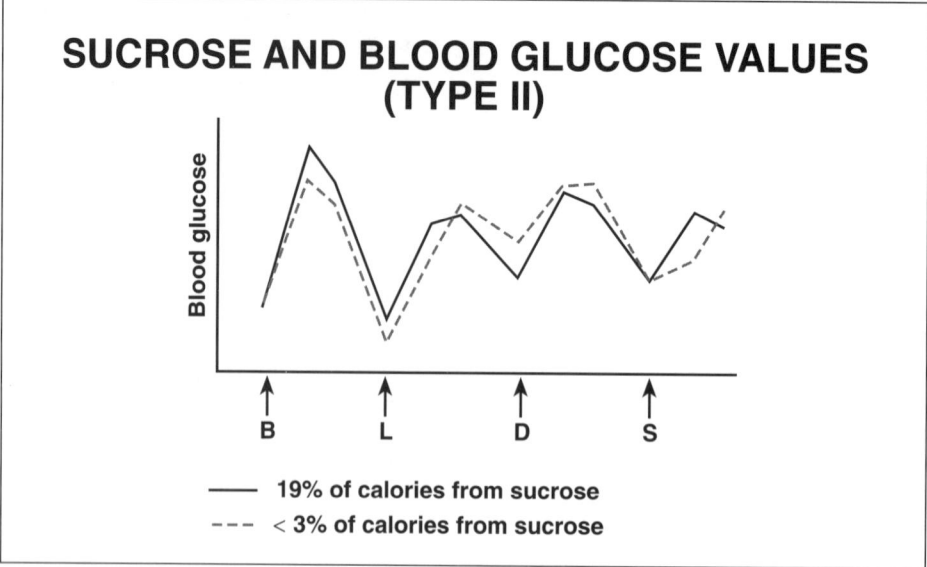

Reprinted with permission from JP Bantle et al, *Diabetes Care,* 1993;16:1302.

Figure 3.5

Sucrose and Blood Glucose Values (Type I)

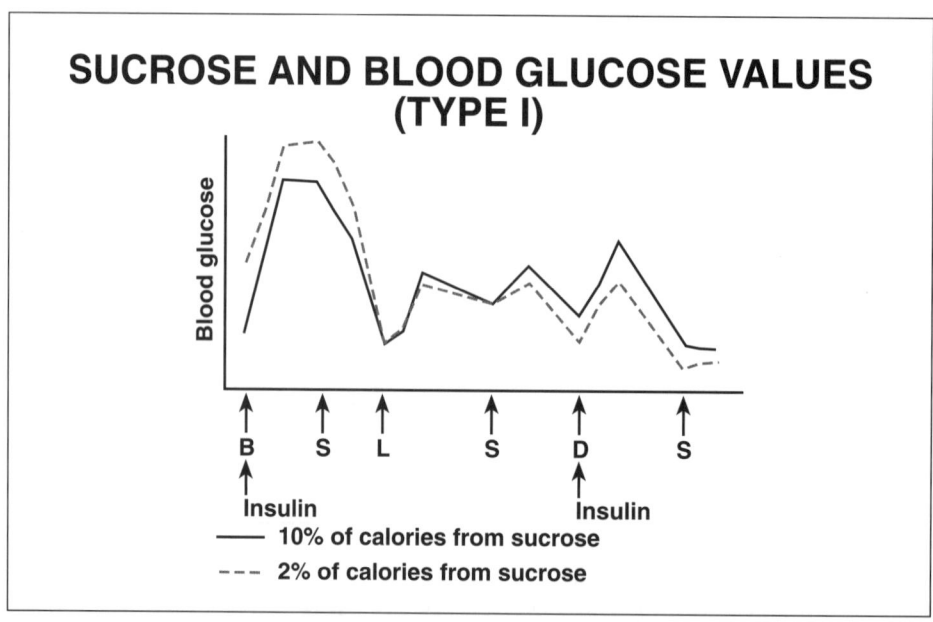

Reprinted with permission from E Loghmani et al, *J Pediatr,* 1991;119:535.

In the second study[18] *(Figure 3.5)* 10 children 7 to 12 years of age with type I diabetes consumed either 10% or 2% of dietary calories from sucrose in a crossover study design with 2-day diet periods. Otherwise the diets were comparable. Again, there were no differences in preprandial and postprandial blood glucose levels, total area under the glucose curve, or insulin doses with either diet.

Nutritive Sweeteners

Nutritive sweeteners include fructose, honey, corn syrup, molasses, fruit juice or fruit juice concentrates, dextrose, maltose, mannitol, sorbitol, xylitol, and hydrogenated starch hydrolysates, as well as sucrose. Research has shown no significant advantage or disadvantage of any of these nutritive sweeteners over sucrose.[19]

Fructose, which occurs naturally in fruits, vegetables, and honey, provides 4 kcal/g—as do other carbohydrates—but causes a smaller rise in plasma glucose than do sucrose and other starches. For this reason, it has been a popular sweetener in meal plans for people with diabetes. In research by Bantle et al,[20] a 28-day diet with 20% of the energy from fructose (ie, double the usual intake) resulted in cholesterol values 6.9% higher and LDL cholesterol values 10.9% higher than did a diet with starch as the only carbohydrate. However, there is no reason to recommend that people avoid consumption of fruits and vegetables, in which fructose occurs naturally, or moderate consumption of fructose-sweetened foods.

Sorbitol, mannitol, and xylitol are common sugar alcohols (polyols) that cause a lower glycemic response than do sucrose and other carbohydrates. They are used as bulking agents and sweeteners in foods. Their energy value is 2–3 kcal/g.[21] The main disadvantage of their use is the osmotic diarrhea effect if consumed in large amounts. Polyols do not appear to have significant advantages over other nutritive sweeteners. When 30 g sorbitol (the amount in 10 pieces of small hard candy) or more is ingested in a single dose, the result may be abdominal gas, discomfort, and osmotic diarrhea, depending on the individual's gastrointestinal sensitivity.[21] An individual's tolerance level may be as low as 10 g.[22] The US Food and Drug Administration (FDA) requires a statement on a food label, "excess consumption may have a laxative effect," if reasonable consumption of that particular food may result in a daily ingestion of ≥ 50 g because of the potential gastrointestinal side effects.

Nonnutritive Sweeteners

Aspartame, acesulfame K, and saccharin are currently approved for use in the United States. Each of these products underwent rigorous testing by the manufacturer and scrutiny from the FDA before it was approved for consumption. All can be used safely by people with diabetes.[19]

The average intake of all the nonnutritive sweeteners is much less than the acceptable daily intake (ADI), which is determined by the FDA. The ADI represents the amount of a food additive that, even if consumed on a daily basis throughout an individual's lifetime, is still considered safe by a 100-fold safety margin. It is not a toxic threshold, and even if an individual occasionally ingested a substance in amounts greater than the ADI, it would not pose a health risk.[21] For example, aspartame consumption (14-day average) in persons with diabetes is 2–4 mg/kg body weight (BW) per day—well below the ADI of 50 mg/kg BW.

Fiber

The American Diabetes Association recommendations for fiber intake for persons with diabetes are the same as recommendations for the general public: approximately 20–35 g/day of dietary fiber from a variety of food sources.[5] Dietary fiber may be beneficial in maintaining normal GI function and in treating or preventing several benign GI disorders and colon cancer, and large amounts of soluble fiber may have a beneficial effect on serum lipids.[23] Although selected soluble fibers are capable of delaying glucose absorption, the effect of dietary fiber on glycemia is probably insignificant.[10] This is in contrast to what many dietetics professionals have been recommending based on earlier research.[24]

Sodium

There is an association between hypertension and both type I and type II diabetes, especially for people with type II diabetes who are obese.[25] There is also evidence that people with type II diabetes are more salt-sensitive than the general population.[26]

Sodium-intake recommendations for people with diabetes are the same as for the general population: less than 3,000 mg/day. For persons with mild hypertension and diabetes, the intake should be reduced to less than 2,400 mg/day.[25,26] In hypertensive clients or edematous clients with nephropathy, sodium restriction is required and sodium intake should not exceed 2,000 mg/day.[10]

Food selection guidelines for a reduced-sodium food plan could include less than 400 mg sodium per single serving of food, or less than 800 mg sodium per entree or convenience meal.

Alcohol

If diabetes is well controlled, moderate use of alcohol is unlikely to adversely affect blood glucose.[27] However, it is important to verify this through blood glucose monitoring. Clients who take insulin should limit their intake to no more than two drinks per day (one drink equals 12 oz beer, 5 oz wine, or 1½ oz distilled alcohol).[5] If alcohol is consumed, it should not be counted as a part of the meal plan, but in addition to the meal plan. In the fasting state, alcohol may produce hypoglycemia. This is because alcohol cannot be converted to glucose, inhibits gluconeogenesis, and augments or increases the effects of insulin by interfering with the counterregulation of insulin-induced hypoglycemia.[10]

Alcohol is metabolized in a manner similar to fat. Even though extra calories are consumed, total food intake should not be reduced. When caloric intake is being restricted, as in individuals trying to reduce their body weight, alcohol is best substituted for fat (one drink equals two fat exchanges, or about 100 kcal that would have been consumed as fat).

Here are some guidelines for alcohol use:

For insulin users:
- Limit to two drinks per day.
- Drink only with food.
- Do not cut back on food.
- Abstain if there is a history of alcohol abuse and during pregnancy and lactation.

For non–insulin users:
- Substitute for fat calories.
- Limit to promote weight loss or maintenance.
- Limit if triglycerides are elevated.
- Abstain if there is a history of alcohol abuse and during pregnancy and lactation.

Micronutrients

The vitamin and mineral needs of clients with diabetes who are healthy appear to be adequately met by the RDAs,[28] which include a generous safety factor. Furthermore, a client's response to vitamin and mineral supplements is largely determined by nutritional state, so only clients with micronutrient deficiencies respond favorably.[10]

People who are at greatest risk of micronutrient deficiency and who may require evaluation for vitamin/mineral supplements include those on extreme weight-reducing diets, strict vegetarians, the elderly, pregnant or lactating women, those taking medications known to alter micronutrient metabolism, clients in poor metabolic control (eg, with glycosuria), clients with a malabsorption disorder or in a critical care environment, and clients with congestive heart failure or myocardial infarction.[10] There appears to be no justification for routine prescription of vitamin and mineral supplements for the majority of clients with diabetes.

Chromium deficiency is associated with elevated blood glucose, cholesterol, and triglyceride levels in animal models. However, it is unlikely that most individuals with diabetes are chromium-deficient. Three double-blind crossover studies of chromium supplementation in people with diabetes did not show any improvement of blood glucose control.[29-31] In people with IGT who consumed a diet deficient in chromium for 4 weeks, chromium supplementation improved glucose tolerance.[32]

Magnesium depletion has been associated with insulin sensitivity, which may improve with oral supplementation.[33] Magnesium should be repleted only if hypomagnesemia is demonstrated.

Clinical Application of 1994 Nutrition Recommendations

The 1994 nutrition recommendations state that a nutrition prescription is based on a nutrition assessment and individual treatment goals. The nutrition intervention should involve modifying *usual* intake based on desired outcomes for blood glucose and lipid levels, body weight, age, and lifestyle considerations, rather than a calculated meal plan.[5,34]

The 1994 nutrition recommendations emphasize the importance of the dietitian's taking an active role in the management of diabetes. They challenge dietitians to become more knowledgeable about current research and more competent and skilled in overall diabetes management. Using the best clinical judgment and thinking creatively about new and different options for nutrition intervention are implicit in these recommendations.

Translation of the 1994 Nutrition Recommendations for Health Care Institutions

Standardized calorie-level meal patterns based on exchange lists have traditionally been used to plan meals for hospitalized patients. Often the nutrition prescription is physician-determined and is ordered as an "ADA diet" with a specified calorie level and percentage of carbohydrate, protein, and fat based on the exchange lists. It is recommended that the term "ADA diet" (American Diabetes Association) no longer be used, since the ADA does not endorse any single meal plan or specified percentages of macronutrients.[35]

The advantages of using a standardized calorie-level meal pattern are that 1) it provides consistency in calories and nutrient distribution of protein, carbohydrate, and fat; 2) it requires minimal dietitian intervention, particularly at time of admission; 3) it provides the patient with examples of types and quantities of foods to be eaten at home (standardized meal patterns are available from many sources for institutional facilities to adopt and many hospital foodservice departments already have this type of system in place); and 4) it is used as the basis for many types of therapeutic diets.

The disadvantages of using standardized meal patterns are 1) inappropriate calorie levels are often ordered and 2) they may not be individualized by a dietitian to meet the needs and requirements of the patient. Unfortunately, this often leads to patient dissatisfaction and a negative bias or opinion that this "diet" or meal plan is unpalatable, too structured, and limited in choice.[36]

Just as there is no one prescription that meets the needs of every patient with diabetes, there is no one type of meal-planning approach that is ideal for every hospital setting. Several approaches can be used effectively in institutional settings to assist in meal planning for persons with diabetes. These include regular hospital menus; incorporation of the *Dietary Guidelines for Americans* or the *Daily Food Guide Pyramid* through use of menus such as "Heart Healthy," "Low-Fat," or "Cardiac" menus using carbohydrate counting; or individualized meal plans developed by the patient and dietitian.[35]

Meal-planning options such as no concentrated sweets, no sugar added, or low sugar are still commonly used in many health care settings as an alternative to a more flexible meal plan than exchange lists. These options are not recommended because they do not reflect the 1994 diabetes nutrition recommendations and unnecessarily restrict sucrose, which may perpetuate the false notion that simply restricting sucrose-sweetened foods will improve blood glucose control.[35] The emphasis should be on limiting the total amount of carbohydrate rather than the source of the carbohydrate.

A preferred method emphasizing the total amount vs source of carbohydrate would be to implement a consistent-carbohydrate diabetes meal plan. In developing menus for this method, a regular or modified-fat menu could serve as the basis. Adjustments would be made in the distribution of carbohydrate-containing foods, so that a consistent amount of carbohydrate is offered at each meal. For hospitals using selective menus, the carbohydrate-containing foods can be identified on the menu and the patient given guidance in selection of the appropriate numbers of these foods to maintain a consistent carbohydrate intake (eg, 4 carbohydrate choices/meal with 15 g carbohydrate equaling 1 carbohydrate choice; would need to be individualized according to the needs of the patient).[36]

Nutrition Practice Guidelines

Nutrition practice guidelines (for definition, see page 7) for type I[37] and type II diabetes[38] can be used by dietitians to anticipate and simplify the decision-making process, increase the quality and consistency of diabetes medical nutrition therapy, and foster improved metabolic control. The guidelines define diabetes medical nutrition therapy and integrate it into systems of total care for management of type I and type II diabetes. The practice guidelines provide a framework that can assist the dietitian in the nutrition assessment, goal setting, intervention, and evaluation of outcomes of medical nutrition therapy for clients with type I and type II diabetes. The guidelines were developed by an expert panel and were submitted for review by peers and opinion leaders in the field of diabetes medical nutrition therapy.

Nutrition practice guidelines for type I and type II diabetes consist of a series of visits with the dietitian. Nutrition practice guidelines for type II diabetes have been developed for initial visits, first follow-up visits, second follow-up visits, and ongoing care. For each of these visits, the guidelines include desired outcomes, nutrition assessment criteria, components of intervention, essential client education topics for nutrition self-management, and communication guidelines.[38]

Summary

Diabetes medical nutrition therapy must be based on the four-pronged approach of nutrition assessment, goal setting, intervention, and evaluation. Medical nutrition therapy for people with diabetes must be individualized, with consideration given to usual eating habits and other lifestyle factors.[5,33] Monitoring metabolic parameters, including blood glucose, glycosolated hemoglobin, lipids, blood pressure, and body weight, as well as quality of life, is crucial to ensuring successful outcomes. Nutrition practice guidelines provide dietitians with a consistent framework in which diabetes medical nutrition therapy can be individualized to the client's needs and goals.

References

1. Diabetes Control and Complications Trial Research Group. The effect of intensive treatment of diabetes on the development and progression of long-term complications in insulin-dependent diabetes mellitus. *N Engl J Med.* 1993;329:977–986.
2. Diabetes Control and Complications Trial Research Group. Expanded role of the dietitian in the Diabetes Control and Complications Trial: implications for clinical practice. *J Am Diet Assoc.* 1993;93:758–767.
3. Delahanty LM, Halford BN. The role of diet behaviors in achieving improved glycemic control in intensively treated patients in the Diabetes Control and Complications Trial. *Diabetes Care.* 1993;16:1453–1458.
4. Pastors JG, Holler HJ, eds. *Meal Planning Approaches for Diabetes Management.* 2nd ed. Chicago, Ill: The American Dietetic Association; 1994:3.
5. American Diabetes Association. Nutrition recommendations and principles for people with diabetes mellitus (position statement). *Diabetes Care.* 1995;18:16–19.
6. The American Dietetic Association and American Diabetes Association. *The Effective Application of "Exchange Lists for Meal Planning."* Chicago, Ill: The American Dietetic Association and American Diabetes Association; 1976:17.
7. Powers MA. Medical nutrition therapy for diabetes. In: Powers MA, ed. *Handbook of Diabetes Medical Nutrition Therapy.* 2nd ed. Gaithersburg, Md: Aspen Publishers, Inc; 1996:33–60.
8. Simkins SW. Lessons from the DCCT: the nutritional challenges of implementing intensive therapy. *Diabetes Spectrum.* 1994;7(5):294–295.
9. Diabetes Control and Complications Trial Research Group. Nutrition interventions for intensive therapy in the DCCT. *J Am Diet Assoc.* 1993;93:768–773.
10. Franz MJ, Horton ES, Bantle JP, Beebe CA, Brunzell JD, Coulston AM, Henry RR, Hoogwerf BJ, Stacpoole PW. Technical review: nutrition principles for the management of diabetes mellitus and related complications. *Diabetes Care.* 1994;17:490–518.
11. American Diabetes Association. Diabetic nephropathy (position statement). *Diabetes Care.* In press.
12. Kontessis P, Jones S, Dodds R, Trevisan R, Nosadini R, Fioretto P, Brosato M, Sacerdoti D, Viberti GC. Renal metabolic and hormonal responses to ingestion of animal and vegetable proteins. *Kidney Int.* 1990;38:136–144.
13. Henkins Y, Kriesberg RA. Dyslipidemia. In: *Therapy for Diabetes Mellitus and Related Disorders.* 2nd ed. Alexandria, Va: American Diabetes Association; 1994:194.
14. Garg A, Bonanome A, Grundy SM, Zhang AJ, Unger RH. Comparison of a high-carbohydrate diet with high-monounsaturated-fat diet in patients with non-insulin-dependent diabetes mellitus. *N Engl J Med.* 1988;391:829–834.
15. Parillo M, Rivellese AA, Ciardullo AV, Capaldo B, Giacco A, Genovese S, Ricardi G. A high-monounsaturated-fat/low-carbohydrate diet improves peripheral insulin sensitivity in non-insulin-dependent diabetic patients. *Metabolism.* 1992;41:1371–1378.
16. Hollenbeck CB, Coulston A, Donner C, Williams R, Reaven GM. The effects of variations in percent of naturally occurring complex and simple carbohydrates on plasma glucose and insulin response in individuals with non-insulin-dependent diabetes mellitus. *Diabetes.* 1985;34:151–155.
17. Bantle JP, Swanson JE, Thomas W, Laine DC. Metabolic effects of dietary sucrose in type II diabetic subjects. *Diabetes Care.* 1993;16:1301–1305.
18. Loghmani E, Rickard K, Washburne L, Vandagriff H, Fineberg N, Golden M. Glycemic response to sucrose-containing mixed meals in diets of children with insulin-dependent diabetes mellitus. *J Pediatr.* 1991;119:531–537.

19. The American Dietetic Association. Appropriate use of nutritive and nonnutritive sweeteners (position statement). *J Am Diet Assoc.* 1993;93:816–821.
20. Bantle JP, Swanson JE, Thomas W, Laine DC. Metabolic effects of dietary fructose in diabetic subjects. *Diabetes Care.* 1992;15(suppl 4):1468–1476.
21. Geil PB. Complex and simple carbohydrates in diabetes therapy. In: Powers MA, ed. *Handbook of Diabetes Medical Nutrition Therapy.* 2nd ed. Gaithersburg, Md: Aspen Publishers, Inc; 1996:308–309.
22. Jain NK, Rosenberg DB, Wahannan MJ, Glasser MJ, Pitchumoni CS. Sorbitol intolerance in adults. *Am J Gastroenterol.* 1985;80:678–681.
23. National Research Council, Committee on Diet and Health, Food and Nutrition Board. *Diet and Health: Implications for Reducing Chronic Disease Risk.* Washington, DC: National Academy Press; 1989:291–310.
24. Nuttall FQ. Dietary fiber in the management of diabetes. *Diabetes.* 1993;42:503–508.
25. American Diabetes Association. Treatment of hypertension in diabetes (consensus statement). *Diabetes Care.* 1996;19(suppl 1):S107–113.
26. Tuck M, Corry D, Trujillo A. Salt-sensitive blood pressure and exaggerated vascular reactivity in the hypertension of diabetes mellitus. *Am J Med.* 1990;88:210–216.
27. Koivisto VA, Tulokas S, Toivonen M, Happa E, Pelkonen R. Alcohol with a meal has no adverse effects on postprandial glucose homeostasis in diabetic patients. *Diabetes Care.* 1993;16:1612–1614.
28. Mooradian AD, Failla M, Hoogwerf B, Isaac R, Maryniuk M, Wylie-Rosett J. Selected vitamins and minerals in diabetes mellitus (technical review). *Diabetes Care.* 1994;17:464–479.
29. Rabinowitz MB, Gonick HC, Levin SR, Davidson MB. Effect of chromium and yeast supplements on carbohydrate and lipid metabolism in diabetic men. *Diabetes Care.* 1983;6:319–327.
30. Rabinowitz MB, Levin SR, Gonick HC. Comparison of chromium status in diabetic and normal men. *Metabolism.* 1980;29:355–364.
31. Abraham AS, Brooks BA, Eylate U. The effects of chromium supplementation on serum glucose and lipids in patients with and without non-insulin-dependent diabetes. *Metab Clin Exp.* 1992;41:768–771.
32. Anderson AS, Polansky MM, Canary JJ. Supplemental-chromium effects on glucose, insulin, glucagon, and urinary chromium losses in subjects consuming controlled low-chromium diets. *Am J Clin Nutr.* 1991;54:909–916.
33. American Diabetes Association. Magnesium supplementation in the treatment of diabetes (consensus statement). *Diabetes Care.* 1996;19(suppl 1):S93–95.
34. Fels-Tinker L, Heins JM, Holler HJ. Commentary and translation: 1994 nutrition recommendations for diabetes mellitus. *J Am Diet Assoc.* 1994;94:507–511.
35. Translation of the diabetes nutrition recommendations for health care institutions (position statement). *Diabetes Care.* 1997;20(1):106–108. *J Am Diet Assoc.* 1997;97:52–53.
36. Translation of the diabetes nutrition recommendations for health care institutions (technical review). *Diabetes Care.* 1997;20(1):96–105. *J Am Diet Assoc.* 1997;97:43–51.
37. Leontos C, Splett PL. Nutrition practice guidelines for type I diabetes mellitus: development and field testing. *Diabetes Spectrum.* 1996;9(2):128–130.
38. Monk A, Barry B, McClain K, Weaver T, Cooper N, Franz M. Practice guidelines for medical nutrition therapy provided by dietitians for persons with non-insulin-dependent diabetes. *J Am Diet Assoc.* 1995;95:999–1006.

Management of Diabetes: Exercise

4

Exercise is an important component of diabetes management because of its physiological and psychological benefits. In addition, exercise can be useful in improving the health and quality of life of clients with diabetes. Before specific recommendations about exercise can be made, it is important to know the metabolic effects, benefits, and risks of exercise in clients with type I and type II diabetes.

Metabolic Effects of Exercise

In all individuals, metabolic response to exercise varies according to nutritional state, age, specific pathology, and work capacity. In clients with type I diabetes, other factors that affect metabolic response to exercise include timing of insulin injections, type of insulin and site of administration, degree of metabolic control, and presence of complications.[1]

In clients with type I diabetes, plasma insulin levels do not decrease to low levels during exercise. The major effects of the normal to high insulin level during exercise are decreased output of hepatic glucose, increased peripheral use of glucose, and decreased effects of counterregulatory hormones.[1,2] For someone whose type I diabetes is not well controlled (inadequate insulin), exercise can have negative results. Hepatic glucose output is increased, peripheral use of glucose is reduced, and the effect of counterregulatory hormones is increased. The resulting insulin deficiency leads to hyperglycemia[1] *(Table 4.1)*.

In type II diabetes, exercise improves blood glucose control via an increase in insulin sensitivity, which results in increased peripheral use of glucose. Exercise also decreases the effect of counterregulatory hormones, which in turn reduces hepatic glucose output[3] *(Figure 4.1)*.

Table 4.1

Metabolic Effects of Exercise in Type I Diabetes

Insulin	Hepatic Glucose Output	Peripheral Glucose Use	Counter-regulatory Hormones	Blood Glucose	Ketone Bodies	Free Fatty Acids
Adequate	↓	↑	↓ →	↓	↓	↓
Inadequate	↑	↓	↑ →	↑	↑	↑

Adapted with permission from *Maximizing Nutrition in Diabetes Management* (Alexandria, Va: American Diabetes Association; 1994).

29

Benefits of Exercise

Exercise has many possible benefits for clients with diabetes, and for most people the benefits outweigh the risks *(Table 4.2)*. Although exercise has not been shown to improve glycemic control in clients with type I diabetes, they should be encouraged to exercise because of the potential to improve cardiovascular fitness and for psychological well-being and recreation.[1]

In clients with type II diabetes, exercise is as important a component as medical nutrition therapy to improve glycemic control, reduce certain cardiovascular risk factors, and increase psychological well-being. Clients who receive the greatest benefit from exercise are those with mildly to moderately impaired glucose tolerance and hyperinsulinemia.[3]

Figure 4.1
Metabolic Effects of Exercise in Type II Diabetes

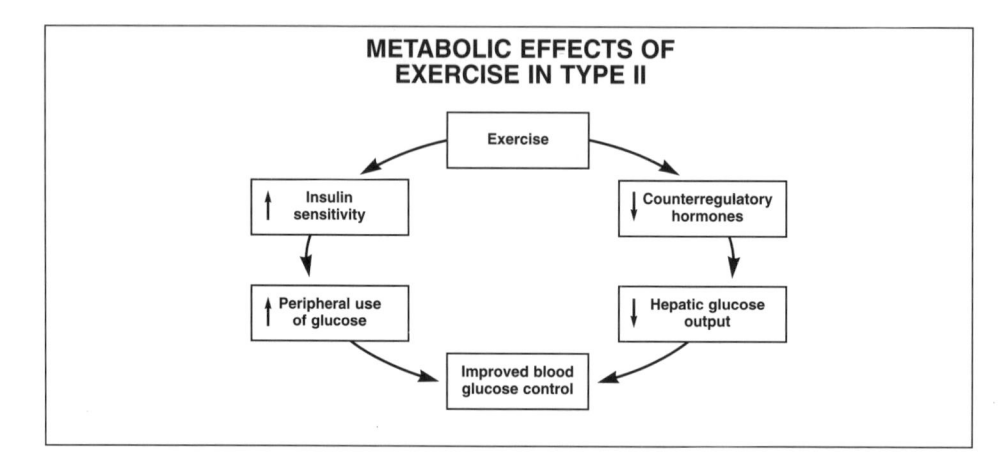

Reprinted with permission from *Maximizing Nutrition in Diabetes Management* (Alexandria, Va: American Diabetes Association; 1994).

Table 4.2
Possible Benefits of Exercise for Persons with Diabetes

	Type I	Type II
Improved cardiovascular and overall fitness	X	X
➤ flexibility		
➤ endurance		
➤ muscle strength		
Improved glucose control		X
➤ decreased blood glucose		
➤ increased insulin sensitivity		
Adjunct to meal planning for weight control and maintenance		X
Decreased cardiovascular risk factors		
➤ hyperlipidemia	X	X
➤ hypertension	X	X
➤ obesity		X
Increased sense of well-being and quality of life	X	X

Risks of Exercise

It is also important to discuss the risks associated with exercise for clients with diabetes *(Table 4.3)*. Hypoglycemia is more common after exercise (for up to 24–36 hours) than during exercise, due to repletion of liver glycogen. Muscle can be sensitive to insulin for up to 24 hours after exercise.[4,5] In type I diabetes, monitoring for hypoglycemia, being prepared to eat more food, and reducing the insulin dose are three important management strategies during exercise.

If fasting blood glucose is >250 mg/dL and ketone bodies are present in the urine, or if fasting blood glucose is >300 mg/dL irrespective of whether ketones are present, it is generally advisable to administer more insulin and delay exercising.[1] When there is insufficient insulin, glucose use by muscle is decreased and the liver will produce or release stored glucose to make up the anticipated muscle deficit, resulting in a further increase in blood glucose. Exercise of higher intensity may also lead to hyperglycemia,[6] as the stress of this type of exercise causes counterregulatory hormones to release glucose from glycogen stores.

Exercise may have additional risks for people with chronic complications associated with diabetes. For example, clients with proliferative retinopathy are at increased risk for retinal or vitreous hemorrhage or retinal detachment during certain types of strenuous exercise; for them, stationary cycling, swimming, and walking can be encouraged. Clients with neuropathy have an increased risk of foot injury, including soft-tissue and joint injury. Although these clients should avoid activities that involve pounding of the lower extremities, they may be able to engage in non–weight-bearing activities such as swimming, stationary cycling, and arm exercises. People who have autonomic neuropathy should avoid all strenuous activities, which could cause a decreased or otherwise abnormal cardiovascular response.

Table 4.3
Possible Risks of Exercise for Persons with Diabetes

Hypoglycemia during or after exercise in persons taking insulin

Increased hyperglycemia in poorly controlled persons and underinsulinized persons with pre-exercise blood glucose levels of 250–300 mg/dL

Myocardial infarction or arrhythmia in persons with diabetes who also have atherosclerotic cardiovascular disease, especially if exercise is not properly paced

Possible worsening of microvascular diabetes complications, particularly retinopathy

Damage to soft tissue and joints, especially if peripheral neuropathy is present

Exercise Recommendations

Several factors affect the blood glucose response to exercise:

- type, amount, and intensity of exercise
- timing and type of previous meal
- timing and type of insulin injection or oral hypoglycemic agent
- pre-exercise blood glucose level
- client's fitness level

For type I diabetes, a uniform recommendation for preventing hypoglycemia and improving the metabolic response to exercise cannot be made. Rather, self-monitoring of blood glucose should be incorporated into the exercise program to provide the information necessary to adjust food intake and/or insulin dosages.[1]

An exercise program for clients with type II diabetes should incorporate the following recommendations:[3]

- type: appropriate to the client's general physical condition and lifestyle
- frequency: at least 3 days per week
- duration: 20–45 minutes
- intensity: 50–70% of the client's maximal heart rate

Clients with type II diabetes taking oral glucose-lowering medications or insulin should self-monitor their blood glucose to determine their glycemic response to exercise.

Exercise Guidelines

The following are important guidelines for clients starting an exercise program:[7]

- Receive a complete medical evaluation or medical clearance from a physician before starting an exercise program.
- Monitor blood glucose before and after exercise to understand how exercise affects blood glucose levels. Self-monitoring of blood glucose (SMBG) is important for deciding when to exercise, as well as for identifying potential hypoglycemia. Exercise may require a decrease in insulin doses, so SMBG is essential.
- Adequate fluid intake is essential.
- Use proper footwear.
- Inspect feet after exercise.
- Avoid exercise in extreme heat or cold.
- Avoid exercise during a period of poor glucose control.
- Carry identification; it may also be necessary to carry a source of carbohydrate, especially for clients engaging in exercise of high intensity and/or long duration.
- The decision regarding the need for and type of additional food intake before or during exercise should be individualized based on the following factors:
    1) blood glucose level;
    2) intensity and duration of the exercise;
    3) preference for or tolerance of solid food vs liquid;
    4) other nutritional factors (osmolality, fiber, and electrolyte supplementation).

➤ Exercise can accelerate absorption of insulin in exercising limbs, especially when it is begun immediately after the insulin injection. Inject insulin into a non-exercising area, such as the abdomen, to minimize the effect of exercise on insulin absorption.

Summary

The response to exercise is so variable and multifactorial that adjustments in medication and food should be based on individual responses to exercise. The use of blood glucose monitoring is important for understanding exercise response patterns and tailoring an exercise program.

References

1. Wasserman DH, Zinman B. American Diabetes Association technical review: exercise in individuals with IDDM. *Diabetes Care.* 1994;17(8):924–937.
2. Maynard T. Exercise: Part I. Physiological response to exercise in diabetes mellitus. *The Diabetes Educator.* 1991;17(3):196–204.
3. Schnieder SH, Ruderman NB. American Diabetes Association technical review: exercise and NIDDM. *Diabetes Care.* 1990;13(7):785–789.
4. Mitchell TH, Abraham G, Schiffrin A, Leiter LA, Marliss EB. Hyperglycemia after intense exercise in IDDM subjects during continuous subcutaneous insulin infusion. *Diabetes Care.* 1988;11(4):311–317.
5. MacDonald MJ. Postexercise late-onset hypoglycemia in insulin-dependent diabetic patients. *Diabetes Care.* 1987;10(5):584–588.
6. Campaigne BN, Wallberg-Henriksson H, Gunnarsson R. Glucose and insulin responses in relation to insulin dose and caloric intake 12 h after acute physical exercise in men with IDDM. *Diabetes Care.* 1987;10(6):716–721.
7. Franz MJ. Exercise benefits and guidelines for persons with diabetes. In: Powers MA, ed. *Handbook of Diabetes Medical Nutrition Therapy.* Gaithersburg, Md: Aspen Publishers; 1996: 116–118, 121–122.

Resources

The Fitness Book: For People With Diabetes. Alexandria, Va: American Diabetes Association; 1994.

Franz M, Barry B. *Diabetes and Exercise: Guidelines for Safe and Enjoyable Activity.* Minneapolis: International Diabetes Center; 1993.

Selected Diabetes and Nutrition Education Resources: For the Diabetes Professional. Chicago, Ill: Diabetes Care and Education Practice Group of The American Dietetic Association; 1995: 44–45.

Stepping Out: A Diabetes Exercise Starter Kit. Chicago, Ill: The American Dietetic Association; 1992.

Management of Diabetes: Medications

5

Diabetes educators need to incorporate medication, in addition to nutrition, exercise, and behavioral assessments, into their evaluation of clients with diabetes. When a medication is needed to lower blood glucose, there are a variety of insulins and oral glucose-lowering medications available to the diabetes care team. This chapter reviews medications that are used in the treatment of clients with diabetes.

Oral Glucose-Lowering Medications

It is estimated that more than half the clients with type II diabetes achieve glycemic control by using oral glucose-lowering medication, often to supplement the preferred treatment methods of diabetes medical nutrition therapy and lifestyle modifications. The effectiveness of oral glucose-lowering medication varies with each individual and is closely linked to residual beta cell function.[1]

Four groups of oral glucose-lowering medication are available: sulfonylureas, biguanides, thiazolidinediones, and an alpha-glucosidase inhibitor. They are described further in *Table 5.1*. Each group is believed to have several different mechanisms of action.

Sulfonylureas

The most significant mechanism of action of sulfonylureas is to enhance insulin secretion at any given glucose level. By reducing serum glucose and correcting "glucotoxicity," sulfonylureas indirectly reduce the accelerated rates of hepatic glucose production and increase the rate of glucose uptake by the muscle.[2]

Because type II diabetes mellitus is a disorder in which insulin secretion is less than that required to overcome insulin resistance, sulfonylureas are useful in controlling hyperglycemia. However, they are ineffective in lowering blood glucose in clients with minimal or no insulin production.

Biguanides

Metformin, a biguanide drug approved for use in this country by the FDA in January 1995, was developed in France in 1959 and has been used worldwide. It has a different mode of action from sulfonylureas in that it works via the liver to decrease hepatic glucose production and on the muscle to increase the glucose uptake, rather than on the pancreas to stimulate insulin secretion. The proposed benefits of using metformin include modest weight loss, decreased risk of hypoglycemia, decreased plasma triglycerides, total

Table 5.1
Time Activity of Oral Glucose-Lowering Medications

Medication	Brand Name	Dosage*	Effective Time
Sulfonylureas			
acetohexamide	Dymelor	250–1500 mg/day	24 hours
chlorpropamide	Diabinese	100–750 mg/day	60 hours
tolbutamide	Orinase	500–3000 mg/day	12 hours
tolazamide	Tolinase	100–1000 mg/day	24 hours
glyburide	DiaBeta, Micronase	1.25–20 mg/day	24 hours
	Glynase	0.75–12 mg/day	24 hours
glipizide	Glucotrol	2.5–40 mg/day	18 hours
	Glucotrol XL	5.0–20 mg/day	24 hours
glimeperide	Amaryl	1–8 mg/day	24 hours
Biguanides			
Metformin	Glucophage	1000–2550 mg/day	24 hours
Thiazolidinediones			
troglitazone	Rezulin	400–800 mg/day	24 hours
Alpha-glucosidase inhibitor			
acarbose	Precose	25–100 mg tid[†]	1 hour

*Higher figure represents maximum daily recommended dose.
[†]Initial dose: 25 mg tid for 4 weeks, maintenance dose: 50–100 mg tid

and LDL-cholesterol, modest elevation of HDL-cholesterol, and decreased insulin levels. Decreased hepatic and renal function increases the risk of developing lactic acidosis, so clients with these conditions should not be treated with metformin. Other conditions that increase the risk of lactic acidosis include cardiac and pulmonary disease, other causes of hypoxia, and alcohol abuse. Contraindications for metformin use include renal failure, hepatic disease, alcohol abuse, history of lactic acidosis, cardiac insufficiency, and other hypoxic conditions.[3] Metformin should be withdrawn during acute illness and before major surgery or angiography because of the potential risk of acute renal failure and increased risk of lactic acidosis.

Thiazolidinediones

Troglitazone is the first available drug of a new class of oral glucose-lowering medications, called thiazolidinediones, that enhance insulin action in the liver, muscle, and adipose tissue by reducing insulin resistance. It binds to receptors on the cell nucleus, leading to actions that are similar to those of insulin. Since insulin resistance is lowered, these compounds may be useful in the treatment not only of diabetes, but of dyslipidemia, hypertension, and even polycystic ovary disease. Because hypoglycemia is not a problem, troglitazone can be used in persons without diabetes. Studies to assess whether lowering insulin resistance with troglitazone can prevent the development of type II diabetes in the high-risk individual are under way.

Alpha-glucosidase Inhibitor

Acarbose is an inhibitor of alpha glucosidase, a digestive enzyme that facilitates the breakdown of starch and disaccharides to glucose in the small intestine.

This agent has been approved by the FDA for use in persons with insulin-requiring type II diabetes. When ingested with the first bite of a meal, it causes a slower and smaller rise in blood glucose levels postprandially. However, since carbohydrate breakdown continues at more distal parts of the small intestine, glucose continues to be absorbed so that total glucose absorption is unchanged. Since there is no decrease in calorie absorption, weight loss does not occur.

The side effects of acarbose are due to the malabsorption of a small amount of carbohydrate, with subsequent metabolism of the carbohydrate by intestinal bacteria. The most common side effects are increased flatulence and abdominal bloating. Some clients also experience diarrhea. Acarbose is most effective when given with a high-fiber, high-carbohydrate meal plan.[4] Hypoglycemia does not occur when acarbose is used alone.

Use of Oral Glucose-Lowering Medications

The use of oral glucose-lowering medications should be based on the duration of action, the range of dose, the client's overall health, and potential side effects. Oral glucose-lowering medications should not be prescribed during pregnancy or when pregnancy is planned because they cross the placenta and may cause congenital malformations. Women taking oral glucose-lowering medications should be transferred to insulin before attempting to become pregnant.

A low dose of oral glucose-lowering medication is initially prescribed for clients with type II diabetes who cannot achieve their blood glucose goals through diabetes medical nutrition therapy alone. If blood glucose control is not initially achieved, the dose can be increased every 1 to 2 weeks until the maximum dose or the desired level of control is obtained.

People with diabetes should be educated about the possible side effects of oral glucose-lowering medications—hypoglycemia, gastrointestinal discomfort, alcohol toxicity, lactic acidosis, hypoxia, and cardiac insufficiency. They also need to know when to take the medication, how to store it, and what the drug interactions are.

Like insulin, the timing and amount of oral glucose-lowering medications can be varied to improve glycemic control. If the maximum dosage is used and elevated blood glucose levels continue, insulin should be considered. This may be the time when the client with diabetes becomes more committed to a meal and exercise plan.

Combination Therapy with Oral Glucose-Lowering Medication

Because sulfonylureas, biguanides, thiazolidinediones, and the alpha-glucosidase inhibitor have different mechanisms of action, combination therapy using different types of oral glucose-lowering medication is possible. Advantages of this treatment approach include delaying the need for insulin therapy, decreasing the dose of each drug, which may reduce the incidence of adverse drug reactions, and improving the lipid profile. In addition, combination therapy achieved by using different therapeutic actions improves glycemic control.[5,6] When acarbose is used in comination with a sulfonylurea or insulin, hypoglycemia may occur. If hypoglycemia occurs, it should be corrected with glucose, a monosaccharide, instead of sucrose, a disaccharide.

Insulin

For clients with type I diabetes who have an absolute deficiency of insulin, daily injections of insulin are needed to survive. The aim of insulin replacement in the treatment of type I diabetes is to simulate as closely as possible the meal-related fluctuations in plasma insulin that are typical in clients without diabetes.

Insulin may also be used to normalize blood glucose levels in clients with type II diabetes when their insulin resistance and/or insufficiency cannot be corrected through changes in eating, exercise, or an oral glucose-lowering medication. The following factors are considered in making the decision to initiate insulin therapy:

- the severity of the diabetes (ie, the degree of hyperglycemia and the presence or absence of clinical symptoms);
- the presence or absence of concurrent diseases and conditions;
- the preferences of the client with diabetes after being informed about the use, expected therapeutic effects, and possible side effects of oral glucose-lowering medications or insulin; and
- the motivation of the client with diabetes.

Insulin should be initiated at least temporarily when the glucose level is over 300 mg/dL and the client is symptomatic or when there is a serious illness accompanied by high serum glucose levels, which, if persistent, may impede recovery from infection or healing. A short course of insulin (2 to 4 weeks), by correcting "glucotoxicity," will lower insulin resistance and improve release of insulin from the pancreas. When this occurs, control with diabetes medical nutrition therapy and/or an oral glucose-lowering medication can be initiated or reinitiated.

When insulin therapy becomes necessary, it can be initiated with a single injection of NPH at bedtime or mixed NPH and Regular insulin at dinner while the use of oral glucose-lowering medications is continued. However, when little or no endogenous insulin remains, the client will need to be progressed to at least twice daily insulin, as described for the client with type I diabetes.

Insulin preparations are characterized by source and duration of action. Insulin was originally derived from the bovine or porcine pancreas. Commercial preparations contain both single mixtures and combinations of beef and pork insulin. In the past decade, human insulin has been commercially produced by recombinant DNA technology. Human and purified pork insulins produce fewer immunological reactions than poorly purified insulin from animal sources.[2]

The time course of action falls into four general categories: rapid-acting (insulin analog—Lispro), short-acting (Regular insulin), intermediate-acting (NPH or Lente insulin), and long-acting (Ultralente).[2] The time course of action of these insulins is illustrated in *Figure 5.1*.

Lispro (Humalog) insulin is absorbed, acts, and disappears very rapidly. This rapidity of action is due to reversal of two amino acids in the B chain of the insulin. It acts quickly with an onset at 15 minutes, a peak at one hour, and a duration of 3½–4½ hours, and is taken before eating. Because its effect is short-lived, Lispro insulin must be combined with an intermediate-acting or long-acting insulin (NPH, Lente, or UltraLente) to avoid low insulin levels and hyperglycemia before the next meal. Lispro, unlike other insulins, is available only by prescription.

Regular or short-acting insulin is clear and may be used independently or in combination with intermediate- or long-acting insulins. It is used in insulin pumps and is the only insulin that can be administered intravenously. The

Figure 5.1

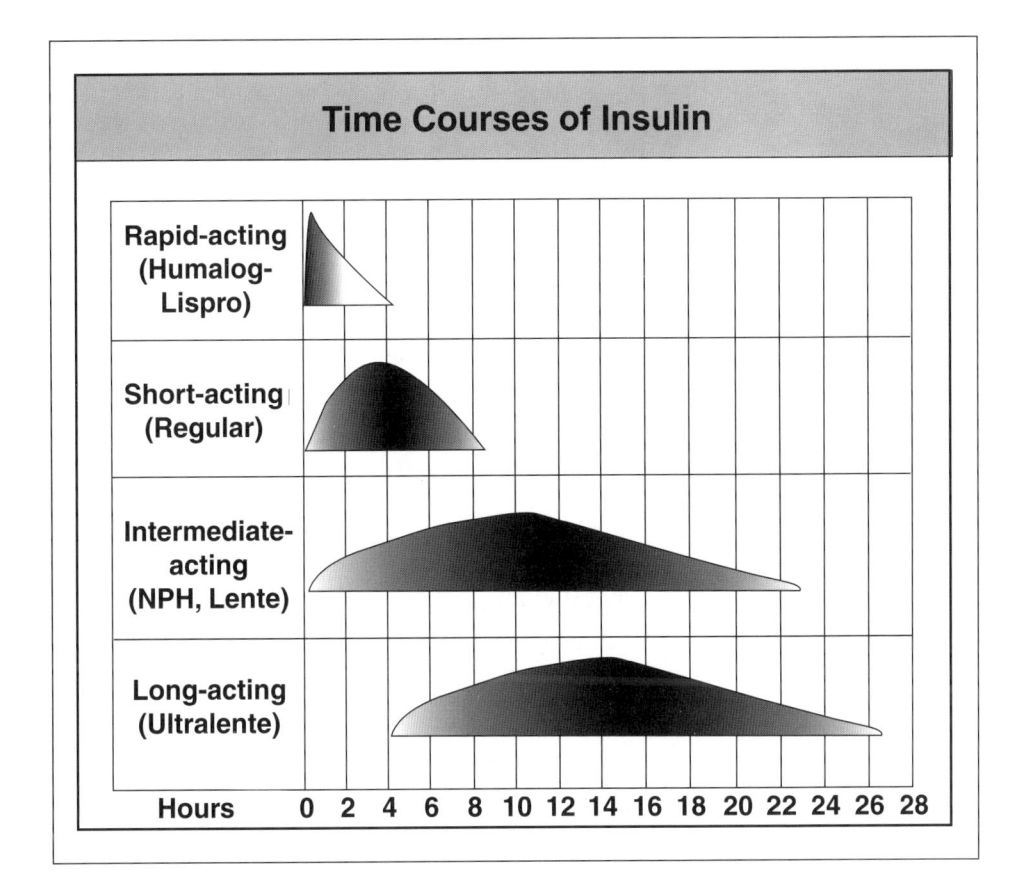

Approximate Time Courses of Insulin

Adapted with permission of Nutrition Dimension Inc, from J Green Pastors, *Nutritional Care of Diabetes,* 2nd ed (San Marcos, Calif: Nutrition Dimension; 1995).

intermediate-acting insulins, NPH and Lente, have a cloudy appearance; their onsets, peaks, and durations are very similar. Regular and intermediate-acting insulins are available in premixed preparations such as 70/30 (70% NPH, 30% Regular) and 50/50 (50% NPH, 50% Regular). Lispro insulin is too unstable for premixed preparations. These mixtures simplify insulin administration, since the user avoids possible errors in drawing up two types of insulin into one syringe. However, they do not allow adjustment of the short-acting regular insulin in response to an elevated blood glucose level or in anticipation of a larger meal or increased exercise. Like NPH and Lente, the long-acting insulin, Ultralente, is cloudy. Ultralente typically has been used to provide a basal, or flat, even dose of insulin, but modern preparations are short-acting and tend to peak. Therefore, Ultralente insulin needs to be used twice daily in most clients. Long-acting insulin analogs that can truly provide "basal insulin" are being developed.

The variation in duration makes it possible to inject insulin in a pattern that is as close to normal insulin activity as possible. An individualized regimen allows insulin to be adjusted to the food intake pattern, rather than adjusting food intake to the insulin dose.

Insulin Regimens

Diabetes educators need to be familiar with the common insulin regimens so they can knowledgeably promote improved blood glucose levels. But, as stated earlier, no attempt should be made to fit a client with diabetes into a particular insulin regimen. The regimen of choice should be individualized, taking into consideration desired eating habits, activities, and motivation, and should be determined by working closely with the client and his or her physician to find the best total treatment regimen.

It is almost impossible in clients with type I or type II diabetes that is no longer controlled with oral glucose-lowering medications to reach target blood glucose goals with only one injection of insulin a day. Four common insulin regimens are discussed below.

Regimen One

One of the most widely used regimens is a split-mixed dose. It consists of twice-daily injections of intermediate- and rapid- or short-acting insulin, administered before breakfast and before dinner *(Table 5.2 and Figure 5.2)*. The amount of rapid- or short-acting insulin can easily be adjusted to accommodate a variation in food intake or physical activity.

Regimen Two

In another common regimen, the predinner intermediate-acting insulin dose is moved to bedtime or before the evening snack and the rapid- or short-acting insulin is given before dinner *(Table 5.2* and *Figure 5.2)*. Moving the intermediate-acting insulin to bedtime will prevent it from peaking when it is least needed (between 0100 and 0300) and cause it to peak when it is most needed (0500–0800), when insulin resistance and insulin needs are at their highest. The increased insulin resistance between 0500 and 0800 is a delayed response to growth hormone surges that occur during sleep. In addition, in some clients NPH taken at dinnertime may "run out" by morning. Another potential and rare cause of high fasting blood glucose levels is the Somogyi effect (or severe hypoglycemia with serum glucose below 50 mg/dL occurring during the night), resulting in the release of counterregulatory hormones and a high fasting glucose. To differentiate between the Somogyi effect and the Dawn phenomenon, the blood glucose level should be checked at 0200. Moving the intermediate-acting insulin to bedtime will also alleviate the Somogyi effect.

Regimen Three

A third regimen involves administering short-acting insulin before breakfast, lunch, and dinner and intermediate-acting insulin before the evening snack *(Table 5.2 and Figure 5.2)*. This regimen is conducive to further individualization of therapy. It can be adjusted to mimic normal insulin secretion at meals. It can be adjusted for intake at each meal, the premeal blood glucose value, and the predicted postmeal activity. Individualized algorithms can be established, based on the client's response to Regular insulin at different times during the day, to provide guidance for the premeal dose (eg, if blood glucose is 70–120 mg/dL before lunch, take the basic dose of Regular; if it is 120–160 mg/dL, add 1 unit of Regular).[7] The intermediate-acting dose before the evening snack covers nighttime and early-morning blood glucose levels, while premeal Regular insulin doses cover postmeal glucose excursions. The use of rapid-acting insulin in this regimen will result in periods of hypoinsulinemia and high glucose levels. To avoid this, intermediate or long-acting insulin should be given twice a day.

Regimen Four

The fourth regimen *(Table 5.2 and Figure 5.2)* involves injection of short-acting insulin before breakfast, lunch, and dinner plus injection of long-acting

Management of Diabetes: Medications

Table 5.2
Sample Multiple Daily Injection Regimens

Regimen	Before Breakfast	Before Lunch	Before Supper	Before Bedtime	Advantage	Disadvantage
1	N/R or L/R		N/R or L/R		Requires only 2 injections	Meal times and sizes less flexible; Fasting AM hyperglycemia
2	N/R* or L/R		R*	N or L	Improved AM fasting BG	Requires 3 injections; Meal times and sizes less flexible
3	R*	R*	R*	N or L	More flexibility with meal times and sizes	Requires 4 injections
4	U/R	R	U/R†		More flexibility with meal times and sizes	Requires 3 injections

R = Regular (short-acting insulin); N = NPH (intermediate-acting insulin); L = Lente (intermediate-acting insulin); U = Ultralente (long-acting insulin); BG = blood glucose.
*In some cases, Lispro may be used in place of Regular insulin.
†In some cases, Ultralente insulin may be given before bedtime rather than before supper.

Source: Diabetes Care and Education Practice Group, *Meal Planning Approaches for Diabetes Management*, 2nd ed (Chicago, Ill: American Dietetic Association; 1994).

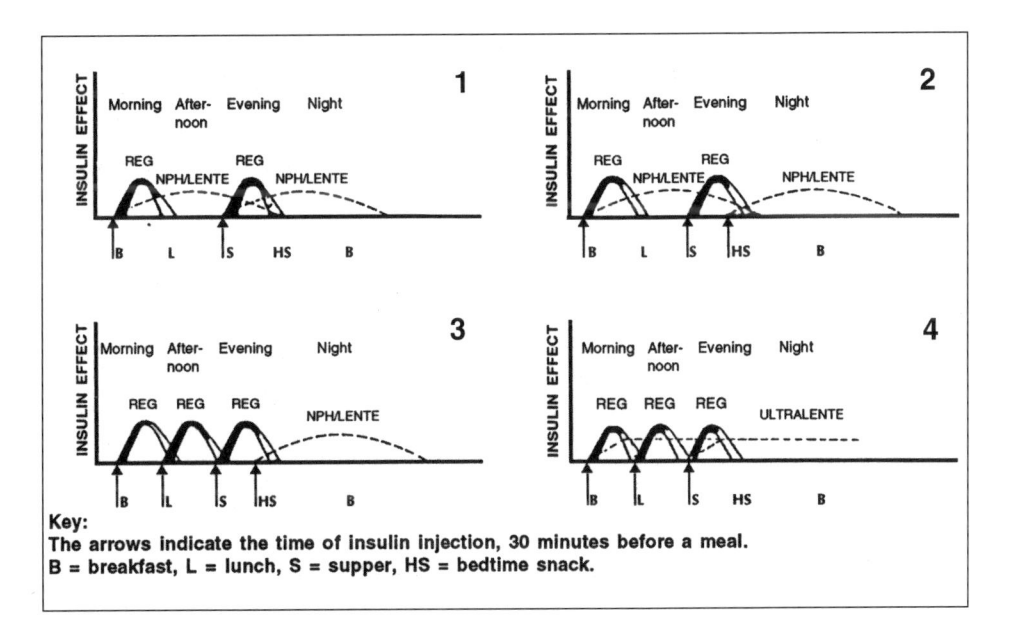

Figure 5.2
Idealized Periods of Insulin Effect in Four Multiple Daily Injection Regimens

Key:
The arrows indicate the time of insulin injection, 30 minutes before a meal.
B = breakfast, L = lunch, S = supper, HS = bedtime snack.

Adapted with permission from DS Schade et al, *Intensive Insulin Therapy* (Princeton, NJ: Excerpta Medica; 1983: 133).

insulin twice daily. Similar to insulin-pump therapy, this regimen mimics the normal, nondiabetic state of insulin at meals, with the slow release of a long-acting insulin providing a constant basal level.

Insulin Pumps

Insulin is administered by very frequent pumping of small amounts of rapid- or short-acting insulin through a subcutaneous catheter every few minutes to establish a steady basal insulin level. Bolus insulin doses are given before meals through the same catheter. Although pump therapy is more expensive than other regimens, it provides another option for flexible, optimal diabetes management.[7,8]

Because of the expense and the need for frequent self-monitoring, pump therapy requires a committed and dedicated client who is willing to perform at least four blood glucose tests a day, keep blood glucose and food records, and learn the technical features of pump use.

Summary

The goal of therapy in patients with diabetes is to normalize blood glucose levels. In patients with type I diabetes several different regimens can be used. For persons with type II diabetes more flexibility and more treatment modalities are available. With the increased availability of glucose-lowering medications and knowledge regarding the etiology of diabetes, we can better tailor treatment options using diabetes medical nutrition therapy, exercise therapy, and pharmacotherapy.

References

1. Lebovitz HE. Sulfonylureas drugs and metformin. In: Lebovitz HE, ed. *Therapy for Diabetes Mellitus and Related Disorders.* 2nd ed. Alexandria, Va: American Diabetes Association; 1994; 116–127.
2. Herman LS, Schersten B, Bitzen PO, Kjellstrom T, Lindegarde F, Melander A. Therapeutic comparison of metformin and sulfonylurea, alone and in various combinations. *Diabetes Care.* 1994;17(10):1100–1109.
3. Bailey CJ. Biguanides and NIDDM. *Diabetes Care.* 1992;15(6):755–772.
4. Bloomgarden ZT. New and traditional treatment of glycemia in NIDDM. *Diabetes Care.* 1996;19(3):295–299.
5. Skyler JS. Insulin treatment. In: Lebovitz HE, ed. *Therapy for Diabetes Mellitus and Related Disorders.* 2nd ed. Alexandria, Va: American Diabetes Association; 1994; 131–141.
6. Thom SL. Diabetes medications and delivery methods. In: Powers MA, ed. *Handbook of Diabetes Medical Nutrition Therapy.* Gaithersburg, Md: Aspen Publishers; 1996; 77–106.
7. Farkas-Hirsch R, ed. *Intensive Diabetes Management.* Alexandria, Va: American Diabetes Association; 1995.
8. Bell DSH. Insulin pump therapy for the 90s. *Endocrinologist.* 1994;4(4):270–278.

Management of Diabetes: Self-Monitoring of Blood Glucose

6

The purpose of self-monitoring of blood glucose (SMBG) in persons with diabetes is to identify treatment needs and then to evaluate the effectiveness of the treatment. SMBG is used to:

- ➤ coordinate the diabetes management plan;
- ➤ accomplish the goals of diabetes medical nutrition therapy;
- ➤ evaluate the effectiveness of the meal plan; and
- ➤ enhance the flexibility of food choices.

Since the first goal of diabetes medical nutrition therapy is to achieve glycemic control, self-monitoring of blood glucose is imperative. Each time blood glucose is tested, the level should be entered on a record *(Figure 6.1)* so that the results can then be reviewed, evaluated, and used by the diabetes care team to determine the person's food, insulin, and exercise needs. This is the best method for evaluating the effects of diabetes medical nutrition therapy on blood glucose control.[1-3]

Diabetes medical nutrition therapy is an involved activity that requires an individualized meal plan and the use of blood glucose monitoring records to be successful. If a person's food consumption and eating pattern is not adjusted based on data in the monitoring records, inappropriate recommendations can be made that can complicate management and compromise adherence.

The diabetes care team should work with each person with diabetes to establish target blood glucose goals. Monitoring records help to evaluate whether goals are being met, whether the existing goals need to be revised, or whether new goals should be developed. It is important to note that out-of-target blood glucose results are not always caused by eating indiscretion. Stress, illness, infection, change in exercise, and incorrect medication dosage are all causes that should be considered. If the cause is food related, the diabetes care team should consider management changes to accommodate the change in food consumption.

Frequency of Monitoring

The frequency of monitoring depends on the type of diabetes and each person's overall therapy. Monitoring up to seven times a day seems excessive, but may be appropriate for the person with newly diagnosed type I diabetes or the pregnant woman. In this schedule, blood glucose would be monitored before breakfast, lunch, and dinner; at bedtime; and 1 to 2 hours after

Diabetes Medical Nutrition Therapy

Figure 6.1

Diabetes Self-Care Daily Record

		Diabetes Self-Care Daily Record					
Day of week _____					Date _____		
Time	Medication	BG Results		Food Intake		Nutrient Information	Physical Activity
	type | amount	am | pm		amount | type of food/drink			type | amount

Comments   Daily Totals

Source: University of Virginia Diabetes Center, Charlottesville, 1995.

meals.[4] Some persons with diabetes may even need to test in the middle of the night (2–4 AM) to help determine if the fasting blood glucose is elevated.

The basic guidelines for frequency of monitoring are listed below. It is important to emphasize that these are guidelines only and individualization will be necessary.[4]

Type I Diabetes

➤ Test before each meal and at bedtime.
➤ If necessary, test again 1 to 2 hours after meals and in the middle of the night (2–4 AM).

Type II Diabetes

➤ If the condition is managed with diabetes medical nutrition therapy and exercise, ideally test daily at random times throughout the day; at a minimum test once or twice a week at random times throughout the day (eg, Sunday—before breakfast; Monday—2 hours after breakfast; Tuesday—before lunch; Wednesday—2 hours after lunch; Thursday—before dinner; Friday—2 hours after dinner; and Saturday—before bedtime).
➤ If the condition is managed with the addition of oral glucose-lowering medication, test at least once a day, at different times each day. If control is good, test one to two times per week.
➤ If the condition is managed with the addition of insulin, test at least twice a day, at different times each day. Random testing is important to determine a 24-hour profile of blood glucose levels, but testing at consistent times is important to determine a pattern in blood glucose levels.

Types I and II Diabetes

Testing more frequently is important when:

➤ schedules change;
➤ exercise is adjusted;
➤ illness occurs;

- a new nondiabetes medication is initiated that will affect blood glucose (eg, prednisone) or will affect the ability to recognize low blood glucose (eg, beta blockers);
- diabetes medication is adjusted;
- the effect of a certain kind or amount of food is being determined;
- the effect of weight loss and/or exercise is being determined.[4]

Monitoring records should be examined at each visit to identify patterns. On the basis of these patterns, medical, nutritional, and lifestyle therapy can be adjusted to meet the identified goals. A three-step process that can be used to review blood glucose records is described in *Table 6.1*.[5]

Reviewing Blood Glucose Monitoring Records

Table 6.1
Framework for Interpreting SMBG Records

SMBG records are used to evaluate the diabetes management triad (food, insulin, and activity), as well as other factors that affect diabetes care, eg, stress, sick days, and treatment of hypoglycemia. Using the following three-step process will provide guidance in interpreting the records. The diabetes educator should involve the client with each question to obtain his or her perspective.

Step 1. Are additional data needed?

- Is food intake consistent from day to day?
- Are changes from the meal plan noted?
- How are low blood glucose levels treated? Are they really low blood glucose levels? Are they being overtreated?
- Are changes in activity noted?
- Are stressful situations noted?
- Has the client made medication adjustments?
- Are possible reasons for glucose excursions written in the comment column of the record book?
- Are more blood tests needed?
- Can the client provide answers to questions or other insight on schedule or lifestyle variations?

Step 2. Are all possible interpretations considered?

- Are the results accurate and are they being correctly recorded?
- Is the meter calibrated? Are the strips fresh? Is user technique acceptable?
- Is diabetes medication being taken appropriately?
- Is there a trend to the results or are fluctuations isolated?
- Could meals be spaced more appropriately?
- Is one meal too large or too small?
- Is the meal plan understood and followed?
- Is activity irregular?
- Is there improper insulin coverage for meals?
- Has the influence of food, activity, and insulin (endogenous and/or exogenous) been considered?

Step 3. Are all possible management changes considered?

- What changes would the client choose to make?
- Should food be distributed differently?
- Should weight reduction be the priority?
- Should changes in type and amount of carbohydrate, fat or alcohol intake, etc, be made?
- Should activity be more regular, increased, or decreased?
- Should the medication regimen be adjusted?
    - Would multiple insulin injections help?
    - Would larger/smaller doses of oral glucose-lowering medication be helpful?

Source: © 1987 Margaret A. Powers. Adapted from *Handbook of Diabetes Medical Nutrition Therapy* (Gaithersburg, Md: Aspen Publishers; 1996), p. 139.

Diabetes Medical Nutrition Therapy

Adjustment of therapy should be based on a pattern, rather than a single blood glucose test result, and changes in medication dosage need to be made gradually. There are several possible solutions to any management problem, and the best answer may not be a change in the eating plan. Common problem patterns of blood glucose monitoring are presented in *Table 6.2*.

The following case studies show how monitoring records are used in diabetes medical nutrition therapy.

Table 6.2
Common Problem Patterns Found from Blood Glucose Monitoring

Problem	Potential Cause	Potential Solutions
High fasting glucose	Insulin resistance, insufficient insulin available overnight, rebound hyperglycemia overnight (Somogyi effect), dawn phenomenon	Adjust PM intermediate- or long-acting insulin dose or time Lose weight to reduce insulin resistance
High glucose after breakfast	Inadequate insulin produced or injected to cover breakfast, peak insulin action not at anticipated time	Adjust time or dose of short-acting AM insulin Decrease size of breakfast, adjust amount of breakfast carbohydrate, or divide breakfast into two smaller morning meals
Insulin reactions (hypoglycemia) before lunch	Insufficient breakfast for AM short-acting insulin or peak action later than anticipated time	Adjust time, type, or dose of AM short-acting insulin Add morning snack or increase breakfast
Insulin reactions (hypoglycemia) in afternoon	Excessive AM intermediate-acting insulin, skipping or inadequate lunch	Adjust time, type, or dose of AM intermediate-acting insulin Add afternoon snack or increase lunch
High glucose in afternoon	Inadequate insulin produced, intermediate-acting AM insulin insufficient, or excessive snack or lunch	Adjust time or dose of PM insulin Decrease or omit afternoon snack or decrease lunch carbohydrate
High glucose at night after evening meal	Inadequate insulin produced, insulin insufficient to cover dinner, or evening meal too large	Adjust time or dose of PM insulin Reduce size of meal or alter meal composition (decrease carbohydrate)
Insulin reactions (hypoglycemia) at night	Excessive amount of insulin or insufficient dinner meal or evening snack	Adjust time, type, or dose of evening or bedtime insulin Increase dinner and/or snack carbohydrate

Adapted from MA Powers et al, *Nutrition Guide for Professionals: Diabetes Education and Meal Planning* (Chicago, Ill: American Dietetic Association; 1989), p 6.

In addition to food and insulin, other factors may affect blood glucose (eg, exercise, sick days, infection). Insulin resistance associated with obesity is likely to result in high glucose levels throughout the day.

Case Study 1A

Evaluation of JB's case *(Table 6.3)* is a good way to begin reviewing blood glucose records using the three-step process presented in Table 6.1.

➤ *Step 1: Determine if more data are needed.*
Three blood glucose tests are within JB's target range and two are above. Breakfast and lunch are 5½ hours apart and lunch and dinner 3½ hours apart. These are interesting data, but they are inadequate for making management changes. More blood glucose tests, especially postprandial blood glucose, are needed to establish a pattern of control, and information on actual food intake and exercise/activity habits is needed. Some records are designed to collect this information along with the blood glucose test results.

➤ *Step 2: Consider possible interpretations.*
The data are too limited for interpretation.

➤ *Step 3: Develop a plan of action and recommendations.*
Discuss the need for additional data. Ask for JB's input; find out what JB is willing to do. Establish specifics about more blood glucose tests (three or more times a day for one week) and recording of food and activity habits.

Case Study 1B

In this case *(Table 6.4)*, JB returns with additional blood glucose monitoring test results.

➤ *Step 1: Determine if more data are needed.*
JB did more than asked and did four blood glucose tests a day to establish whether there was a pattern. Assuming that the food and activity records are consistent and are not unusual, one would look closely at the monitoring record for clues as to why the predinner blood glucose tests were elevated.

➤ *Step 2: Consider possible interpretations.*
Knowing JB's meal times provides valuable information. He has type II diabetes and takes no diabetes medication; thus, the meal spacing most likely is the cause of the elevation before dinner.

➤ *Step 3: Develop a plan of action and recommendations.*
Moving lunch earlier would be ideal; however, JB probably has this eating pattern for a reason. If eating lunch earlier is not a possibility due to lack of access to food, lack of time, or another reason, other options should be

Table 6.3
JB Blood Glucose Record

	Breakfast	*Lunch*	*Dinner*	*Evening Snack*
Wed	110	—	153	—
Thurs	80	—	—	—
Fri	—	182	—	—
Sat	—	—	91	—

Diabetes: type II
Medications: none
Target Goals: 80–120 mg/dL premeal
Meal Times: B—8:30 AM; L—2:00 PM; D—5:30 PM; S—9:30 PM

Reprinted with permission from *Maximizing the Role of Nutrition in Diabetes Management* (Alexandria, Va: American Diabetes Association, Inc; 1994).

Table 6.4
JB Blood Glucose Record

	Breakfast	Lunch	Dinner	Evening Snack
Tues	90	100	215	110
Wed	110	90	190	85
Thurs	100	115	185	90

Diabetes: type II
Medications: none
Target Goals: 80–120 mg/dL premeal
Meal Times: B—8:30 AM; L—2:00 PM; D—5:30 PM; S—9:30 PM

Reprinted with permission from *Maximizing the Role of Nutrition in Diabetes Management* (Alexandria, Va: American Diabetes Association, Inc; 1994).

explored. Perhaps two small snacks could replace the lunch, one at 11:30 AM or noon and the other at 2:00 PM. The earlier snack could be food that could be planned in the morning and would not require special care or preparation. The diabetes care team needs to be sure the plan is acceptable to JB and can realistically be achieved. In addition to meal/snack timing changes, the plan would also recommend continuing the additional blood glucose testing.

Case Study 2

CW *(Table 6.5)* has type I diabetes and is on two injections of split-mixed insulin a day (before breakfast and before dinner; Regular and NPH intermediate-acting insulin). In order to intensify her care and improve glycemic control, the types, times, and amounts in the insulin regimen need to be examined.

▶*Step 1: Determine if more data are needed.*
CW is willing to change her current insulin regimen; the dietitian needs to carefully assess the consistency of her meal plan, current level of physical activity, timing of insulin injection, activity, and meals, and knowledge of nutrition and hypoglycemia. Also, CW's accuracy in the blood glucose testing procedure and insulin-administration skills need to be assessed to exclude errors that may have resulted in the elevated blood glucose tests.

▶*Step 2: Consider possible interpretations.*
▶ Elevated glucose levels — fasting, before lunch, and before bedtime snack.
▶ Evaluate meal spacing, size of breakfast and bedtime snack, and patterns of exercise.

▶ *Step 3: Develop a plan of action and recommendations.*
▶ Consider switching NPH intermediate-acting insulin injection to before bedtime instead of before dinner meal.
▶ Consider increasing amount of evening intermediate insulin.
▶ Consider increasing Regular insulin in the morning.
▶ Consider adding Regular insulin in the evening.
▶ Consider injecting insulin more than 30 minutes before meals.
▶ Consider switching from short-acting (Regular) insulin to rapid-acting (Lispro) insulin.

Table 6.5
CW Blood Glucose Record

	Breakfast	Lunch	Dinner	Evening Snack
Wed	180	165	90	146
Thurs	192	227	70	160
Fri	174	150	140	184

Diabetes: type I
Medications: 22 NPH, 6 Reg before breakfast; 12 NPH, 4 Reg before dinner
Target Goals: 80–120 mg/dL premeal
Meal Times: B—6:30 AM; L—11:30 AM; D—6:30 PM; S—10:00 PM

Reprinted with permission from *Maximizing the Role of Nutrition in Diabetes Management* (Alexandria, Va: American Diabetes Association, Inc; 1994).

Summary

Blood glucose response patterns are very useful in initial meal planning and subsequent adjustments of food, medication, and exercise regimens. Careful review of SMBG records by the diabetes educator is necessary to evaluate the client's management of diabetes.

References

1. American Diabetes Association Consensus Statement: self-monitoring of blood glucose. *Diabetes Care.* 1996;19(suppl 1); S62–S66.
2. Diabetes Control and Complications Trial Research Group. Expanded role of the dietitian in the Diabetes Control and Complications Trial: implications for clinical practice. *J Am Diet Assoc.* 1993;93:758–767.
3. Monk A, Barry B, McClain K, Weaver T, Cooper N, Franz M. Practice guidelines for medical nutrition therapy provided by dietitians for persons with non-insulin-dependent diabetes. *J Am Diet Assoc.* 1995;95:999–1006.
4. Franz M, Kulkarni K, Leontos C, Maryniuk M, McLaughlin S, Powers M. *Maximizing the Role of Nutrition in Diabetes Management.* Alexandria, Va: American Diabetes Association; 1994.
5. Wylie-Rosett J, Walker EA, Engel SS. Comprehensive monitoring for evaluating diabetes therapy. In: Powers MA, ed. *The Handbook of Diabetes Medical Nutrition Therapy.* 2nd ed. Gaithersburg, Md: Aspen Publishers, Inc; 1996: 134–149.

For Further Reading

American Diabetes Association. Self-monitoring of blood glucose (consensus statement). Diabetes Care. 1995;18:47–52.
Delahanty L, Richardson MG. Blood glucose monitoring for nutrition focused care. In: Powers MA, ed. *The Handbook of Diabetes Medical Nutrition Therapy.* 2nd ed. Gaithersburg, Md: Aspen Publishers, Inc; 1996: 150–161.
Diabetes Care and Education Practice Group/The American Dietetic Association. Applying new technology in diabetes management: meters, insulin and insulin delivery. *On the Cutting Edge.* Summer 1992.
Powers MA. Self-monitoring of blood glucose. *Top Clin Nutr.* 1988;3(1):25–31.
Skyler SJ. Insulin treatment. In: Lebovitz HE, ed. *Therapy for Diabetes Mellitus and Related Disorders.* 2nd ed. Alexandria, Va: American Diabetes Association; 1994: 1131–1141.

Management of Diabetes: Intensive Insulin Therapy

7

In the 1990s we are witnessing the emergence of the concept of "empowerment." Clients now can become masters of self-management using therapeutic tools developed during the 1980s. Technological advances include improvements in blood glucose monitoring equipment and supplies, oral glucose-lowering medications, insulin, and insulin delivery systems. Self-management tools, which include a variety of meal-planning approaches, exercise programs, and stress-management skills, are combined with technology for improved diabetes care.

For complete understanding of the relationship between diabetes technology and state-of-the-art management of type I diabetes, including carbohydrate-to-insulin ratios, a review of intensive insulin therapy is included here.

Intensive insulin therapy (IIT) is a comprehensive system of diabetes management.[1] The treatment goals are improved glycemia and client well-being. IIT includes multiple daily injections (MDI) using combinations of insulin analog (rapid-acting), Regular (short-acting), NPH or Lente (intermediate-acting), or Ultralente (long-acting) insulin, as well as continuous subcutaneous insulin infusion (CSII) of Regular insulin or insulin analog using a pump.

Researchers in the 1980s determined that the best way to approximate normal physiologic insulin delivery for people with type I diabetes was through IIT, using either MDI or CSII. Many diabetes care team members believe that IIT is the best way to achieve normoglycemia or near normoglycemia and prevent or delay the chronic complications of diabetes, as demonstrated in the Diabetes Control and Complications Trial (see Chapter 3).[2]

Elements of ITT include:

- A multiple-component insulin regimen,
- Frequent self-monitoring of blood glucose (SMBG),
- Individualized target blood glucose levels (Appendix 1),
- Balance of food, activity, and insulin,
- Client self-management training in adjusting food, insulin, and activity,
- Strong support from a diabetes care team experienced in IIT, with 24-hour availability. The team usually includes a physician, nurse, and dietitian and may also include an exercise specialist and mental health professional.

An insulin program is selected for optimal control and the ability to coordinate with the client's meal plan and lifestyle.

Selecting Insulin Regimens

Diabetes Medical Nutrition Therapy

Table 7.1

Sample Multiple Daily Injection Regimens

REGIMEN	BEFORE BREAKFAST	BEFORE LUNCH	BEFORE DINNER	BEFORE BEDTIME	ADVANTAGE	DISADVANTAGE
A	N/R or L/R		R	N or L	Improved AM fasting BG	Requires 3 injections. Meal times and sizes are less flexible
B	R	R	R	N or L	More flexibility with meal times and sizes	Requires 4 injections
C	R or U/R	R	U/R*		More flexibility with meal times and sizes	Requires 3 injections

R = Regular (short-acting insulin); N = NPH (intermediate-acting insulin); L = Lente (intermediate-acting insulin; U = Ultralente (long-acting insulin). In some cases, insulin analog may be used in place of R.
*In some cases, Ultralente insulin may be given before bedtime rather than before dinner.

Source: Diabetes Care and Education Practice Group, *Meal Planning Approaches for Diabetes Management*, 2nd ed (Chicago, Ill: American Dietetic Association; 1994: 103).

Figure 7.1

Idealized Periods of Insulin Effect in Three MDI Regimens

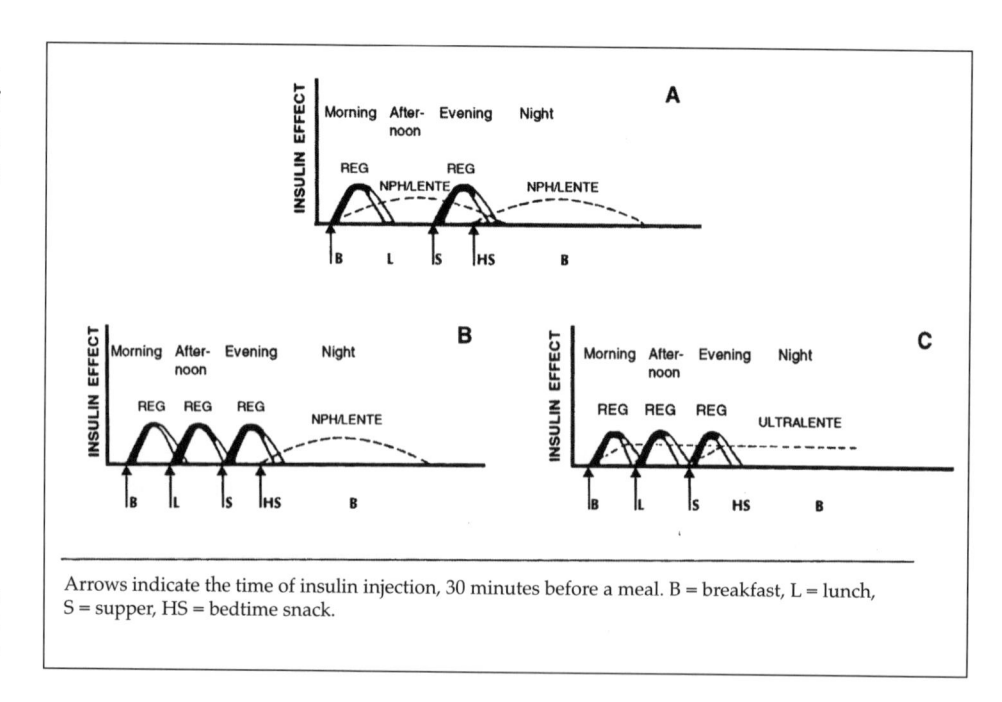

Arrows indicate the time of insulin injection, 30 minutes before a meal. B = breakfast, L = lunch, S = supper, HS = bedtime snack.

Adapted with permission from *Intensive Diabetes Management* (Alexandria, Va: American Diabetes Association; 1995).

MDI regimens are summarized in *Table 7.1* and *Figure 7.1*. Some devices for administering insulin can facilitate MDI therapy:

➤ Ultrafine needles, lubricated and honed to precision sharpness, minimize discomfort at injection sites.
➤ Low-dose syringes increase accuracy at smaller dose levels.
➤ Insulin pens (injection devices that look like a pen and use insulin cartridges) provide added convenience.
➤ Jet injectors do not puncture the skin, but instead force a tiny stream of insulin through the skin (these devices are expensive and must be well cleaned).

Continuous subcutaneous insulin infusion (CSII or insulin pump) regimens involve an insulin pump that is smaller (about the size of a pager) and easier

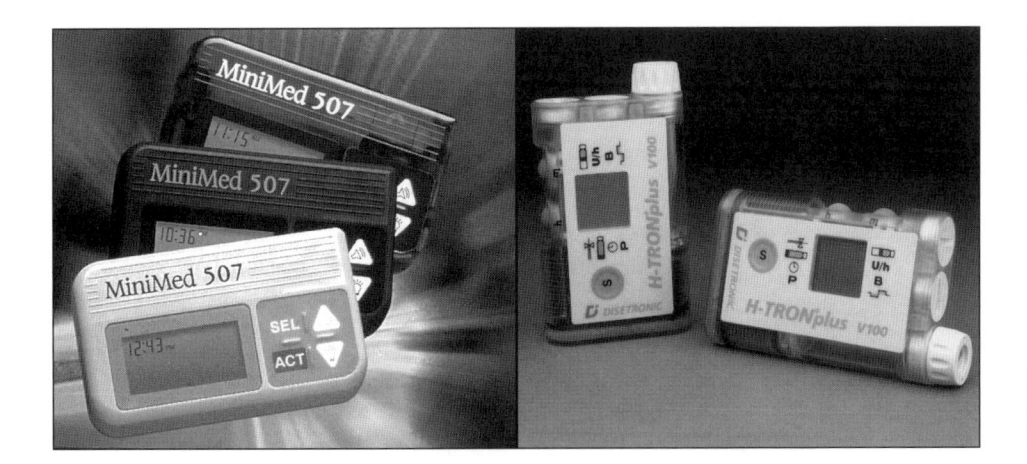

Figure 7.2
Insulin Pumps

Reprinted with permission from MiniMed and Disetronic Medical Systems, Inc.

to use and has better safety features than earlier models *(Figure 7.2)*. The pump is worn externally (clipped to a belt, for example) or carried in a pocket or customized case or pouch. The insulin pump delivers a continuous flow of basal regular insulin through a flexible, plastic infusion line that ends in a small needle or flexible plastic cannula inserted under the skin, usually in the abdomen, and secured with bio-occlusive tape. The basal insulin rate is individualized to a client's need for varying amounts of insulin throughout the day and night. The user can command the pump to deliver a bolus of insulin whenever needed, as before a meal or snack (meal dose), or to counteract a high blood glucose value. The latter is referred to as a supplemental dose.[3]

Glucose Monitoring

In comparing studies of IIT regimens, researchers noted that excellent glycemic control could be achieved with all regimens.[2] Two key factors in attaining optimal glycemic control were noted: frequent SMBG (four or more times per day) and taking action on the information obtained from SMBG.

Improvements in blood glucose meters facilitate making insulin adjustments based on SMBG results. These improvements include increased accuracy, greater ease of use, built-in data management systems, and telemetry (sending records via modem over phone lines to a computer for access by the diabetes care team).

Insulin Adjustment

Insulin adjustments can be made retrospectively based on information obtained from SMBG and careful recording of results. Basic daily doses are adjusted based on patterns seen in several days of blood glucose records. The effects of changes in food, activity, and stress are considered before insulin doses are increased or decreased to achieve target blood glucose ranges. Generally, using the retrospective method for insulin adjustment and using a target blood glucose range of 80 to 150 mg/dL, the following calculations are made:

➤ Raise insulin dose by 1–2 units for corresponding blood glucose values of > 150 for 2 or more days.
➤ Lower insulin dose by 1–2 units for corresponding blood glucose values of < 80.

Many algorithms and record forms have been developed to simplify these adjustments. A sample of an algorithm for insulin adjustment and supple-

Figure 7.3

Algorithm/Record for Insulin Adjustment and Supplementation

Name: _____ Phone: H( )_____ W( )_____ Fax ( )_____
Current Insulin Dose: Breakfast: _____ Lunch: _____ Dinner: _____ Bedtime: _____
BG Target Range: _____ mg/dL to _____ mg/dL   Supplement Formula: $\dfrac{BG - Y}{X}$

DATE	3 AM	Pre-Breakfast				Pre-Lunch				Pre-Dinner					Bedtime		Remarks
	BG	BG	NPH/UL	REG	SUP	TOT	BG	REG	SUP	TOT	BG	NPH/UL	REG	SUP	TOT	BG	NPH/UL	

Key:
BG = blood glucose
NPH/L = NPH or Lente: intermediate-acting insulin (basal)
UL = Ultralente: long-acting insulin (basal)
REG = Regular: short-acting insulin (meal dose)
SUP = supplemental Regular insulin: based on BG value obtained prior to injection and using personal supplement formula:
$$\dfrac{BG - Y}{X}$$
Y = specific target BG established by diabetes team (usually midpoint of target BG range, eg, 120 mg/dL for target range of 80–150 mg/dL)
X = estimated BG drop per 1 unit insulin [X can be estimated by dividing 1500 by total number of units of insulin per day (REG + NPH/L or UL)]
TOT = total units REG + SUP to be given at the meal

Steps for using algorithm and calculating insulin adjustment and supplement
1. Record results of self-monitored BGs and units of insulin taken.
   a. Use a * symbol to indicate a low BG value (usually <60 mg/dL) or a BG that corresponds with symptoms of an insulin reaction. Include specific comments about the event under remarks section.
   b. Use a # symbol to indicate a low BG value that was the result of exercise. Include specific comments about the type and duration of exercise under remarks section.
   c. Use a + symbol to indicate a high BG value that is the result of eating more than your usual amount. Include specific comments about the event under remarks section.
2. Adjust daily insulin doses based on patterns seen in BGs resulting from usual daily activities and usual meals and snacks:
   Raise insulin dose by 1–2 units for corresponding BGs >150 for 2 days.
   Lower insulin dose by 1–2 units for corresponding BGs <80.
   a. Pre-Breakfast and 3 AM BGs correspond to Pre-Dinner or Bedtime NPH
   b. Pre-Lunch BG corresponds to Breakfast Regular
   c. Pre-Dinner BG corresponds to Pre-Breakfast NPH/L or Pre-Lunch Regular
   d. Bedtime BG corresponds to Pre-Dinner Regular
3. You may find it helpful to highlight BGs >150 with a yellow marker and BGs <80 with a pink marker.
4. Determine Regular insulin supplement, based on current BG value, using personal supplement formula and add or subtract (if BG is low, you will get a negative number) number of units of insulin supplement to/from meal dose Regular.

Based on algorithm/record developed by Paul C. Davidson, MD. Used by permission.

Source: Diabetes Care and Education Practice Group, *Meal Planning Approaches for Diabetes Management*, 2nd ed (Chicago, Ill: American Dietetic Association; 1994: 103).

---

mentation appears in *Figure 7.3*, and an example using the retrospective method of insulin adjustment is detailed in *Figure 7.4*.

Prospective adjustments, often referred to as insulin supplements, are used for altering doses of Regular insulin. Prospective adjustments are either compensatory or anticipatory.[4] Compensatory adjustments are based on the blood glucose value obtained just prior to injection. Using an individualized formula or dose schedule based on the blood glucose value, the client with diabetes can increase or decrease the usual amount of Regular insulin to compensate for the current blood glucose value.

The formula for calculating individualized compensatory Regular insulin adjustment is[5]:

Figure 7.4
Algorithm/Record for Insulin Adjustment and Supplementation (Retrospective Adjustment)

Name: __Marianne__ Phone: H( ) W( ) Fax ( )
Current Insulin Dose: Breakfast: __6 U R__ Lunch: __7 U R__ Dinner: __8 U R__ Bedtime: __15 U NPH__
BG Target Range: __80__ mg/dL to __150__ mg/dL   Supplement Formula: $\frac{BG - 120}{40}$

DATE	3AM BG	Pre-Breakfast BG	NPH/UL	REG	SUP	TOT	Pre-Lunch BG	REG	SUP	TOT	Pre-Dinner BG	NPH/UL	REG	SUP	TOT	Bedtime BG	NPH/UL	Remarks
7/1		58		6			182	7			80		8			200	13	
7/2	62*	163		6			176	7			220		8			250	11	
7/3	80	112		8			148	7			318		10			160	11	
7/4	120	64		8			80	9			168		10			247+	9	+BBQ Supper Ate too much
7/5		172		8			100	9			60#		10			140	9	# Cycling in afternoon
7/6	72	138		8			90	9			118		10			147	9	

Key:
BG = blood glucose
NPH/L = NPH or Lente: intermediate-acting insulin (basal)
UL = Ultralente: long-acting insulin (basal)
REG = Regular: short-acting insulin (meal dose)
SUP = supplemental Regular insulin: based on BG value obtained prior to injection and using personal supplement formula:
$$\frac{BG - Y}{X}$$
Y = specific target BG established by diabetes team (usually midpoint of target BG range, eg, 120 mg/dL for target range of 80–150 mg/dL)
X = estimated BG drop per 1 unit insulin [X can be estimated by dividing 1500 by total number of units of insulin per day (REG + NPH/L or UL)]
TOT = total units REG + SUP to be given at the meal

Steps for using algorithm and calculating insulin adjustment and supplement
1. Record results of self-monitored BGs and units of insulin taken.
  a. Use a * symbol to indicate a low BG value (usually <60 mg/dL) or a BG that corresponds with symptoms of an insulin reaction. Include specific comments about the event under remarks section.
  b. Use a # symbol to indicate a low BG value that was the result of exercise. Include specific comments about the type and duration of exercise under remarks section.
  c. Use a + symbol to indicate a high BG value that is the result of eating more than your usual amount. Include specific comments about the event under remarks section.
2. Adjust daily insulin doses based on patterns seen in BGs resulting from usual daily activities and usual meals and snacks:
   Raise insulin dose by 1–2 units for corresponding BGs >150 for 2 days.
   Lower insulin dose by 1–2 units for corresponding BGs <80.
  a. Pre-Breakfast and 3 AM BGs correspond to Pre-Dinner or Bedtime NPH
  b. Pre-Lunch BG corresponds to Breakfast Regular
  c. Pre-Dinner BG corresponds to Pre-Breakfast NPH/L or Pre-Lunch Regular
  d. Bedtime BG corresponds to Pre-Dinner Regular
3. You may find it helpful to highlight BGs >150 with a yellow marker and BGs <80 with a pink marker.
4. Determine Regular insulin supplement, based on current BG value, using personal supplement formula and add or subtract (if BG is low, you will get a negative number) number of units of insulin supplement to/from meal dose Regular.

Based on algorithm/record developed by Paul C. Davidson, MD. Used by permission.

Source: Diabetes Care and Education Practice Group, *Meal Planning Approaches for Diabetes Management*, 2nd ed (Chicago, Ill: American Dietetic Association; 1994: 106).

$$\frac{BG - Y}{X} = \text{Regular insulin (units) for adjustment}$$

where
BG = blood glucose value;
Y = specific target BG established by diabetes care team (usually midpoint of target BG range, eg, 120 mg/dL for target range of 80 to 150 mg/dL); and
X = estimated BG drop for 1 unit Regular insulin (sensitivity factor).

The sensitivity factor or estimated BG drop for 1 unit of Regular insulin is 1,500 divided by the total units insulin per day. The "1,500 rule" is based on clinical observation of 15 years of use in a practice of 10,000 persons with diabetes.[5] Estimated BG drop also can be determined based on the client's history.

Total units of insulin per day include intermediate- or long-acting insulin plus Regular insulin if on MDI or basal plus meal dose regular if on CSII. There are two different methods for estimating total daily insulin requirements:

➤ Divide actual body weight in pounds by 4.[5]
➤ Multiply reasonable body weight (RBW) in pounds by 0.3 (0.2 if new to insulin treatment).[5] According to this method, a client with a RBW of 120 lb would need an estimated 36 units of insulin per day (120 × 0.3 = 36).

Total daily insulin would be increased or decreased as insulin adjustments are made over time, changing the estimated BG drop for 1 unit of Regular insulin. The X value may need to be recalculated from time to time.

The following is an example for calculating compensatory insulin adjustment (insulin supplement). A client with diabetes has an actual BG of 200 mg/dL and takes 36 units of insulin per day. The first calculation is to determine X, since the actual BG value (200 mg/dL) and Y (120 mg/dL) are already known. $X = 1,500 \div 36$ units of insulin per day = 41.6 (round off to 40 for ease in calculating supplement). Therefore, the compensatory insulin adjustment can be determined as follows:

$$\frac{200 - 120}{40} = 2 \text{ units of Regular insulin}$$

An example using the prospective compensatory method for insulin supplementation in a sample client for several days in a variety of situations (eg, insulin reaction, exercise, overeating) is shown in *Figure 7.5*. The figure combines retrospective adjustments and prospective, anticipatory compensatory adjustments (insulin supplements) as used in actual clinical practice.

Anticipatory adjustments can be accomplished through two different methods. First, they can be based on the amount of food (primarily carbohydrate) to be eaten at the meal. Regular insulin doses are increased or decreased depending on whether one is consuming larger or smaller amounts of carbohydrate than normal at the meal. This method of insulin adjustment is also called *carbohydrate counting: using carbohydrate/insulin ratios* and is discussed in further detail in Chapter 20.

The second method of anticipatory adjustment is based on the amount of exercise to be performed. The NPH and/or Regular insulin dose is adjusted up or down depending on the anticipated activity level during the duration of insulin action.

Both of these types of anticipatory adjustments need to be individualized and involve both the client and the diabetes team.

Candidates for IIT

Candidates for IIT include clients with type I diabetes who are seeking improved glycemic control and/or increased flexibility in lifestyle. If the client with type I diabetes is a child* or older adult and needs assistance with diabetes management, a caregiver must be available for training and supervision.

---

* There currently exists controversy about use of intensive insulin therapy for infants, toddlers, and children with diabetes because of the increased risk of hypoglycemia. The decision to use IIT should be individualized based on the family's support and intellectual, emotional, financial, and domestic status.[3]

Figure 7.5

Algorithm/Record for Insulin Adjustment and Supplementation (Retrospective Adjustments Plus Supplements)

Name: __Marianne_____ Phone: H( )_____ W( )_____ Fax ( )_____
Current Insulin Dose: Breakfast: __6 UR__ Lunch: __7 UR__ Dinner: __8 UR__ Bedtime: __15 U NPH__
BG Target Range: __80__ mg/dL to __150__ mg/dL   Supplement Formula: $\frac{BG - 120}{40}$

DATE	3AM BG	Pre-Breakfast BG	NPH/UL	REG	SUP	TOT	Pre-Lunch BG	REG	SUP	TOT	Pre-Dinner BG	NPH/UL	REG	SUP	TOT	Bedtime BG	NPH/UL	Remarks
7/1		58		6	-2	4	182	7	+2	9	80		8	0	8	200	13	
7/2	62*	163		6	+1	7	176	7	+1	8	220		8	+2	10	250	11	
7/3	80	112		8	0	8	148	7	+1	8	318		10	+5	15	160	11	
7/4	120	64		8	-1	7	80	9	0	9	168		10	+1	11	247+	9	+BBQ Supper Ate too much
7/5		172		8	+1	9	100	9	0	9	60#		10	-1	9	140	9	# Cycling in afternoon
7/6	72	138		8	0	8	90	9	0	9	118		10	0	10	147	9	

Key:
BG = blood glucose
NPH/L = NPH or Lente: intermediate-acting insulin (basal)
UL = Ultralente: long-acting insulin (basal)
REG = Regular: short-acting insulin (meal dose)
SUP = supplemental Regular insulin: based on BG value obtained prior to injection and using personal supplement formula:
$$\frac{BG - Y}{X}$$
Y = specific target BG established by diabetes team (usually midpoint of target BG range, eg, 120 mg/dL for target range of 80-150 mg/dL)
X = estimated BG drop per 1 unit insulin [X can be estimated by dividing 1500 by total number of units of insulin per day (REG + NPH/L or UL)]
TOT = total units REG + SUP to be given at the meal

Steps for using algorithm and calculating insulin adjustment and supplement
1. Record results of self-monitored BGs and units of insulin taken.
   a. Use a * symbol to indicate a low BG value (usually <60 mg/dL) or a BG that corresponds with symptoms of an insulin reaction. Include specific comments about the event under remarks section.
   b. Use a # symbol to indicate a low BG value that was the result of exercise. Include specific comments about the type and duration of exercise under remarks section.
   c. Use a + symbol to indicate a high BG value that is the result of eating more than your usual amount. Include specific comments about the event under remarks section.
2. Adjust daily insulin doses based on patterns seen in BGs resulting from usual daily activities and usual meals and snacks:
      Raise insulin dose by 1-2 units for corresponding BGs >150 for 2 days.
      Lower insulin dose by 1-2 units for corresponding BGs <80.
   a. Pre-Breakfast and 3 AM BGs correspond to Pre-Dinner or Bedtime NPH
   b. Pre-Lunch BG corresponds to Breakfast Regular
   c. Pre-Dinner BG corresponds to Pre-Breakfast NPH/L or Pre-Lunch Regular
   d. Bedtime BG corresponds to Pre-Dinner Regular
3. You may find it helpful to highlight BGs >150 with a yellow marker and BGs <80 with a pink marker.
4. Determine Regular insulin supplement, based on current BG value, using personal supplement formula and add or subtract (if BG is low, you will get a negative number) number of units of insulin supplement to/from meal dose Regular.

Based on algorithm/record developed by Paul C. Davidson, MD. Used by permission.

Source: Diabetes Care and Education Practice Group, *Meal Planning Approaches for Diabetes Management*, 2nd ed (Chicago, Ill: American Dietetic Association; 1994: 108).

Additional characteristics of candidates for IIT include:

➤ Responsible and motivated to be the key player on the management team,
➤ Capable of performing the technical and cognitive skills of frequent SMBG and administration of either multiple injections or insulin pump therapy in response to blood glucose information, food intake, and activity level,
➤ Psychologically stable,
➤ Financially able to manage the expense of IIT,
➤ Access to knowledgeable health care professionals.

Blood glucose targets must be individualized for each client's needs and must be clearly defined to aid in self-adjustment of insulin. Special precautions must be used for those at increased risk for hypoglycemia—clients with hypoglycemia unawareness (hypoglycemic unresponsiveness or desensitization to the usual early warning signs of hypoglycemia) and/or counterregulatory insufficiency (decreased activity of the body's natural defenses against low blood sugar levels).[6] Age is also a factor. Young children and older adults may not sense or respond to hypoglycemia as well as other age groups. Blood glucose targets may need to be higher for people at increased risk for hypoglycemia, if they are candidates for IIT.

Clinical Setting

Self-management skills may be introduced in either the inpatient or ambulatory care setting. The inpatient setting offers the advantage of frequent observation of response to insulin doses and the opportunity to make adjustments with the 24-hour supervision of the diabetes care team. The outpatient setting offers the advantage of experiencing the effects of living in the "real world" while making adjustments to the new regimen, and requires 24-hour access to a knowledgeable diabetes team member.

Length of Time to Teach

The length of time required to teach IIT skills varies according to age, current diabetes self-management skills, and ability to master new skills. Clients on MDI may need two to six visits over 4 to 6 weeks, with additional telephone contact and weekly or semiweekly reporting of blood glucose records. Clients on CSII may need daily visits or contact for the first week, followed by weekly visits for the following 2 to 3 weeks, with additional telephone contact and weekly or semiweekly reporting of blood glucose levels.

Advantages/ Disadvantages

Advantages associated with IIT are:

➤ *Increased lifestyle flexibility.* Insulin can be adjusted for greater flexibility with exercise, meal timing, and food portions.
➤ *Improved diabetes control.* Clients can more closely duplicate the body's normal physiologic insulin secretion than with standard or conventional insulin therapy (see Figure 7.1).[3] In pregnancy, tight blood glucose control prior to conception will reduce the frequency of congenital anomalies in infants of mothers with diabetes.[7] Preprandial blood glucose levels less than 100 mg/dL or 1-hour postbreakfast blood glucose levels that are less than 130 mg/dL (7.2 mmol) during pregnancy can reduce the risk of macrosomia to that of the nondiabetic population.[8]
➤ *Potentially fewer complications.* The benefits of IIT on prevention and delay of other diabetic complications have been established in the DCCT results (see Chapter 3).

Disadvantages associated with IIT include:
➤ *Hypoglycemia.* The DCCT's feasibility phase showed that IIT was accompanied by a threefold increase in severe hypoglycemia. These findings led to the exclusion of potential volunteers with a high risk

of hypoglycemia.[9] Because of this risk, clients on IIT need a comprehensive review of the prevention and treatment of hypoglycemia. Family members and caregivers also need a working knowledge of hypoglycemia treatment, including glucagon administration. Skipping and/or delaying meals, reducing carbohydrate intake at meals, and increasing activity without adjusting insulin are the major causes of hypoglycemia. Alcohol consumption also may induce hypoglycemia. Certain medications, such as beta blockers, reduce hypoglycemia awareness and therefore increase risk.

➤ *Weight gain.* After instituting intensive insulin therapy, people may experience weight gain because fewer calories are lost from glycosuria as glycemic control improves. Experimenting with new foods and larger meals may contribute to weight gain. Frequency of hypoglycemia and the extra calories used for treatment may also add unwanted pounds. Decreasing calories overall and closely monitoring fat intake may compensate for this tendency to gain weight.

Summary

Clients on IIT require close monitoring and encouragement. Clients may become discouraged and frustrated when target blood glucose levels are not met. However, diabetes educators can provide encouragement and support as well as reminders that progress, not perfection, is the treatment goal.

References

1. Hirsch IB, Farkas-Hirsch R, Skyler JS. Intensive insulin therapy for treatment of type I diabetes. *Diabetes Care.* 1990;13:1265–1283.
2. DCCT Research Group. The effect of intensive treatment of diabetes on the development and progression of long-term complications in insulin-dependent diabetes mellitus. *N Engl J Med.* 1993;329(4):977–986.
3. Farkas-Hirsch R, ed. *Intensive Diabetes Management.* Alexandria, Va: American Diabetes Association; 1995.
4. Davidson MB. How to get the most out of insulin therapy. *Clinical Diabetes.* 1990;8: 65–73.
5. Davidson PC. Bolus and supplemental insulin. In: Fredrickson L, ed. *The Insulin Pump Therapy Book: Insights from the Experts.* Los Angeles, Calif: MiniMed Technologies; 1995: 59–71.
6. Cryer PE, Fisher JN, Shamoon H. Hypoglycemia (technical review). *Diabetes Care.* 1994;17:734–755.
7. Kitzmiller JL, Buchanan TA, Kjos S, Combs CA. Preconception care of diabetes, congenital malformations, and spontaneous abortions (technical review). *Diabetes Care.* 1996;19(5):514–541.
8. Jare JW. Gestational diabetes mellitus: levels of glycemia as management goals. *Diabetes.* 1991; 40(suppl 2): 193–196.
9. Lorenz RA, Santiago JV, Siebert C, et al. Epidemiology of severe hypoglycemia in the diabetes control and complications trial. *Am J Med.* 1991;90:450–459.

Resources

Hollander P, Castle G, Ostrom-Joynes J, Nelson J. *Intensified Insulin Management for You: A Personal Program for Advanced Diabetes Self-Care.* Minneapolis: Chronimed Publishing; 1990.

Walsh J, Roberts R. *Pumping Insulin: Everything in a Book for Successful Use of an Insulin Pump.* San Diego, Calif: Torrey Pines Press; 1994.

For Further Reading

Applying new technology in diabetes management to nutrition counseling: meters, insulin, and insulin delivery systems. *On the Cutting Edge.* 1992;13:1-34.

Gokey D. Improving adherence: getting patients to stick to an intensive insulin regimen. *Diabetes Spectrum.* 1992;5:140-145.

Powers M. Facilitating nutritional changes in "difficult" patients. *Diabetes Spectrum.* 1991; 4:186-192.

Strowig SM. Initiation and management of insulin pump therapy. *Diabetes Educator.* 1993; 19:50-58.

Management of Diabetes: Different Life Stages

8

The role of diabetes medical nutrition therapy can influence the growth and development of children and adolescents, the outcome of pregnancy, and the quality of life of older adults. This chapter reviews the special situations in which nutritional intake is particularly critical for managing diabetes in these three life stages. As with adult clients with diabetes, using the four-pronged approach to diabetes medical nutrition therapy (assessment, goal setting, intervention, and evaluation), discussed in detail in Chapter 12, is crucial to achieving the individualized goals of diabetes self-management.

Children and Adolescents

Teamwork is particularly critical for optimal diabetes management in children and teens. The management process is complex and time-consuming and is best handled by a diabetes care team, which should include at least a physician, dietitian, and nurse trained in pediatric diabetes. However, the most important team members are the child and his or her family; their goals and concerns should be a priority.

Nutrition Assessment

A thorough nutrition assessment is the basis for the development of a meal plan for children and adolescents with diabetes (see Chapter 12 for more detail).

Clinical Data

A major goal in the nutritional care of children and adolescents with type I diabetes is maintenance of normal weight gain and growth. Five to 10 percent of all children with type I will not grow optimally. Possible causes of poor weight gain or linear growth include poor glycemic control, inadequate insulin, and overrestriction of calories.[1] The last may be a consequence of the common erroneous belief that restricting food, rather than adjusting insulin, is the way to control blood glucose. Reasons unrelated to diabetes also need to be considered, such as thyroid abnormalities, growth hormone deficiency, or malabsorption.

Excessive weight gain can be due to excessive calorie intake, overtreatment of hypoglycemia, or overinsulinization. Possible causes unrelated to diabetes include low activity level and hypothyroidism, which is always accompanied by poor linear growth.

The calorie level and a nutrition care plan for a child or adolescent are based on the nutrition assessment, as with other clients with diabetes. There are various ways to calculate the appropriate calorie needs for a child. The

Table 8.1
Estimating Needs for Calories in Youth

1. Base calories on nutrition assessment
2. Validate caloric needs
   - ► Method 1: National Academy of Sciences/Recommended Dietary Allowances guidelines
   - ► Method 2: 1,000 kcal for first year
     Toddlers between 1–3 years, 40 kcal per inch length
     Add 100 kcal per year up to age 11
     Girls 11–15 years, add 100 kcal or less per year after age 10
     Girls > 15 years, calculate as an adult
     Boys 11–15 years, add 200 kcal per year after age 10
     Boys > 15 years, 23 kcal/lb very active
                         18 kcal/lb usual
                         16 kcal/lb sedentary
   - ► Method 3: 1,000 kcal for first year
     Add 125 kcal × age for boys
     Add 100 kcal × age for girls
     Up to 20% more kcal for activity

Reprinted with permission from *Maximizing the Role of Nutrition in Diabetes Management* (Alexandria, Va: American Diabetes Association; 1994).

best method is probably to ascertain what the child usually eats to maintain his or her weight, because children have a natural ability to know just how much to eat for normal growth and development. As previously mentioned, adolescents and parents of young children need to learn to adjust insulin intake, rather than restrict food to control blood glucose levels.

Several formulas that can be used to confirm that a child is receiving the minimum number of necessary calories are shown in *Table 8.1*; also see Appendix 2, Table 4. Whatever the method, it is essential that the meal plan provide sufficient calories. If children are hungry, they must be allowed to eat.[2]

Nutrition History

An assessment of usual nutrition and food intake is important in developing or revising the meal plan.[3] A nutrition history for an infant should include types of foods/formulas consumed, amount consumed, usual feeding schedule, consistency of feeding schedule, and time/duration of naps and bedtime. For older children, there are several methods of obtaining information, including the following.

24-Hour Recalls and Food Records

The difficulty of obtaining food recalls or records may be increased if many people are involved in the care and feeding of the child. For a toddler, it is often hard to assess food eaten because as much ends up on the floor or the bib as actually gets swallowed.

Food History/Preferences

A food history should include questions about trying new foods, food aversions, food jags (cycles of eating the same food day after day), the place(s) where the child eats his or her meal, and the way food is obtained (eg, in a self-service kitchen, by trading lunches with others, from vending machines, or at fast-food restaurants).

All the factors in a child's life that will give a clear picture of usual activities and influences on eating should be included in the nutrition history. In evaluating the history, the dietitian must differentiate between what is offered and what is actually eaten. The following questions are helpful for exploring usual food intake:

➤ *School Routine:* What is the class schedule? Where is lunch eaten? Is food purchased from a cafeteria or vending machines? How are birthday parties/special events handled?
➤ *Weekend Routine:* Is there participation in after-school activities? Is a snack provided? How does this differ from the weekday routine?
➤ *Relationships with Siblings/Friends:* Is food part of the social life? Does the child go to a mall with friends on the weekend? If everyone else orders a milkshake at a fast-food restaurant, what does the child choose?
➤ *Factors That Influence Food Choices:* What are family food preferences and traditions? Is Friday night "pizza night"? What are the small child's self-feeding skills? Is the child making appropriate progress in the consumption of a variety of foods?
➤ *Self-Care Skills:* Is the child responsible for any part of his or her diabetes management? Does the child get his or her own breakfast or make lunch?

Since this assessment can be particularly challenging with a child, parents and caregivers play an important role.

➤ *Role of Parents and Caregivers.* Ideally, the dietitian should have data from all the people who are involved in the child's feeding, which may include parents, older siblings, grandparents, day-care workers, and teachers. Information about the purchasing and preparation of food and supervision of meals should be gathered.
➤ *Previous Nutrition Education.* Whatever nutrition education parents and other caregivers have had may prove to be either a help or a hindrance. What they know and where they learned it must be ascertained. Concerned parents tend to be enthusiastic learners and sometimes obtain as much nutrition misinformation as nutrition fact. If there are misconceptions, they will need to be corrected. Additionally, other family members who have food restrictions should be identified, so that all nutrition needs can be blended together.

Goal Setting

Blood glucose goals used for adults may not be realistic for most children, especially infants and toddlers (see Appendix 1 for blood glucose goals). Many pediatric endocrinologists aim for higher blood glucose levels to reduce the risk of hypoglycemia. Although the DCCT confirmed the relationship between control of glucose levels and the development of complications, the youngest participants in the study entered at the age of 13 years, and this study was not designed to evaluate the benefits or risks of tight control in prepubertal subjects. Moreover, there is evidence that the prepubertal years of diabetes may contribute minimally to progression of long-term complications.[4]

"Good control" is defined in the broader context of achievable goals, which include prevention of hypoglycemia and diabetic ketoacidosis, elimination of the symptoms of hyperglycemia, achievement of a sense of physical and emo-

Table 8.2
NCEP Treatment Guidelines for Ages 2–19 Years[5]

	Total Cholesterol (mg/dL)	LDL Cholesterol (mg/dL)
Desirable	< 170	< 110
Borderline high	170–199	110–129
High	≥ 200	≥ 130

tional well-being, maintenance of normal physical growth, and sexual maturation.

Young persons with diabetes are more likely than their age- and sex-matched counterparts without diabetes to experience morbidity and mortality from cardiovascular disease. Therefore, it is critical to reduce the risk factors associated with cardiovascular disease in children with type I diabetes. One method is to monitor and evaluate their lipid levels. Treatment guidelines established by the National Cholesterol Education Program (NCEP) for children (2 years of age and older) and teenagers are shown in *Table 8.2*. For children, the NCEP Step I meal plan of approximately 30% of total calories from fat is an appropriate therapy goal.[5]

Intervention

Most pediatric diabetes educators agree that it is better to start with a more precise meal plan and then teach flexibility than to start out too flexible and try to "tighten up" later. Chapters 17–21 present information about in-depth meal-planning resources.

Evaluation

Continuous assessment is more important for children than for adults because children's lives tend to be more variable. Changes in growth and development, changes in school routines, seasonal sports, and new child-care arrangements are just some of the factors that may necessitate a change in calorie requirements and meal plans. Blood glucose records help the dietitian determine the types of changes that will result in improved control and that will be easy to incorporate. Achieving optimal blood glucose control is a gradual process, and the family should be advised not to react to a single high blood glucose level on a particular day.

Summary (Children and Adolescents)

Successful outcomes in children and adolescents with type I diabetes are the result of a combination of factors:

➤ teamwork,
➤ frequent contact, with praise and reinforcement,
➤ flexibility and fun,
➤ healthful eating just as for children without diabetes,
➤ recognition that children are children *first!*

Pregnancy

Normalization of blood glucose levels during pregnancy is extremely important for women with diabetes. Glycemic goals for women with previously

Table 8.3
Blood Glucose Goals in Pregnancy[6,10]

	Preexisting Diabetes (mg/dL)	GDM (mg/dL)
Fasting	—	≤ 105
Premeal	70–100	—
1 hour postprandial	≤ 140	≤ 120
2 hours postprandial	≤ 120	≤ 120

Table 8.4
Preconception Planning[7]

	Blood Glucose Goals
Fasting and premeal	70–100 mg/dL
1 hr postprandial	≤ 140 mg/dL
2 hr postprandial	≤ 120 mg/dL
Hemoglobin A_{1c}	At or near upper limit of normal range

diagnosed diabetes and those who develop gestational diabetes mellitus (GDM) are shown in *Table 8.3*. Inadequate glycemic control affects the health and well-being of both the mother and her unborn child. This exciting time can be trying, yet some women become more committed to the management demands because of the influence on the unborn child.

Preconception Counseling for Women with Preexisting Diabetes

Several studies conducted over the last 10 years have compared the percentage of anomalies in infants born to mothers who had undergone preconception counseling and had achieved optimal blood glucose control with those in infants of mothers who had not received such counseling and who had poor metabolic control.[6] In every study, a larger percentage of anomalies occurred in infants with mothers with poor metabolic control. Thus, preconception counseling and the ability to achieve near-normal blood glucose levels can effectively reduce the incidence of anomalies to nearly that of the general population.[7]

Ideally, a woman with type I diabetes should have begun to receive preconception counseling at the onset of puberty, and it should continue throughout her childbearing years.[7] Blood glucose goals for preconception counseling are shown in *Table 8.4*. The implication of this table is that reaching these blood glucose goals leads to a decreased incidence of anomalies similar to those in the general population. The American Diabetes Association recommends that this level of glycemic control be achieved 1 to 2 months before contraception is discontinued.[6]

Metabolic Changes in Pregnancy
First Trimester

As a result of hormonal changes during the first trimester of pregnancy, blood glucose levels are often erratic for women with preexisting diabetes, making metabolic control difficult. Although caloric needs during the first trimester do not differ from those preceding pregnancy, the meal plan may need to be adjusted to accommodate these metabolic changes.

Increased Risk of Hypoglycemia

During the first trimester, the incidence of hypoglycemia increases. The two major reasons why hypoglycemia is more likely at this time are 1) an overall lowering of basal blood glucose levels of 14 to 18 mg/dL because of the con-

Figure 8.1
Insulin Requirements
Increase During
Pregnancy

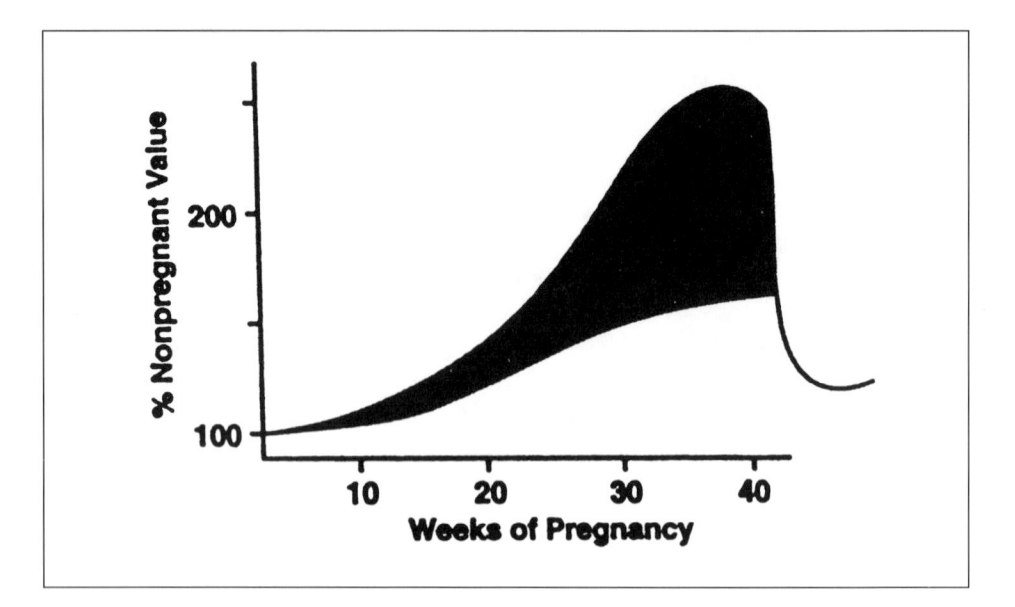

Reprinted with permission from
N Freinkel, *Diabetes*, 1980;29:1025.

tinuous fetal demand, placental glucose consumption, and urinary glucose losses, and 2) an increased sensitivity to insulin.[8,9] Women should be educated about the possibility of hypoglycemia and cautioned against overtreatment. The importance of between-meal snacks should be stressed.

Gastrointestinal Disturbances

Gastrointestinal upsets, including "morning sickness," may occur at any time during the day and can make blood glucose control a challenge. Sick-day guidelines—with liberal fluid intake to prevent dehydration—should be followed on days when nausea and vomiting are present. Insulin adjustments are likely to be needed, and more frequent blood glucose monitoring is essential. If hyperemesis (excessive vomiting) occurs, hospitalization may be required.

Second and Third Trimesters

Figure 8.1 illustrates the increase in insulin demands that occurs during the second and third trimesters of pregnancy. This is why screening for GDM occurs in pregnant women who do not have preexisting diabetes between the 24th and 28th weeks of pregnancy.[10]

Insulin requirements peak at two to three times the prepregnancy level at 38 to 40 weeks postconception. This increase occurs in response to elevated blood glucose levels caused by increased production of pregnancy-associated hormones. These hormones antagonize the action of insulin and result in postreceptor target-cell resistance.

For women with preexisting diabetes, either type I or type II, this increased insulin need must be met by exogenous insulin. Women with type II diabetes who take an oral glucose-lowering medication must replace it with injected insulin because these oral medications cross the placenta.

Meal plan adjustments are necessary to provide the additional calories needed to support the growth of the fetus. Regular follow-up is needed to monitor calorie and nutrient intake, weight gain, and blood glucose control and to prevent starvation ketosis.[10]

Table 8.5
Frequency of Testing for Pregnant Women

Blood Glucose
Ideal: 8 tests/day
➤ before each meal
➤ 1–2 hours after each meal
➤ at bedtime
➤ in the middle of the night
Minimum: 4 tests/day
➤ before each meal
➤ at bedtime

Urine Ketones
Test fasting daily
Test when meals are delayed or missed
Test during illness
Test when blood glucose is > 200 mg/dL

Reprinted with permission from *Maximizing the Role of Nutrition in Diabetes Management* (Alexandria, Va: American Diabetes Association; 1994).

Monitoring for Preexisting Diabetes

The monitoring of blood glucose and urine ketones is another important component of the medical management of preexisting diabetes during pregnancy. To achieve recommended blood glucose goals, intensive insulin therapy is needed, and careful attention must be paid to diabetes meal-planning principles.

The frequency and timing of blood glucose testing for pregnant women with preexisting diabetes should be individualized. A suggested schedule can be found in *Table 8.5*.

Monitoring for Gestational Diabetes Mellitus

Diagnosis of GDM is discussed in Chapter 2. Those who develop GDM should immediately begin to monitor their blood glucose levels to ensure the best pregnancy outcome. Self-monitoring of blood glucose (SMBG) is the only way for a woman to determine her individual glycemic response to meals and individual foods, and is thus important in the prevention or correction of ketosis.[8] Testing times for glucose and ketones are similar to those for women with preexisting diabetes: four times a day for glucose and every day for ketones (see Table 8.5). At this frequency, SMBG provides timely feedback about response to both the types and amounts of food the woman is eating. It also enables her to participate actively in the management of her own care. By reviewing the food, blood glucose, and urine ketone records together, the dietitian and the woman can identify problem areas where modification of the meal plan can help to achieve normoglycemia and prevent starvation ketosis.[8]

Starvation Ketosis

Ketonuria in pregnancy is a signal that starvation ketosis is occurring. This condition can be caused by one or more of the following: inadequate calorie intake, inadequate carbohydrate intake, omission of meals or snacks, and prolonged intervals between meals (eg, more than 10 hours between bedtime snack and breakfast). The more time that elapses between eating episodes, the greater the chance that starvation ketosis will occur. This is why pregnant women are directed to test for ketones before breakfast. The concern over ketonuria stems from the results of studies that suggest that high levels of blood ketones during pregnancy may be related to reduced IQ scores in children.[12]

Table 8.6

Medical Nutrition Therapy for Preexisting Diabetes and Gestational Diabetes

Nutrient Composition
- Individualized on the basis of nutrition history, prepregnancy weight, activity level, and nutritional needs of pregnancy.
- Vitamin and mineral supplement-diabetes does not alter requirements

Weight Gain
- Plot weight gain on a graph (using the weight gain grid from *Nutrition During Pregnancy*[11])

Meals and Snacks
- Should be based on individual eating habits and blood glucose goals

Monitoring
- Use food, blood glucose, and urine ketone monitoring records to meet glycemic control goals and prevent or correct ketosis

Source: C Fagan et al, *J Am Diet Assoc*, 1995;95:460–467.

Summary (Pregnancy)

Table 8.6 summarizes the components of medical nutrition therapy for preexisting diabetes and GDM (ie, nutrient composition, weight gain, meals and snacks, and monitoring). Much is yet to be learned about the best way to manage diabetes in pregnancy to improve outcomes for both mothers and infants. More research is needed to provide firm recommendations regarding weight gain, nutrient intake, calorie and carbohydrate distribution, ketone prevention, and exercise.

On the other hand, we have learned that diabetes medical nutrition therapy is essential for a successful pregnancy outcome. We know that intensive management of blood glucose makes a difference. Women with gestational diabetes who maintain a reasonable body weight postpartum and exercise on a regular basis have a decreased incidence of developing type II diabetes in the future.

Older Adults

There is a dramatic increase in the prevalence of diabetes and impaired glucose tolerance as people age. In fact, of the people in the United States known to have type II diabetes, nearly one half are over 55 years old.[13]

Special challenges confront older adults who have diabetes, and some of the strategies for prevention and treatment of diabetes-related problems must be adapted to their needs. As with all age groups, nutrition interventions are necessary to improve glycemic control and meet nutritional needs, as well as to improve quality of life.

Insulin resistance and other factors predispose the older adult to diabetes (*Figure 8.2*).[14] Most investigators agree that the major reason for the glucose intolerance associated with aging is insulin resistance. Controversy exists as to whether the insulin resistance is itself a primary change or is due to the more inactive status of many older adults and the accompanying increase in adipose tissue. Medications used to treat coexisting diseases may complicate diabetes therapy in older adults.[14]

Older adults differ in their responses to illness. Multiple chronic diseases, multiple medications, and increased physical disabilities make older people

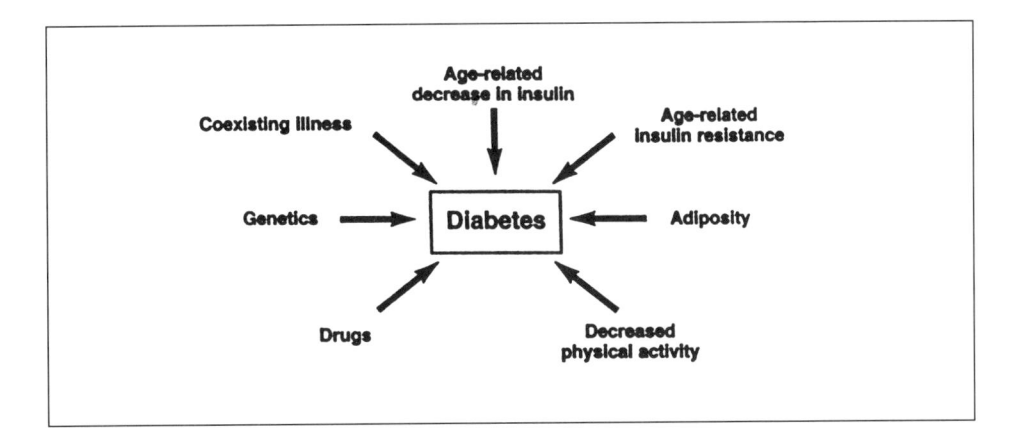

Figure 8.2

Factors Predisposing the Elderly to Diabetes

Reprinted with permission from JB Halter, *Diabetes Update* (Kalamazoo, Mich: The Upjohn Co; 1990).

with diabetes more vulnerable to both biologic and emotional stresses.[3,15] They have greater risks from both acute illnesses and complications of chronic illnesses. Also, recovery from physiologic insults, such as bone fractures and acute illness, is slower in the older adult and is further impaired by diabetes.

Despite the increase in glucose intolerance with age, aging per se should not be a reason for suboptimal control of blood glucose.[3] Goals should be established that ensure the older adult's safety, independence, and quality of life. Achieving blood glucose control is the first and foremost goal of diabetes therapy for all age groups, and for the same reason—to avoid acute and long-term complications. In the older adult, acute hyperglycemia and dehydration can lead to hyperglycemic hyperosmolar nonketotic syndrome (HHNS), a serious complication of diabetes (see Chapter 9 for more details).

Special Problems of the Older Adult

Special problems may be encountered by older adults with diabetes. The diabetes educator needs to be aware of them in order to maximize the nutrition intervention. They include the following:

➤ Age-related changes in thirst perception, total body water, renal concentrating ability, and vasopressin effectiveness predispose to dehydration. Dehydration is the most common fluid and electrolyte problem in the older adult.
➤ Decreased physical activity and difficulty carrying out activities of daily living affect diabetes self-management.
➤ Altered renal and hepatic functions affect response to oral glucose-lowering medications.
➤ Cognitive dysfunction and depression can interfere with compliance with diabetes self-management plans.
➤ Medications needed to treat coexisting diseases can complicate diabetes self-management. See *Table 8.7* regarding medications that affect blood glucose levels.
➤ The impact of disease processes on metabolism can alter blood glucose control.
➤ Social and financial changes may impair access to services related to diabetes self-management.

Table 8.7
Medications Affecting Blood Glucose

May increase hyperglycemia
Diuretics
Glucocorticoids
Nicotinic acid
Lithium and other antidepressants

May increase hypoglycemia
Beta blockers
Monoamine oxidase inhibitors
Phenylbutazone
Aspirin in large doses
Cimetidine

Reprinted with permission from *Maximizing the Role of Nutrition in Diabetes Management* (Alexandria, Va: American Diabetes Association; 1994).

➤ The need for optimal nutrition is highlighted by the fact that the incidence of protein-energy malnutrition (PEM) in the older adult ranges from 35% to 65%. The condition often remains subclinical or unrecognized because its result—excessive loss of lean body mass—is associated with the aging process. Until a primary disease develops or chronic problems are exacerbated by illness or some other stress, PEM may remain unrecognized.

Malnutrition and diabetes are interrelated in several ways. Both conditions have deleterious effects on wound healing and defense against infection. Malnutrition is associated with depression and cognitive deficits that alter an older person's ability to comply with therapeutic regimens to control diabetes.[16]

Because of the concern about malnutrition, it is essential that older adult residents in long-term-care (LTC) settings be provided with a meal plan that meets their nutritional needs, that enables them to attain or maintain a reasonable body weight, that helps control blood glucose, and that is palatable. Ultimately, the primary goal for older adults in LTC settings is to provide a good quality of life. Therefore, it is questionable whether strict adherence to a "diabetic" meal plan is necessary in this environment.

Although LTC residents with diabetes have traditionally been offered set-calorie (eg, 1,200, 1,500, 1,800) "no added sugar" meal plans, a better approach is to offer a regular meal plan that incorporates the basic nutrition guidelines for people with diabetes. This approach is often better accepted by residents and has been shown to result in glycemic control similar to that achieved with the more traditional meal plan limitations.[3,15]

Figure 8.3 shows results of a study conducted by Coulston et al,[17] who monitored 18 residents of LTC facilities with type II diabetes for glycemic control on diabetic and regular meal plans. Weekly fasting blood glucose and food intake were followed for 16 weeks, which included 4 weeks on the diabetes meal plan before and after an 8-week regular meal plan period. The results indicated that the short-term substitution of a regular meal plan for diabetes meal plans did not result in deterioration of glycemic control in these residents. It should be noted that glycemic control of the subjects was good when the study was initiated. For LTC residents with poor glycemic control, an increase in medication requirements may be a better option than imposing a stricter meal plan.

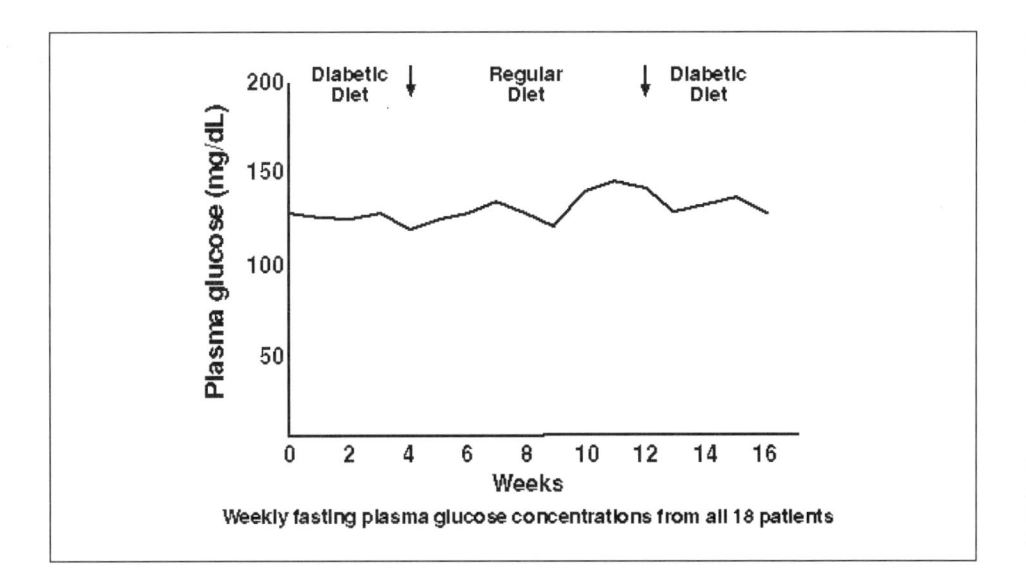

Figure 8.3

Is Strict Adherence to a "Diabetic" Diet Necessary?

Weekly fasting plasma glucose concentrations from all 18 patients

Reprinted with permission from AM Coulston et al, *Am J Clin Nutr*, 1990;51:67. ©*Am J Clin Nutr*, American Society for Clinical Nutrition.

If an older adult is unable to meet his or her nutritional needs through a normal solid-food meal plan, nutritional support may be indicated. The following four steps should be considered for clients who are unable to meet their nutritional needs through a regular meal plan.

Nutrition Intervention for the Older Adult

➤ *Step 1: Modification of usual food intake by changing nutrient content or density.*

Examples include incorporating nutrient-dense foods into the meal plan of someone who has little appetite or who may refuse to eat meals large enough or nutrient-dense enough to meet nutritional needs, and increasing the number of times a day that a person eats.

➤ *Step 2: Modification of food consistency and use of medical nutritional supplements.*

Clients who may benefit include those who are not eating well because of tooth loss or painful teeth or gums, who have difficulty swallowing, or who have anorexia or depression.

➤ *Step 3: Consideration of enteral nutrition support*

Enteral nutrition support, provided by feeding tube, may be either supplemental to the meal plan or a total replacement for solid foods, when needed. Partial or total liquid enteral nutrition support provides energy and nutrients to maintain nutritional status in persons unable to ingest adequate amounts by mouth.

➤ *Step 4: Consideration of parenteral nutrition support.*

Candidates for parenteral nutrition are those who can not meet their nutritional goals by the more physiologic oral or tube-feeding routes that use the GI tract.

Effective diabetes self-management for older adults includes the following components:

Summary (Older Adults)

➤ determination of target blood glucose levels—elevated levels should be taken seriously;

71

- recognition of accompanying psychological, socioeconomic, and emotional changes;
- provision of a nutritionally adequate meal plan for special needs;
- blood glucose monitoring;
- medication, if needed;
- prevention of acute complications; and
- physical activity, as appropriate.

References

1. Wise JE, Kolb EL, Sauder SE. Effect of glycemic control on growth velocity in children with insulin-dependent diabetes mellitus. *Diabetes Care.* 1992;15(7):826–830.
2. Birch LL, Johnson SL, Anderson G. The variability of young children's energy intake. *N Engl J Med.* 1991;324:232–235.
3. Franz MJ, Horton ES, Bantle JP, Beebe CA, Brunzell JD, Coulston AM, Henry RR, Hoogwerf BJ, Stacpoole PW. Nutrition principles for the management of diabetes mellitus and related complications (technical review). *Diabetes Care.* 1994;17:490–518.
4. Diabetes Control and Complications Trial Research Group. The effect of intensive treatment of diabetes on the development and progression of long-term complications in insulin-treated diabetes mellitus. *N Engl J Med.* 1993;329:977–986.
5. National Cholesterol Education Program. *Report of the Expert Panel on Blood Cholesterol Levels in Children and Adolescents.* Bethesda, Md: US Department of Health and Human Services; 1991. National Heart, Lung and Blood Institute publication 91-2732.
6. American Diabetes Association. *Medical Management of Pregnancy Complicated by Diabetes Mellitus.* 2nd ed. Alexandria, Va: American Diabetes Association; 1994.
7. American Diabetes Association. Preconception care of women with diabetes (position statement). *Diabetes Care.* 1996;19(suppl 1):S25–28.
8. Fagan C, King JD, Erick M. Nutrition management in women with gestational diabetes mellitus: a review by ADA's Diabetes Care and Education dietetic practice group. *J Am Diet Assoc.* 1995;95:460–467.
9. Metzger BE. Pregnancy and diabetes. In: Powers MA, ed. *Handbook of Diabetes Medical Nutrition Therapy.* 2nd ed. Gaithersburg, Md: Aspen Publishers, Inc; 1996:503–526.
10. American Diabetes Association. Gestational diabetes mellitus (position statement). *Diabetes Care.* 1996;19(suppl 1):S29.
11. Food and Nutrition Board, Institute of Medicine. *Nutrition During Pregnancy—Weight Gain and Nutrient Supplements,* Washington, DC: National Academy of Science; 1990:63–95.
12. Rizzo T, Metzger BE, Burns WJ, Burns KC. Correlations between antepartum maternal metabolism in child intelligences. *N Engl J Med.* 1991;325:911–916.
13. National Institutes of Health. *Diabetes in America.* 2nd ed. Washington, DC: National Institute of Diabetes Mellitus and Digestive and Kidney Diseases; 1995. NIH publication 95-1468.
14. Halter JB. *Diabetes Update: Elderly Patients with Non-Insulin Dependent Diabetes Mellitus.* Kalamazoo, Mich: The Upjohn Co; 1990.
15. McLaughlin S. Considerations in caring for older persons with diabetes. In: Powers MA, ed. *Handbook of Diabetes Medical Nutrition Therapy.* 2nd ed. Gaithersburg, Md: Aspen Publishers, Inc; 1996:527–546.
16. Kerstetter JE, Holthausen BA, Fitz PA. Malnutrition in the institutionalized older adult. *J Am Diet Assoc.* 1992;92:1109–1116.
17. Coulston AM, Mandelbaum D, Reaven GM. Dietary management of nursing home residents with non-insulin-dependent diabetes mellitus. *Am J Clin Nutr.* 1990;51:67–71.

For Further Reading
Children and Adolescents

Connell JE, Thomas-Dobersen D. Nutritional management of children and adolescents with insulin-dependent diabetes mellitus: a review by the Diabetes Care and Education dietetic practice group. *J Am Diet Assoc.* 1991;91:1556–1566.

DCCT Research Group. Effect of intensive diabetes treatment on the development and progression of long-term complications in adolescents with insulin-dependent diabetes mellitus. *J Pediatrics.* 1994;125(2):177–188.

Drash A. Clinical care of the patient with diabetes: what is the role of the diabetes professional? *Diabetes Care.* 1994;17(1):40-44.

LaGreca AM, Hanson CL. Adolescents and diabetes. *Diabetes Spectrum.* 1995;8(1):27-48.

Lawlor M, Laffel L, Anderson B, Bertorelli A. *Caring for Young Children Living with Diabetes: A Professional Manual.* Boston, Mass: Joslin Clinic; 1996.

Loghmani E, Rickard KA. Alternate snack system for children and teenagers with diabetes mellitus. *J Am Diet Assoc.* 1994;94:1145-1148.

Pregnancy

Durnin JVGA. Energy requirements of pregnancy. *Diabetes.* 1991;40(2):152-156.

Fagen C, King JD, Erick M. Nutrition management in women with gestational diabetes mellitus: a review by ADA's Diabetes Care and Education dietetic practice group. *J Am Diet Assoc.* 1995;95:460-467.

Institute of Medicine, National Academy of Science. *Nutrition During Pregnancy.* Washington, DC: National Academy Press; 1990.

Jovanovic-Petersen L. *Medical Management of Pregnancy Complicated by Diabetes.* 2nd ed. Alexandria, Va: American Diabetes Association; 1995.

Ramus RM, Kitzmiller JL. Diagnosis and management of gestational diabetes. *Diabetes Review.* 1994;2(1):43-52.

Older Adults

Diabetes Care and Education dietetic practice group. Diabetes in the older person. *On the Cutting Edge.* 1990;11:1-19.

Glasgow RE, Toobert DJ, Hampson SE, et al. Improving self-care among older patients with type II diabetes: the "sixty something..." study. *Patient Educ Couns.* 1992;19(1):61-74.

Kiley LE, Dwyer J. Helping older adults control their diabetes. *Top Clin Nutr.* 1993;8(2):32-39.

Kohrt WM, Kirwan JP, Staten MA, Bbourey RD, King DS, Holloszy JO. Insulin resistance in aging is related to abdominal obesity. *Diabetes.* 1993;42:273-281.

Mooradian AD, ed. Diabetes in the elderly. *Diabetes Spectrum.* 1994;7(6):357-381.

Management of Diabetes: Complications

9

The various forms of glucose intolerance have a tremendous impact on the health status and health care costs of millions of Americans.[1] Although these syndromes differ in etiology and pathology, they all result in abnormal glucose tolerance and can lead to acute and/or chronic complications if not appropriately managed. Because medical and nutritional intervention priorities must be established, the dietitian should consult with other members of the diabetes care team to ensure that nutrition goals and priorities are incorporated into the total care plan.

Acute Complications

The major acute complications of diabetes are hypoglycemia, hyperglycemia, diabetic ketoacidosis (DKA), and hyperglycemic hyperosmolar nonketotic syndrome (HHNS).

Hypoglycemia

Hypoglycemia is defined as an abnormally low blood glucose level. It can also be referred to as an *insulin reaction.* It can result from administration of excessive insulin or oral glucose-lowering medications, too little food intake, delayed or missed meals or snacks, unusual exercise, or alcohol intake without food (especially in clients who take insulin). A blood glucose level of 70 mg/dL or below indicates the presence of hypoglycemia and should be rapidly corrected.[2]

Hypoglycemia frequently occurs in individuals taking insulin, less frequently for those taking sulfonylureas, and almost never in individuals taking Metformin, Troglitazone, or Acarbose or treatment using diabetes medical nutrition therapy alone.

Signs and symptoms of hypoglycemia, its recognition, and its prevention and treatment should be reviewed with all persons taking insulin or sulfonylureas. Initial symptoms of hypoglycemia are due to the release of catecholamines, which cause sweating, tremors, palpitations, and fearfulness. Later symptoms, which occur when glucose is lower and affects the central nervous system, include headache, blurred vision, lack of coordination, confusion, anger, and numbness around the mouth and in the hands and feet. (See *Table 9.1.*)

Individuals who have very tight glycemic control may not recognize hypoglycemia. This is because, with frequent hypoglycemic episodes, the brain adapts by increasing glucose transporter activity so that it is protected from hypoglycemia. Because the brain is protected, the expected acute response

Table 9.1

Causes, Symptoms, and Treatment of Hypoglycemia

Causes

Excessive insulin or oral hypoglycemic agents
Too little food intake
Delayed or missed meals or snacks
Excessive exercise or physical activity
Alcohol intake without food (for clients using insulin)

Symptoms

Shakiness
Sweating
Confusion
Irritability

Treatment for Blood Glucose < 70 mg/dL

Treat with 15 grams of carbohydrate
Wait 15 minutes
Retest blood glucose and monitor symptoms

Reprinted with permission from *Maximizing the Role of Nutrition in Diabetes Management* (Alexandria, Va: American Diabetes Association, Inc; 1994).

---

with release of catecholamines is not initiated. In addition, persons who have had diabetes for more than 10 years and those who have severe neuropathy often lose the ability to release catecholamines in response to hypoglycemia. In both groups the lack of catecholamine response results not only in hypoglycemic unawareness, but also in failure to rapidly correct the hypoglycemia.[3]

The treatment goal for hypoglycemia is to increase the blood glucose level, and immediate treatment is essential. The procedure outlined in Table 9.1 should be used: each 5 grams of carbohydrate raises the blood glucose level approximately 15 mg/dL.[4] A repeat blood test is necessary to confirm if blood glucose has risen or if there is a need for additional treatment. See Chapter 10 for further information on the treatment of hypoglycemia.

If the individual with diabetes develops severe hypoglycemia and becomes unconscious, an injection of Glucagon can be administered by someone trained in its use. All at-risk persons with type I diabetes should be provided with Glucagon, and training on its administration should be given to significant others.

Severe hypoglycemia is a much greater problem in the person with type I diabetes than it is in the individual with type II diabetes. Hypoglycemia does not occur with Metformin, Troglitazone, or Acarbose. However, the risks of chronic complications due to hyperglycemia in both type I and type II diabetes mandate that even in older persons the best possible glycemic control should be obtained, which will put the individual at risk for occasional hypoglycemia.

Hyperglycemia

Hyperglycemia is an excessive amount of glucose in the blood caused by too little insulin, insulin resistance (either inherited or induced by infection, anxiety, depression, or medication), or excessive food intake. When blood glucose is high, exercise can actually aggravate hyperglycemia (see Chapter 4). The symptoms vary with the degree of severity and the causes, which are outlined along with treatment in *Table 9.2*.[2,5]

Persistent hyperglycemia has deleterious effects on the body's defense mechanisms against infection. It also increases the pain threshold, thereby

Table 9.2
Causes, Symptoms, and Treatment of Hyperglycemia

Causes
Too little insulin
Insulin resistance
Increased food intake

Symptoms
Polyuria
Polydipsia
Dry mouth
Weight loss
Fatigue

Treatment (depends on the severity)
Oral glucose-lowering medications or supplemental insulin
Replacement of fluids and electrolytes
Medical monitoring

exacerbating neuropathic pain, and has a detrimental effect on the outcome of cerebrovascular accidents and myocardial infarctions. Hyperglycemia associated with dehydration, which results in the kidneyís being unable to excrete glucose, can cause the development of hyperglycemic hyperosmolar nonketotic syndrome (HHNS).

Hyperglycemic Hyperosmolar Nonketotic Syndrome

Hyperglycemic hyperosmolar nonketotic syndrome (HHNS) is a serious condition that is frequently found in older adults and persons on hyperalimentation or peritoneal dialysis. Ketones are usually not elevated, but the blood glucose level is extremely high (> 600 mg/dL and generally between 1,000 and 2,000 mg/dL).[6] The dietitian needs to carefully review the fluid intake of older adults with diabetes, since dehydration is the precipitating cause. For persons in long-term-care facilities, prevention includes provision of adequate fluids and documentation that they are being taken, as well as control of blood glucose.

Prior to the development of HHNS, most persons have had polyuria for days or weeks. As long as the person has access to fluid, blood glucose does not rise. In a well-hydrated individual who has normal renal function, excess glucose will be excreted and serum glucose will not rise above 500 mg/dL. However, after 2 to 3 weeks mineral deficiencies occur, the person becomes weak, fluid intake decreases, dehydration occurs, and there is a rapid rise in blood glucose.

Treatment involves rehydration and administration of small amounts of insulin.[7] Because of the severity of dehydration, there is a tendency for excessive blood clotting to occur and mortality is high. However, most persons after recovery have little difficulty controlling their diabetes.

Diabetic Ketoacidosis (DKA)

Diabetic ketoacidosis (DKA) is a life-threatening but reversible condition in which there is an absolute lack of insulin so that ketoacids are produced in excess. Persons with type I diabetes who have utilized all available serum buffers become acidotic.[2]

Table 9.3

Causes, Symptoms, and Treatment of Diabetic Ketoacidosis

Causes

Insulin deficiency relative to counterregulatory hormones
Failure to take insulin
Excess hormones due to stress from infection, tissue injury, or surgery

Warning Symptoms

Nausea
Vomiting
Stomach pains
Thirst
Fruity breath

Treatment

Administration of insulin
Administration of fluids and electrolytes

DKA occurs in persons with type I diabetes who are unable to absorb enough insulin to overcome the effects of excessive counterregulatory hormones. Counterregulatory hormones are produced in excess with infection, tissue injury, depression, or anxiety.[6] The clinical indicators of DKA are high blood glucose levels (above 250 mg/dL), the presence of ketones, and acidosis. Because of the almost total lack of insulin, dangerously high levels of blood glucose occur due to the inability of glucose to enter the cells. In addition, with very low insulin levels, there is an excessive release of fatty acid from adipocytes, which are used as a substrate for excessive ketoacid production by the liver. DKA can be prevented by self-monitoring of blood glucose, self-testing for urine ketones, ensuring an adequate fluid intake, controlling vomiting, and taking extra insulin.

The person with DKA is not comatose but is often stuporose, nauseated, and short of breath due to the acidosis. DKA is a medical emergency treated by the administration of insulin, fluids, and electrolytes. If untreated or inadequately treated or if treatment is delayed, death may occur from ketoacidosis (see *Table 9.3*).

Chronic Complications

Chronic complications of diabetes account for much more morbidity and mortality than do acute complications.

The microvascular complications of diabetes (retinopathy, neuropathy, and nephropathy) are undoubtedly related to hyperglycemia and can be prevented with good glycemic control. The presence of hypertension will worsen both the retinal and renal complications and should be energetically treated.

The macrovascular complications of diabetes (ischemic heart disease, cerebrovascular disease, and peripheral vascular disease) are related not only to glycemic control but also to the factors associated with insulin resistance (hypertension, dyslipidemia, and obesity), which must also be treated.

All of the microvascular and macrovascular complications of diabetes are worsened by smoking. Energetic treatment of hypertension is mandatory, and the use of antihypertensive agents that do not worsen insulin resistance is indicated. Since 85% of individuals with type II diabetes die from cardiovascular causes and 60% from ischemic heart disease, aggressive treatment of dyslipidemia is indicated. The dyslipidemia seen with insulin resistance is characterized by high triglycerides and low HDL. While the total LDL level is normal or slightly elevated, the LDL is made up of small, dense particles that are increased in number and highly atherogenic. The first step in treating dyslipidemia in the person with diabetes is improved glycemic control accompanied by medical nutrition therapy and physical activity.[8,9] Diabetes medical nutrition therapy includes caloric restriction for gradual, moderate weight loss if the individual is overweight and decreased intake of saturated fat and cholesterol. Drug therapy is a component of treatment when lipid goals are not achieved through medical nutrition therapy and physical activity.

Retinopathy

Retinopathy is preventable, detectable, and treatable. It can be prevented by glycemic control, detected by annual eye exams through a dilated pupil, and treated with panretinal photocoagulation (laser treatment). Retinopathy occurs as a result of disease of the small blood vessels, which leak and collapse, causing retinal ischemia. When leakage occurs, there is usually no loss of vision. However, especially in the person with type II diabetes, when leakage occurs in the area of high visual acuity (the macula), vision can be lost. Loss of blood supply to the retina results in retinal infarction, new blood vessel formation (neovascularization), and bleeding from these new vessels into the vitreous (vitreous hemorrhage), causing a loss of vision. In addition, contraction of the collagen support tissue of the new blood vessels puts traction on the retina, which can buckle and even separate its layers (retinal detachment).[10] New vessel formation can even occur in the anterior chamber of the eye, where, by blocking fluid drainage, it causes hemorrhagic glaucoma, which is the terminal stage of diabetic retinopathy.

Laser treatment by destroying some of the retinal tissue ensures a good blood supply and viability of the remaining retinal tissue. Visual acuity is maintained at the expense of loss of color discrimination, night vision, and peripheral vision. A vitrectomy, in which vitreous hemorrhages and scar tissue is removed and, if necessary, the retina repaired, can potentially save or restore vision.

Diseases of the Nervous System

Chronic hyperglycemia is associated with diabetic neuropathy. Peripheral neuropathy usually affects the nerves controlling sensation in the feet and in severe cases the hands. Autonomic neuropathy affects nerve function control in various organs supplied by the sympathetic and parasympathetic nervous systems.[10,11] This includes the digestive system, the cardiovascular system (causing postural hypotension and painless or silent ischemic heart disease), and the urogenital system (causing sexual dysfunction, with erectile impotence being the most common manifestation), and bladder emptying problems. Diabetic neuropathy occurs in both type I and type II diabetes.

Gastrointestinal Neuropathy

Neuropathy involving the nerves supplying the gastrointestinal tract can cause a variety of problems, which are outlined in *Table 9.4* and *Figure 9.1*. One of the most important is gastroparesis. Neurogenic delayed gastric emptying or gastroparesis has a detrimental effect on blood glucose level. As

Table 9.4

Gastrointestinal Neuropathy[5]

Location	Effect
Esophagus	Possible nausea Esophagitis
Stomach	Unpredictable emptying Formation of bezoars
Small bowel	Nutrient loss
Large bowel	Diarrhea, constipation

Reprinted with permission from *Maximizing the Role of Nutrition in Diabetes Management* (Alexandria, Va: American Diabetes Association, Inc; 1994).

Figure 9.1

Neurogenic Delayed Gastric Emptying

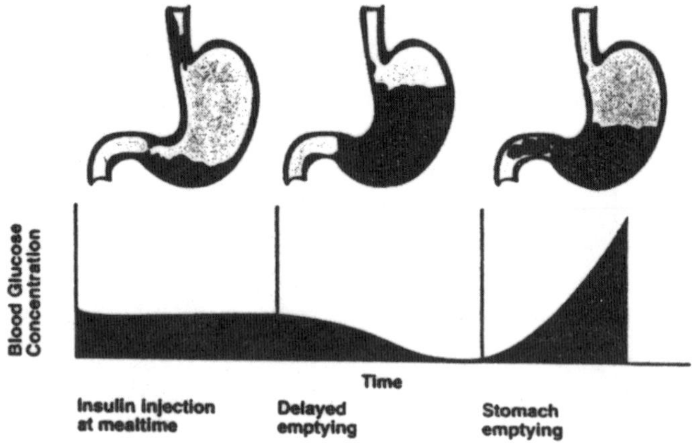

Reprinted with permission from M Pfeifer and D Greene, Diabetic neuropathy, *Current Concepts* (Kalamazoo, Mich: Upjohn Company; 1986).

Figure 9.1 illustrates, when absorption is normal (left side of figure), the blood glucose response is also normal. But if glucose from a meal is not being released into the small intestine, the blood glucose will drop (center of figure). When the movement of nutrients is delayed through the gut and then absorbed, the delay may result in higher than normal blood glucose (right side of figure). This is because the insulin that was administered to cover the meal has now passed its peak activity and there is no longer adequate insulin available to cover the late glycemic effect.

Minimizing gastric distention is a primary goal of therapy. The aim is to control early satiety, nausea, and vomiting so that the person with diabetes can tolerate adequate food and fluids.[13] First and foremost, small frequent meals may be better tolerated than three full meals a day. If solid foods are not well tolerated, liquid meals can be recommended. Lowering the fat content of meals will help improve the slow gastric emptying, but relief of symptoms varies from person to person and symptoms can be episodic. Because of the potential for gastric bezoar (a mass of indigestible material found in the stomach), high-fiber foods should be limited or avoided altogether.[13] If the individual cannot consume sufficient calories and nutrients, the dietitian may suggest oral nutrition supplements or tube feeding. A feeding jejunostomy may have to be used in severe cases.

As much as possible, the timing of insulin administration should be adjusted to match the usually delayed nutrient-absorption pattern. This may mean giving the insulin injection with a meal or after the meal to cover the delayed glycemic peak. Frequent blood glucose monitoring will guide the dietitian and the diabetes care team in making recommendations for insulin administration.

Medications that stimulate gastric emptying independent of the autonomic nervous system are helpful in the treatment of gastroparesis.

Kidney Disease (Nephropathy)

Although nephropathy more frequently complicates type I than type II diabetes, there are many more persons with type ll diabetes in the general population. The majority of individuals with nephropathy will have type II diabetes. In addition, ethnic groups such as African Americans, Mexican Americans, and Native Americans have a higher incidence of nephropathy associated with type II diabetes. Preventing nephropathy in diabetes is important since, in addition to renal decompensation, persons with type I diabetes who have nephropathy are at a 140-fold greater risk of myocardial infarction than the general population. They have a 35-fold greater risk than other persons with diabetes who do not have nephropathy.

Chronic hyperglycemia results in an increase in growth hormone and other counterregulatory hormones, which causes an increase in renal blood flow and glomerular hypertension. With glycemic control this reverses, but in persons in whom glomerular hypertension persists, growth factors are released locally and over time cause glomerular damage and later loss of glomerular function.[13] The first clinical sign of nephropathy is the appearance of microalbumin (30 to 300 mg albumin per 24 hours) with little or no change in the glomerular filtration rate. Subsequently 80% of these individuals will develop macroalbuminuria (over 300 mg albumin per 24 hours) or overt nephropathy. At this stage, due to loss of albumin in the urine and low serum albumin, edema is present and the glomerular filtration rate starts to decline. With overt nephropathy, virtually all persons with diabetes eventually progress to end-stage renal disease (ESRD). With the treatment of hypertension, including the use of ACE inhibitors and a lower protein intake, progression to ESRD can be decelerated.[13]

Persons with type II diabetes can have a substantially different clinical course, due in part to failure to recognize the presence of diabetes for a prolonged period before diagnosis and the presence of hypertension.[13] Proteinuria is often present at the time of diagnosis.

Hypertension must also be energetically treated as in type II diabetes with ACE inhibitors. If retinopathy is not present and the diagnosis of nephropathy is in doubt, this must be proven by biopsy. However, only 75% of persons with type II diabetes will have retinopathy accompanying the nephropathy.

To avoid nephropathy, good glycemic and hypertension control are essential. The same factors apply with microalbuminuria as with macroalbuminuria. The use of ACE inhibitors will not only treat systemic hypertension, but also lower intraglomerular pressure, decrease proteinuria, and decelerate the decline in renal function. Decrease in the protein intake as described in Chapter 3 is also helpful. Prompt treatment of urinary tract infections and wherever possible avoiding the use of radiocontrast material and other medications with the potential for further renal damage is also helpful.

Summary

Just as the DCCT has shown the value of nutrition self-management in attaining and maintaining glycemic control, so diabetes medical nutrition therapy is essential in the treatment of complications. Referral for diabetes medical nutrition therapy for improved nutrient intake and glycemic control is essential in the prevention and delay of these conditions. Dietitians need to define their services in terms of improving the quality of life as well as reducing the cost of health care.

References

1. *Diabetes in America.* 2nd ed. Washington, DC: National Institutes of Health, National Institute of Diabetes and Digestive and Kidney Diseases; 1995. NIH Publication No. 95-1468.
2. *Medical Management of Insulin-Dependent Diabetes Mellitus.* 2nd ed. Alexandria, Va: American Diabetes Association; 1994.
3. Clarke WL, Gonder-Frederick LA, Richards FE, Cryer PE. Multifactorial origin of hypoglycemic unawareness in IDDM: association with defective glucose counterregulation and better glycemic control. *Diabetes.* 1991;40:680–685.
4. *Intensive Diabetes Management.* Alexandria, Va: American Diabetes Association; 1995.
5. American Diabetes Association consensus statement: the pharmacological treatment of hyperglycemia in NIDDM. *Diabetes Care.* 1996;19(1):S54–S61.
6. Schade DS, Eaton RP. Pathogenesis of diabetic ketoacidosis: a reappraisal. *Diabetes Care.* 1979;2:296–306.
7. *Medical Management of Non-Insulin-Dependent Diabetes Mellitus.* 3rd ed. Alexandria, Va: American Diabetes Association; 1994.
8. American Diabetes Association consensus statement: detection and management of lipid disorders in diabetes. *Diabetes Care.* 1996;19(1):S96–S102.
9. *Prevention and Treatment of Complications of Diabetes: A Guide for Primary Care Practitioners.* Atlanta, Ga: Centers for Disease Control, National Center for Disease Prevention and Health Promotion; 1991.
10. American Diabetes Association consensus statement: screening for diabetes. *Diabetes Care.* 1996;19(1):520–522.
11. Molitch ME. Complications of diabetes mellitus and implications for nutrition therapy. In: Powers MA, ed. *Handbook of Diabetes Medical Nutrition Therapy.* Gaithersburg, Md: Aspen Publishers, Inc; 1996: 15–30.
12. American Diabetes Association consensus statement: diabetic neuropathy. *Diabetes Care.* 1996;19(1):S67–S71.
13. Parrish CR. Gastrointestinal issues in persons with diabetes. In: Powers MA, ed. *Handbook of Diabetes Medical Nutrition Therapy.* Gaithersburg, Md: Aspen Publishers, Inc; 1996: 618–637.
14. American Diabetes Association consensus statement: diagnosis and management of nephropathy in patients with diabetes mellitus. *Diabetes Care.* 1996;19(1):S103–S106.

For Further Reading

Cronin B. Nutritional concerns in gastrointestinal neuropathy. *Diabetes Educator.* 1992; 18(6):531–535.

Garg A, Grundy SM. Management of dyslipidemia of NIDDM. *Diabetes Care.* 1990; 13(2):153–169.

Garg A. Management of dyslipidemia in IDDM patients. *Diabetes Care.* 1994;17(3):224–234.

McLaughlin S. Nutritional considerations for other complications of diabetes. *Diabetes Educator.* 1992;18(6):527–529.

Modification of Diet and Renal Disease (MDRD) Study Group. The effects of dietary protein restriction and blood pressure control on the progression of chronic renal disease. *N Engl J Med.* 1994;330(13):877–884.

Thom S. Nutritional concerns in diabetic nephropathy. *Diabetes Educator.* 1992; 18(6): 537–539.

White N, ed. The risk of hypoglycemia during intensive therapy of IDDM. *Diabetes Spectrum.* 1994;7(4):232–265.

10 Special Topics in Meal Planning

One of the primary goals of diabetes nutrition therapy is to integrate positive nutrition changes into the eating habits of clients with diabetes without disrupting their lifestyles. This chapter addresses some of these lifestyle issues and gives guidelines for producing maximal change toward positive nutrition habits while causing a minimal change in lifestyle. Additional reading should be done by diabetes educators to expand understanding of these guidelines. A suggested reading list is included at the end of this chapter.

Alcohol

Alcohol is absorbed rapidly by the stomach and small intestine and appears in the bloodstream within 5 minutes after ingestion. The alcohol concentration in the blood reaches its highest level 30 to 90 minutes after ingestion. Foods high in fat and protein delay gastric emptying time and, when consumed with alcohol, may slow down the rate at which alcohol is absorbed.[1]

Alcohol is metabolized by the liver via three different pathways. The main pathway is the alcohol dehydrogenase system. The second pathway is the microsomal ethanol oxidizing system. The third pathway involves the enzyme catalase, but an insignificant amount of alcohol is metabolized this way.[1]

The initial step in the alcohol dehydrogenase system is the conversion of alcohol to acetaldehyde by the enzyme alcohol dehydrogenase. Acetaldehyde is further reduced by acetaldehyde dehydrogenase to carbon dioxide, water, and acetyl coenzyme A (CoA). Both carbon dioxide and water are eliminated from the body, whereas acetyl CoA is subsequently converted to fatty acids that are stored by the body.[1]

Because both alcohol and fats are metabolized through common intermediates—two carbon units and acetyl CoA—alcohol can be substituted for fat in a meal plan for clients who need to monitor their calorie intake.

Alcohol intake may cause hypoglycemia in clients who take insulin because alcohol dehydrogenase inhibits gluconeogenesis in the liver. In a fasting person, 2 oz liquor may result in hypoglycemia. In a fed person with well-controlled diabetes, moderate alcohol intake does not seem to affect the blood glucose level dramatically.[2]

Clients with diabetes who have had only minimal food intake may experience hypoglycemia within 6 to 36 hours after alcohol ingestion. Self-monitoring of blood glucose before and after alcohol intake enables the client to predict potential hypoglycemia and prevent it from occurring.[3]

Alcohol has been shown to cause hyperglycemia in the fed state due to glycogenolysis in the liver and peripheral insulin resistance.[4] The rise in blood glucose is dependent on the quantity of alcohol consumed and the amount of liver glycogen stores available.[5]

Effects of Alcohol on Triglycerides

High triglyceride levels are more common in persons with diabetes than in those without diabetes and may play a significant role in cardiovascular disease. Alcohol may have the following effects on triglyceride metabolism[1]:

> Alcohol ingested with food may cause plasma triglycerides to be higher;
> Alcohol may cause a slight transient rise in plasma triglycerides in persons who are fasting;
> In some people with hypertriglyceridemia, even moderate amounts of alcohol can further elevate triglycerides for some time after cessation of alcohol intake (it is not clear how long this elevation lasts)[1];
> Stopping alcohol ingestion can decrease triglyceride levels.

It appears that alcohol ingestion has the potential to raise triglycerides, especially in susceptible persons, and should be discouraged for those with hypertriglyceridemia regardless of whether they have diabetes.

Alcohol and Oral Glucose-Lowering Medication

With regard to the concurrent use of alcohol and an oral glucose-lowering medication, two medications should be discussed. The first, a sulfonylurea, is chlorpropamide. A disulfiram (antabuse-like) reaction has been reported in clients with diabetes who consume alcohol and are taking this medication. The symptoms mimic a heart attack and can include headache, nausea, vomiting, thirst, sweating, flushing, a feeling of warmth, syncope, palpitations, chest pain, confusion, vertigo, difficulty breathing, and/or hypotension. The severity of symptoms, which can last from 30 minutes to several hours, depends on the amount of alcohol consumed. Clients using chlorpropamide need to be counseled about discontinuing or moderating alcohol intake.[1]

The second medication is metformin, a biguanide. A rare, but severe, side effect of therapy with metformin is lactic acidosis. One of the factors that can increase the blood concentration of lactic acid, and thus increase the risk of lactic acidosis, is the concurrent use of alcohol and metformin.[6]

Nutritional Composition of Alcoholic Beverages

Alcohol is a concentrated source of calories that yields 7 kcal/g (carbohydrates and protein yield 4 kcal/g and fat yields 9 kcal/g). Alcohol provides energy but no essential nutrients. The calorie and carbohydrate content of liquors should not be overlooked; otherwise, total daily calorie intake will be seriously underestimated.

Alcoholic beverages vary in carbohydrate content; distilled spirits have virtually no carbohydrate content, whereas sweet wines, beers, and cordials may contain considerable quantities. Because of their carbohydrate content, mixers (such as tonic, carbonated beverages, fruit juices, and premade mixes) can be an additional source of carbohydrates and calories. *Table 10.1* contains information on alcoholic beverage composition.[7]

If a client with diabetes is planning to incorporate alcohol into a calorically defined meal plan, the type and quantity of alcohol should be calculated. One drink is defined as 1.5 oz distilled liquor (gin, whiskey, rum, vodka, scotch,

Table 10.1
Composition of Alcoholic Beverages

Beverage	Serving (oz)	Alcohol (g)	Carbohydrate (g)	Kcal	Exchanges
Beer					
Regular	12	13	13	150	1 starch, 2 fat
Light	12	12	5	100	2 fat
Nonalcoholic	12	1.5	12	60	1 starch
Distilled Spirits					
80 proof*	1.5	14	trace	100	2 fat
Whiskey (86 proof)	1.5	15	trace	105	2 fat
Wine					
Dry white	5	14	2	105	2 fat
Red or rosé	5	14	2.5	105	2 fat
Cocktails					
Bloody Mary	5	14	5	115	1 vegetable, 2 fat
Daiquiri	4	28	8	220	½ starch, 4 fat
Manhattan	4	35	4	255	5 ½ fat
Martini	4	18.5	trace	250	5 ½ fat
Tom Collins	7.5	16	3	120	2 ½ fat

* gin, rum, vodka

Reprinted with permission from JA Pennington, *Bowes and Church's Food Values of Portions Commonly Used*, 16th ed (Philadelphia, Pa: JB Lippincott Co, 1994).

cognac, or dry brandy), 5 oz wine, or 12 oz beer.[2] Dry wines and low-calorie wines that are lower in carbohydrate should be recommended over sweeter wines, as should reduced-calorie beer. Labels on distilled liquor indicate the proof, which is equal to twice the alcohol percentage. Mixers used in mixed alcoholic beverages can also add significant calories and carbohydrate and thereby increase the blood glucose level. Calorie-free mixers can be used in place of regular mixers.[1]

For some clients with diabetes, ingestion of an alcoholic beverage will probably not cause problems. Educators should teach their clients to drink responsibly, rather than forbidding alcohol altogether. Educators should give their clients a clear understanding of what constitutes responsible drinking and should not leave them wondering and feeling guilty every time they have a drink.

Clients who should be advised to abstain from alcohol use include those with a history of alcohol abuse; clients with pancreatitis, gastritis, hypertriglyceridemia, frequent hypoglycemic reactions, and certain types of kidney and heart disease; and all pregnant women. Alcohol can interact with barbiturates, tranquilizers, and numerous other drugs. Clients with diabetes should check with their physician to see if any of these contraindications apply to them.

Guidelines for alcohol use for insulin users and non-insulin users[2] are outlined in Chapter 3. Additional and more specific guidelines about consuming alcohol that could be discussed with a client are included in *Table 10.2*.

Table 10.2

Guidelines for Alcohol Use

- Alcoholic beverages should be used only upon the advice of the diabetes care team.
- Alcohol should be used in moderation. It is best to limit the amount to no more than two drinks each day.
- If the client requires insulin and his or her weight is normal, two drinks can occasionally be used as an "extra." No food should be omitted because even this amount of alcohol can cause hypoglycemia.
- For all clients with diabetes whose weight is a concern, calories from alcohol must be counted into the meal plan. Calories are best substituted for fat calories (each drink is equal to 90 calories or 2 fat exchanges).
- Hypoglycemia the morning after drinking alcohol can be avoided by waking at the usual time, testing blood glucose levels, and eating a regular breakfast.
- Alcohol should not be consumed on an empty stomach or after vigorous exercise, and should only be consumed directly before or shortly after meals.
- Drinks that contain large amounts of carbohydrate (eg, liqueurs, sweet wines, and sweet mixers) should be substituted into the meal plan, based upon advice from the diabetes care team.
- Avoid alcohol if hypertriglyceridemia is present.
- Never drink before driving.
- Do not jeopardize your health by giving in to social pressures to drink.

Delay of Meals

Clients with diabetes are usually encouraged to eat their meals at regular times because of the following:

- For those taking insulin (especially intermediate-acting insulin), meal times are coordinated with peak action times.
- For those not taking insulin, regular meal times may help prevent hunger and, perhaps, prevent eating more than their meal plan recommends. Some people taking oral glucose-lowering medications may experience hypoglycemia with a delay in meals.[7]

Clients on intensive insulin therapy have more flexibility in the timing of meals, but even these clients often report that the more consistent they can be with the timing and composition of their meals, the easier it is to control blood glucose levels.[8] However, there will be times when meals are unavoidably delayed. If a meal must be delayed for approximately 1 hour and changing the insulin injection time is not an option, eating approximately 15 grams of carbohydrate at the usual meal time should be sufficient to prevent hypoglycemia. It also may be possible to switch a meal with a later snack if a meal must be delayed for longer than 1 hour.

Eating Out

Following a meal plan at home prepares clients with diabetes to enjoy eating out. They can eat out with less hesitation if they know which foods they should eat, the portion sizes, and how to substitute appropriately. Teaching clients with diabetes to be assertive and curious regarding the foods they order prepares them to make appropriate food selections. Suggestions such as calling the restaurant in advance to obtain more information about the menu and how the food is prepared may make the actual experience of eating out easier.[7]

Table 10.3
Dining Out Guidelines

- Order salad dressing, butter, margarine, or sour cream on the side and control the amount used.
- Order reduced-calorie or fat-free salad dressing, or use vinegar and a small amount of oil.
- Request that entrees be prepared with minimal fat (eg, grilled, broiled, or baked with minimal oil or butter).
- Request that vegetables be cooked in reduced amounts or without butter/margarine.
- Order "free foods" (raw vegetables, lettuce salad) as fillers.
- Share an entree to reduce the portion size and order a side salad or vegetable.

Eating out usually results in a higher fat intake. It may be helpful to recommend that calories or fat be "banked" and used at the meal that the client plans to eat out. Restaurant-prepared foods are often high in saturated fat, salt, and sugar and low in fiber. *Table 10.3* describes ways to eat less fat when dining out.[7] *Single-Topic Diabetes Resources,* described in Chapter 16, includes an educational resource, "Eating Out: From Burger to Burritos," which can be used with clients to provide recommendations for eating out.

More restaurants are beginning to offer healthier dessert selections. Examples of acceptable dessert choices include fresh fruit, frozen yogurt or light ice cream, and plain pumpkin pie, custard, pudding, or cake (eg, order carrot cake and remove the icing). Another option is to stop at a frozen yogurt shop for a dessert after dining out.

The key to reducing calories and fat in a fast-food restaurant is to buy small serving sizes and eat only at meal times. The average calorie content of a fast-food meal is 685 calories, which is not outrageously high for a meal, but is usually too many calories for a snack. Words on a menu like "jumbo," "giant," or "deluxe" should signal caution. Larger serving sizes mean not only additional calories but more fat, cholesterol, and sodium. Clients should be taught to make wise food choices and order items without toppings, with special sauces, cheese, and mayonnaise served on the side. They should ask about preparation methods whenever possible.[7]

Snacking

For children, adolescents, and adults requiring insulin, snacks may help prevent fluctuations in blood glucose levels.

The timing of meals and snacks and nutrient distribution need to be individualized, rather than patterned using the antiquated practice of dividing food into three meals and three snacks, with the snacks each containing one ninth of the total carbohydrate. To promote optimal metabolic control and to meet caloric needs, most children with type I diabetes on conventional insulin regimens (ie, 2 injections per day) need three snacks—midmorning, midafternoon, and before bed. When children reach adolescence, conformity with peers is of utmost importance and may provide additional challenges in coordinating the insulin schedule with meal/snack patterns. Insulin adjustments must be made to accommodate desired changes in eating patterns. For example, the morning regular insulin can be decreased to allow for omission of the morning snack.

A controversial issue with snacking and diabetes is the necessity of including a protein-containing bedtime snack, particularly for clients requiring insulin. Protein is a good source of long-term energy, which can cause a sustained rise in blood glucose concentration and help prevent nocturnal hypoglycemia. Adding 10 to 20 g protein to the bedtime snack of clients experiencing nocturnal hypoglycemia is worth trying. Although there is little scientific research to support it, it often seems to help. Encouraging clients with diabetes to monitor their blood glucose before bedtime, especially if they are prone to hypoglycemia, may be the best advice in making the decision about the amount and composition of the snack.

For clients with type II diabetes, snacking should be discouraged if it is not needed for blood glucose control. First, clients with type II diabetes have a delayed response to insulin secretion. A 4- to 5-hour period after meals is usually needed to return glucose levels to baseline. Snacking between meals prevents normalization of glucose levels during the day. Also, most clients with type II diabetes are overweight, and recommending an eating pattern of three meals per day generally encourages healthier food choices and lower caloric intake. In contrast to the above recommendations, there is growing evidence that in some clients with type II diabetes smaller and more frequent meals may actually improve glucose and lipid levels. More research is needed to evaluate the long-term effects of this type of meal patterning.[9]

Individualization is important in promoting permanent behavior change, especially for clients who have a long history of snacking. When clients are not willing to change their usual pattern of eating, snacks that contain less than 20 calories would be recommended. Examples of low-calorie snack choices are shown in *Table 10.4*.[7]

Clients with type II diabetes who are on insulin, especially multiple and mixed doses of insulin, may require between-meal snacks, as suggested for clients with type I diabetes.

For clients with type I and type II diabetes, the decision about when and how much to eat for a snack should be based on the client's blood glucose level. Self-monitoring of blood glucose should be promoted in all clients with diabetes to provide them with flexibility and to give them independence in making these daily self-management decisions.

Hypoglycemia

Eating an adequate amount of food at recommended times is important to help avoid hypoglycemia, especially in clients with diabetes on insulin who have insulin deficiency. Meals and snacks should be matched with the anticipated rise and fall of the client's insulin dose to help prevent hypoglycemia. In the Diabetes Control and Complications Trial (DCCT), severe hypoglycemia occurred approximately three times more often during intensive therapy than during conventional therapy.[10]

Increased physical activity lowers blood glucose levels, and the insulin dose may need to be reduced by one third or more, depending on the client's insulin sensitivity. If the insulin dose is not adjusted and physical activity is increased, then the blood glucose level should be tested after the activity. If it is 70 mg/dL or less, the low blood glucose should be treated appropriately. The effect of exercise can sometimes last up to 24 hours. Therefore, frequent blood glucose monitoring can help the client avoid hypoglycemia.[1]

Table 10.4
Low-Calorie Snacks and Beverages (≤ 20 Calories)

Beverages

Club soda with 2 tbsp fruit juice
Diet soda
Iced tea with artificial sweetener
Coffee or hot tea (use artificial sweetener and skim or 1% milk if desired)
Hot chocolate (use hot water and ½ packet of sugar-free hot cocoa mix)
Fat-free broth or bouillon

Foods

Raw vegetables (eg, celery, cucumber, green and red pepper, broccoli, cauliflower, lettuce, mushrooms)
7 pretzel sticks
1 cup air-popped popcorn
3 mini-rice cakes

Hypoglycemia must be treated immediately with some form of glucose. Fifteen grams of carbohydrate is recommended for treatment; this amount raises the blood glucose by 50 to 100 mg/dL in 15 to 30 minutes. The response to carbohydrate varies from person to person and is possibly influenced by how low the blood glucose actually is and the cause of the reaction.[1] Foods and glucose replacement sources that provide approximately 15 grams of carbohydrate are listed in *Table 10.5*.

Another blood glucose level check is recommended 15 minutes after treatment. If the blood glucose level is at or below 50 to 80 mg/dL, the carbohydrate should be followed by an additional 15 g carbohydrate and another blood glucose test 15 minutes after treatment. After treatment, if the blood glucose has risen to a normal range of 80 to 120 mg/dL and it is still an hour or more until the next meal or snack, 15 g carbohydrate should be consumed.[1]

Some research conducted to determine the optimal treatment for hypoglycemia found varying results with different oral carbohydrate solutions.[11] The researchers investigated the effectiveness of seven types of orally administered carbohydrates in correcting blood glucose levels—glucose in solution, tablets, and gel; sucrose in solution and tablets; a hydrolyzed polysaccharide solution; and orange juice—each of which provided 15 g carbohydrate. Mean blood glucose levels 10 minutes after ingestion were found to be similar whether correction was dispensed with the tablets or the solution of glucose, sucrose, or the polysaccharide preparation. However, glycemic responses were consistently lower with glucose gel and orange juice. The authors concluded that glucose gel and orange juice cannot be recommended for treatment of hypoglycemia.

Given these results and the varying individual responses to different types of carbohydrates, clients with diabetes should be encouraged to keep a record of how they treat their reactions so that they can determine which treatment method is best for them.

Overtreatment of hypoglycemia can occur very easily if a client relies only on symptoms and not on blood glucose results. Overtreating with additional food can result in weight gain, as well as a great increase in blood glucose levels.

Table 10.5
Carbohydrate Sources for Treatment of Hypoglycemia

	Gm CHO	Kcal
Starch List		
6 saltine-type crackers	15	80
3 graham crackers	15	80
8 animal crackers	15	80
Fruit List		
⅓ cup cranberry, grape, or prune juice	15	60
½ cup apple, pineapple, grapefruit, or orange juice	15	60
2 tbsp raisins	17	75
Milk List		
1 cup skim milk	12	90
1 cup low-fat milk	12	120
¾ cup skim milk plain yogurt	12	90
¾ cup low-fat milk plain yogurt	12	120
⅓ cup regular low-fat fruited yogurt	12	100
1 cup skim milk fruited yogurt, sweetened with aspartame	12	100
½ cup regular pudding	12	70
½ cup light ice cream	15	125
Other Carbohydrates		
½ cup regular gelatin	17	80
¼ cup sherbet	15	80
4 ounces cola	13	55
6 ounces ginger ale	16	60
1 tbsp honey	17	60
1 tbsp brown sugar	13	50
1 tbsp corn syrup	15	45
Commercial Products		
3 Glucose Tablets™	15	60
40 gm Glutose™	16	64
18 gm Insta Glucose™	15	60
1½ packets (25 g each) Insulin Reaction Gel™	17	68

Adapted with permission from J Green Pastors, *Nutritional Care of Diabetes*, 2nd ed, San Marcus, Calif: Nutrition Dimension, Inc; 1995: 111.

Some clients with diabetes may want to eat foods such as ice cream or chocolate to treat hypoglycemia. These foods are high in fat, which slows the absorption of glucose and adds extra calories. They therefore are not an appropriate form of treatment for hypoglycemia because low blood glucose has to be treated immediately with a food source that is primarily glucose.

To assist the client with diabetes in preventing hypoglycemia, self-management training should include discussions of[1]:

- ➤ timing of meals and snacks,
- ➤ eating planned meals and snacks,
- ➤ adjusting insulin and/or food before activity change,
- ➤ understanding onset, peak, and duration of insulin dose or oral glucose-lowering medication,

- self-monitoring of blood glucose as part of daily regimen,
- developing survival kit for treatment of hypoglycemia,
- teaching significant others about use of glucagon.

Sick-Day Management

The main rules for sick-day management that clients with diabetes should follow include[1]:

- take diabetes medications,
- self-monitor blood glucose,
- test urine ketones,
- eat the usual amount of carbohydrate, divided into smaller meals and snacks if necessary (if blood glucose is 250 mg/dL or higher, all of the usual amount of carbohydrate is not necessary),
- drink fluids frequently,
- call the diabetes care team.

Ketones in the urine and an elevated blood glucose level indicate that additional insulin, particularly regular or short-acting insulin, may be needed. If the blood glucose level is 250 mg/dL or higher continuously for 24 hours, the physician should be informed. When the body is unable to utilize glucose, it breaks down fats for energy, and the byproducts of the fat breakdown are ketones. Along with elevated blood glucose levels, the presence of ketones in the urine indicates the potential for diabetic ketoacidosis (DKA).[1]

Consuming fluids and taking adequate insulin are critically important during an illness. Soft, semisolid foods and frequent, small meals may be better tolerated by the client with diabetes during illness.[1]

Vomiting and diarrhea cause loss of fluid and electrolytes (potassium and sodium). Adequate rehydration is extremely important because it helps restore and maintain the depleted vascular volume and enhances the kidney's ability to excrete glucose, thus lessening hyperglycemia.[12] Broth or bouillon and tomato juice help replace some of the lost sodium. If unable to tolerate solids or semisolid foods, the client should drink liquids with appropriate amounts of calories and carbohydrate. A list of sick-day foods, including sugar-containing items (eg, soft drinks, gelatins) not routinely purchased by clients with diabetes, should be provided.

References

1. Kulkarni KD. Adjusting nutrition therapy for special situations. In: Powers MA, ed. *Handbook of Diabetes Medical Nutrition Therapy*. 2nd ed. Gaithersburg, Md: Aspen Publishers, Inc; 1996; 437–457.
2. American Diabetes Association. Nutrition recommendations and principles for people with diabetes mellitus (position statement). *Diabetes Care*. 1994;17(5):519.
3. Franz MJ. Alcohol and diabetes. Part 2: Its metabolism and guidelines for its occasional use. *Diabetes Spectrum*. 1990;3:210–216.
4. Menze R, Metel DC, Brunstein U, Heinke P. Effect of moderate ethanol ingestion on overnight diabetes control and hormone secretion in Type I diabetic patients. *Diabetologia*. 1991;34:A188.
5. American Diabetes Association. Nutrition principles for the management of diabetes and related complications (technical review). *Diabetes Care*. 1994;17(5):490–518.
6. Thom SL. Diabetes medications and delivery systems. In: Powers MA, ed. *Handbook of Diabetes Medical Nutrition Therapy*. 2nd ed. Gaithersburg, Md: Aspen Publishers, Inc; 1996: 77–106.

7. Green Pastors J. Special topics for meal planning. In: Green Pastors J, ed. *Nutritional Care of Diabetes*. 2nd ed. San Marcus, Calif: Nutrition Dimension, Inc; 1995: 103–116.
8. Diabetes Control and Complications Trial Research Group. Expanded role of the dietitian in the Diabetes Control and Complications Trial: implications for clinical practice. *J Am Diet Assoc.* 1993;93:758–767.
9. Bertelsen JC, Thomsen C, et al. Effect of meal frequency on blood glucose, insulin, and fatty acids in NIDDM subjects. *Diabetes Care.* 1993;16:4–7.
10. Diabetes Control and Complications Trial Research Group. Epidemiology of severe hypoglycemia in the DCCT. *Am J Med.* 1991;90:450–459.
11. Slama G, et al. The search for an optimized treatment of hypoglycemia. *J Intern Med.* 1990;150:589–593.
12. Genuth S. Diabetic ketoacidosis and hyperosmolar hyperglycemic nonketotic syndrome in adults. In: *Therapy of Diabetes Mellitus and Related Disorders*. 2nd ed. Alexandria, Va: American Diabetes Association, Inc; 1994.

For Further Reading

Alcohol

Franz MJ. Alcohol and diabetes, part I. *Diabetes Spectrum.* 1990;3(3):136–144.
Franz MJ. Alcohol and diabetes, part II. *Diabetes Spectrum.* 1990;3(4):210–216.
Gaziano JM, et al. Moderate alcohol intake, increased levels of high-density lipoprotein and its subfractions and decreased risk of myocardial infarction. *N Engl J Med.* 1993;329(25):1829–1834.
Glasgow AM, et al. Alcohol and drug use in teenagers with diabetes mellitus. *J Adol Health.* 1991;12(1):11–14.
Koivisto VA, et al. Alcohol with a meal has no adverse effects on postprandial glucose homeostasis in diabetic patients. *Diabetes Care.* 1993;16(12):1612–1614.

Eating Away from Home

DeBakey ME, Gotto AM, Scott LW. *The Living Heart Guide to Eating Out*. New York: Master Media Books; 1993.
Natow A, Heslin J. *Fast Food Nutrition Counter*. New York: Pocket Books; 1994.
Warshaw HS. America eats out: nutrition in the chain and family restaurant industry. *J Am Diet Assoc.* 1993;93(1):17–20.
Warshaw HS. Eating away from home: teaching creatively and successfully. *Diabetes Educator.* 1992;18(1):21–28.
Warshaw HS. *The Restaurant Companion: A Guide to Healthier Eating Out*. 2nd ed. Chicago, Ill: Surrey Books; 1995.

Hypoglycemia

Diabetes Control and Complications Trial Research Group. Epidemiology of severe hypoglycemia in the Diabetes Control and Complications Trial. *Am J Med.* 1991;90(4):450–459.
White N, ed. The risk of hypoglycemia during intensive therapy of IDDM. *Diabetes Spectrum.* 1994;7(4):232–265.

Part 2

Diabetes Nutrition Education

From Philosophy to Practice

11

Whether we are fully aware of it or not, our behavior is guided by a philosophy.[1,2] Our beliefs about the nature and purpose of human behavior guide our actions in our personal lives and in our professions. A philosophy is both a viewpoint (a perspective about how things are) and a system of values (a perspective about how things should be). Our philosophy about helping relationships is important because it shapes our professional behavior, attitudes, satisfaction, and effectiveness. If the nutrition education programs and approaches we develop are guided by a consistent, well-articulated philosophy, those programs and activities will be more cohesive, coherent, and satisfying for both our clients and ourselves. New guidelines for diabetes medical nutrition therapy and the expanding list of meal-planning resources for its management call for us to examine our philosophy of care, as well as update our understanding and knowledge of diabetes and nutrition. The assumptions that we have about how, when, and why people change behavior will influence our ability to serve our clients as much as or even more than the information we provide them.

Much has been written about the philosophy of client empowerment and its particular relevance to diabetes self-management.[3-7] The empowerment approach is based on the recognition that persons with diabetes are responsible for their own control and decision making regarding diabetes self-management. This philosophy is also based on the recognition that diabetes affects the cognitive, emotional, physical, social, and spiritual fabric of clients' lives. Diabetes self-management, especially changes in eating behavior, must be tailored to the values, culture, needs, perceptions, goals, and resources of our clients if we are to be effective in helping them maximize their well-being. Clients must feel that whatever changes they make are reasonable, possible, and worthwhile when considered within the framework of their own values, needs, and experiences. Because clients provide the great majority of their own daily diabetes self-management and must live with the consequences, they have both the right and the responsibility to be active participants in the design of their diabetes treatment plans.

If our practice is to be consistent with our beliefs and values, it is important to reflect carefully on our own underlying philosophy of diabetes care and education. A traditional philosophy of client care views the dietitian as the one responsible for teaching, persuading, and/or motivating clients to follow the nutritional recommendations and guidelines provided by diabetes care professionals. The empowerment philosophy views the role of the dietitian as helping clients improve their ability to make informed choices about their nutritional self-care. The ability to make informed choices grows as

Table 11.1
Comparison of Traditional and Empowerment Viewpoints Regarding Diabetes Medical Nutrition Therapy

Traditional Viewpoint	Empowerment Viewpoint
Food choices affect physical health including diabetes management.	Food choices affect psychosocial quality of life as well as physical health.
The dietitian is the expert in nutrition and diabetes and is therefore in charge of developing an appropriate meal plan.	The dietitian is the expert in nutrition and diabetes and clients are the experts about themselves and their life circumstances.
The dietitian is responsible for assessing client needs, providing information, and designing a meal plan based on assessed needs.	Both the dietitian and the client are responsible for sharing information and collaborating to develop a meal plan that is acceptable to the client.
The dietitian's role is to motivate or stimulate adherence to the meal plan.	The dietitian's role is to help the client discover what changes he or she is willing and able to make at this time. The client's right to choose is acknowledged, even if the dietitian disagrees with the client's choices.
The dietitian provides advice often phrased as "You should ...," "The best thing for you to do is...," or "You need to...."	The dietitian provides information and makes recommendations about sound nutrition. The dietitian helps the client to clarify the costs and benefits of employing various nutritional options.
The focus is on metabolic goals such as weight and blood glucose levels.	Desired metabolic outcomes shape behavior change plans but are not in themselves behaviors that clients can control. The focus is on behavioral goals, ie, specific action steps that clients can control.
The dietitian does most of the talking in an effort to provide all the information clients will need during the limited time available.	The dietitian does most of the listening in an effort to help clients identify nutrition changes that most closely fit their needs, lifestyle, and personal goals.
The dietitian provides instruction on an appropriate meal plan and teaches clients how to follow it.	The dietitian teaches behavior-change skills so that clients can achieve their own nutritional goals.
The dietitian provides praise/reinforcement when clients succeed in following their meal plan.	The dietitian provides nonjudgmental support to clients as persons and helps them learn from their choices and apply that learning to the development of subsequent meal plans.
The dietitian feels effective and successful when clients follow nutrition recommendations.	The dietitian feels effective and successful when clients become skilled at making informed choices and solving problems.

clients gain knowledge about nutrition (the potential consequences of a variety of food choices and nutritional approaches) and about themselves (their level of self-awareness and insight about their own habits, goals, needs, and resources). Both of these philosophies are defensible and, in practice, diabetes care and education often involve a blending of the two approaches.

Review *Table 11.1* and carefully consider your own approach to diabetes medical nutrition therapy. Which of the above descriptions of a dietitian's role most closely matches your approach? Are you clearly in one camp or the other, or do you combine the elements of both points of view in your approach? Should you employ different philosophies with different clients? Which approach do you think is most likely to support sustained lifestyle changes? The answers to these questions reflect your philosophy of care and will shape your practice in important ways. A high degree of awareness about your philosophy of helping people change behavior to improve their well-being will serve to make your professional relationships and practice more coherent, effective, and satisfying.

References

1. Anderson RM. Diabetes educators as philosophers. *Diabetes Educator.* 1987;13:259–261.
2. Feste C, Anderson RM. Empowerment: from philosophy to practice. *Patient Education and Counseling.* 1995;26:139–144.
3. Anderson RM, Funnell MM, Butler P, Arnold MS, Fitzgerald JT, Feste C. Patient empowerment: results of a randomized control trial. *Diabetes Care.* 1995;18:943–949.
4. Arnold MS, Butler PM, Anderson RM, Funnell MM, Feste C. Guidelines for facilitating a patient empowerment program. *Diabetes Educator.* 1995;21:308–312.
5. Anderson RM. Patient empowerment and the traditional medical model: a case of irreconcilable differences? *Diabetes Care.* 1995;18:412–415.
6. Funnell MM, Anderson RM, Arnold MS. Empowerment: a winning model for diabetes care. *Practical Diabetology.* 1991;10:15–18.
7. Funnell MM, Anderson RM, Arnold MS, Barr PA, Donnelly MB, Johnson PD, Taylor-Moon D, White N. *Diabetes Educator.* 1991;17:37–41.

For Further Reading

Pryor K. *Don't Shoot the Dog.* New York: Bantam Books; 1984.
Rogers C, Freiberg HJ, eds. *Freedom to Learn.* 3rd ed. New York: Macmillan College Publishing Company; 1994.

Process of Diabetes Medical Nutrition Therapy 12

As explained earlier, diabetes medical nutrition therapy is a four-step model that includes assessment of the client's metabolic, nutrition, and lifestyle parameters, identification and negotiation of nutrition goals, intervention designed to achieve individualized goals, and evaluation of outcomes.[1] The purpose of diabetes medical nutrition therapy is to assist clients in acquiring and maintaining the knowledge, skills, attitudes, behaviors, and commitment to meet the challenges of daily diabetes self-management successfully. This is not accomplished during a single counseling session, but rather occurs over a longer period using the process of diabetes medical nutrition therapy.

Promoting changes in personal eating habits for clients with diabetes constitutes one of the greatest challenges in diabetes self-management training. One of the reasons that clients with diabetes have difficulty with "diet-related issues" may be because they are not referred to dietitians or diabetes educators for diabetes nutrition self-management training.[2] They may instead experience one of the following scenarios:

➤ They are given a "diet sheet" that provides only very basic information about food exchanges, a meal plan, and a sample menu.
➤ They are given a list of "good" and "bad" foods.
➤ They are told to avoid sugar or limit fat and to lose weight.
➤ They are given an exchange list booklet for a prescribed calorie level with minimal education or individualized instruction just prior to hospital discharge.

Without adequate nutrition advice or an individualized meal plan based on the client's lifestyle, "dietary nonadherence" will continue to be reported as a primary inhibitor to optimal blood glucose control.

The four-step model of diabetes medical nutrition therapy is the basis of *Facilitating Lifestyle Change: A Resource Manual,* published in 1996 by the American Diabetes Association and The American Dietetic Association. This manual contains resource forms to be used with clients for the purposes of nutrition assessment, goal setting, intervention, and evaluation. These four steps not only define diabetes medical nutrition therapy, but form the basis for promoting lifestyle change.

Nutrition Assessment
Definition

Even though assessment is the initial step of the four-step model, beginning the relationship or establishing rapport with the client is an important preliminary step. Usually this begins during the assessment phase and continues throughout the self-management training, with a genuine and trusting relationship developing between the diabetes educator and the client.

Nutrition assessment is the most crucial step in diabetes medical nutrition therapy. The main purpose of an assessment is to gather information needed to assist in the development of individual nutrition goals and subsequently establish an appropriate nutrition intervention.[3]

Preliminary Data

Before the diabetes educator can conduct a comprehensive nutrition assessment, preliminary data need to be collected, either from a hospital or clinic medical record or a referring physician. The data needed for review include health service utilization, type of diabetes, current treatment regimen, laboratory values, current medications, risk assessment for complications, previous diabetes education, current diabetes medical nutrition therapy, guidelines for exercise, the physician's diabetes management goals, and the client's self-management needs. *Table 12.1* provides more detail about these preliminary data. Appendix 1 provides laboratory values for diabetes mellitus.

In some clinical circumstances, information about previous diabetes education and current diabetes medical nutrition therapy, guidelines for exercise, physician's goals for the client, and specific self-management needs is not available in the medical record or may not be included in a referring letter from the physician. These preliminary data would then need to become part of the data gathered in the nutrition assessment.

Components of a Nutrition Assessment

The major components of a nutrition assessment are collection of clinical data, nutrition history, weight history, physical activity history, monitoring psychosocial and economic information (including stress and social support), diabetes knowledge and skill level, and readiness to change. *Table 12.2* contains the nutrition assessment components and specific data that can be considered at the initial assessment visit.

Information from all these components must be obtained and utilized to develop achievable goals and workable interventions appropriate to the client. Assessment is an ongoing process that needs to be continuously modified and updated.

The amount of time it takes to do an assessment varies widely and depends on the dietitian, the client, and other factors, such as the client's ability to provide information, as well as the complexity of the information needed.

Clinical Data

The information needed to gather clinical data such as body mass index (BMI), determine reasonable body weight, and estimate daily energy needs is well known and is readily available in many resources. See Appendix 2 for further details; also see the sources listed in For Further Reading at the end of this chapter.

Nutrition History

A nutrition history gives the diabetes educator an idea of the client's usual personal food habits and enables the educator to determine the client's nutrition needs. This information is used to determine the appropriate approach for meal planning and to individualize the meal plan. Specific information that should be collected when completing a nutrition history includes the following:

Table 12.1
Preliminary Data Needed for Diabetes Medical Nutrition Therapy Assessment

Factor	Data Needed
Health services utilization	Primary care physician
	Location of usual diabetes care
Type of diabetes (see Chapter 2)	Type I/type II/gestational/other
Current treatment regimen (see Chapters 3, 5 & 7)	DMNT* alone
	DMNT* & oral glucose-lowering medications
	DMNT* & insulin
	DMNT* & combination therapy
Laboratory values (see Appendix 1)	Glycosylated hemoglobin
	Fasting/nonfasting blood glucose
	Blood lipid panel
Current medications (type and amount)	Diabetes medications (see Chapter 5)
	Antihypertensive medications
	Lipid-lowering medications
	Gastrointestinal medications
	Others
Risk assessment for complications (see Chapter 9)	Hyperlipidemia
	Hypertension
	Nephropathy
	Neuropathy
	Retinopathy
Previous diabetes education	Specify when, where, who, what
Current diabetes medical nutrition therapy	Specify when, where, who, what
Guidelines for exercise	Medical clearance for exercise
	Exercise limitations, if any
Diabetes management goals	Target blood glucose and lipid levels
	Target glycosylated hemoglobin level

*Diabetes Medical Nutrition Therapy

Adapted with permission from M Peyrot, Evaluation of patient education programs: how to do it and how to use it, *Diabetes Spectrum*, 1996;9(2):86–93.

- past nutrition intervention,
- previous meal-planning methods used and assessment of comprehension and compliance,
- household/family situation,
- food preparation/shopping,
- approach to eating away from home,
- use of alcohol,
- use of vitamin/mineral/nutrition supplements,
- issues with compulsive eating.

Table 12.2
Initial Nutrition Assessment

Components	Assessments
Clinical data (see Appendix 2)	Height and weight* Reasonable body weight Daily energy needs
Nutrition history	Current diabetes medical nutrition therapy (if not available from preliminary data) Who does food prep/shopping Frequency/choices for dining out Alcohol intake Use of vitamin/mineral/nutrition supplements Eating disorders Nutrition history (using one or a combination of the following methods: 24-hour recall, usual food intake, food frequency, food records) Energy intake and macronutrient composition (type and amount)
Weight history	Weight history, recent weight changes, and weight goals
Physical activity history	Activity types and frequency Energy expenditure Limitations that hinder exercise Willingness and ability to become more physically active
Monitoring	Knowledge of target blood glucose levels SMBG method/frequency of testing Other types of record keeping being conducted (food, physical activity, etc) Client benefits from monitoring
Psychosocial/economic	Living situation, finances, educational background, employment
Knowledge and skill level	Survival or continuing education knowledge level
Expectations and readiness to change	Willingness to change

*BMI and waist-to-hip ratio are additional clinical measured that can be assessed.

Adapted with permission from M Peyrot, Evaluation of patient education programs: how to do it and how to use it, *Diabetes Spectrum*, 1996;9(2):86–93.

The Lifestyle Questionnaire, a resource included in *Facilitating Lifestyle Change*, includes a nutrition history form that can be used to gather the information described above. A completed nutrition history is used in the case study at the end of this chapter.

In addition, it is important to collect information about common trends in the client's food intake. This can be done using several different methods (24-hour recall, usual food intake, food frequency, and/or food record). Appendix 3 contains examples of two food record forms for collecting this information. The first form, the Food Record Form, focuses on type, quantity, and preparation of food. The second form, the Diabetes Self-Care Record, assists in assessment of food intake, timing of meals, type of medication, amount of physical activity, and blood glucose results.

After collecting the nutrition history and typical food intake information from the client, the diabetes educator can evaluate energy intake and macronutrient composition. Several methods can be used to evaluate nutritional adequacy, including software programs and *Exchange Lists for Meal Planning*. A worksheet using a simplified method to assess nutritional adequacy is also contained in Appendix 3.

Information that is important to collect specific to weight includes: *Weight History*

➤ usual weight, weight history, and healthy weight goals,
➤ assessment of interest/readiness to change current weight,
➤ expectations regarding weight change.

The case study at the end of this chapter includes an example of a completed weight history resource form from *Facilitating Lifestyle Change* that can be used to gather information. This form is most useful with a client for whom weight loss is the primary desired clinical outcome. The components discussed above could also be incorporated into a nutrition history form.

Because physical activity is an important component of diabetes self-management, it should be addressed when completing an assessment. The diabetes educator should ask the client questions concerning his or her previous and current activity levels, readiness to become more physically active, limitations that might hinder exercise, and types of physical activities of interest. See the case study at the end of this chapter for an example of a completed physical activity record (a resource from *Facilitating Lifestyle Change*) that could be used to assess this information.   *Physical Activity History*

An assessment of the client's monitoring practice could include self-monitoring of blood glucose, food, and/or physical activity, usually in the form of written records. It is important to assess the client's previous and/or current practices, as well as interest level regarding record-keeping and self-monitoring. This will help the diabetes educator determine the level of complexity of the nutrition self-management plan and promote his or her participation in self-monitoring. The case study in this chapter includes a resource form from *Facilitating Lifestyle Change* that was used to assess the client's self-monitoring practices.   *Monitoring Information*

Psychosocial and economic information includes the client's living situation, finances, educational background, employment status, ethnic or religious beliefs, family/social support, and level of stress. This type of information could be included on a nutrition history form. Often it is included in a medical chart or as part of a more general diabetes assessment form. The Lifestyle Questionnaire in *Facilitating Lifestyle Change* includes an example of a resource form that can be used to assess a client's history of stress; this is   *Psychosocial and Economic Information* shown in the case study. Other resources that can be used to determine stress level can be found in For Further Reading at the end of this chapter.

Knowledge and Skill Level

Many diabetes educators have developed their own checklists or surveys to assess a client's knowledge of nutrition. See Appendix 4 for an example of a knowledge checklist specific to diabetes medical nutrition therapy. Another method to assess knowledge is to compare client information collected from nutrition questionnaires or a verbal nutrition history with established goals or standards for education.[4]

Readiness to Change

The transtheoretical model for behavioral change developed by Prochaska and colleagues[5] provides a framework for assessing readiness to change using a five-stage model. These stages include:

1. *Precontemplation*—no intention to change in the foreseeable future,
2. *Contemplation*—aware that a problem exists; thinking about making a change,
3. *Preparation*—decision making; seriously considering change in the near future,
4. *Action*—making changes,
5. *Maintenance*—working to prevent relapse.

These stages of change have been applied to a variety of health behavior interventions, including fat reduction, exercise, smoking cessation, alcohol treatment, self-monitoring of blood glucose, and weight management.[6]

Movement through the five stages often involves a move in either direction. Focusing intervention to the appropriate stage can facilitate tailoring intervention to the client's needs, thus improving likelihood of success. Assessment of readiness to change can guide the diabetes educator in negotiating with the client to establish behavior change goals.

There are several readiness-to-change questions included in *Facilitating Lifestyle Change* in three forms of the Lifestyle Questionnaire:

➤ "Do You Want to Change Your Lifestyle?"
➤ "Weight History"
➤ "Physical Activity History"

All of these forms are included in the case study at the end of this chapter, which demonstrates how to use these assessment forms.

Collection of Assessment Data

The two barriers most commonly faced in clinical practice for obtaining assessment data are time limitations and reluctance of the client to provide the information.[7] Some solutions to consider that may help to maximize time more efficiently include:

➤ utilize data previously collected by other staff;
➤ focus on assessment information that is the most pertinent to the client;
➤ prioritize information by obtaining the most crucial information first.

In an ambulatory care setting, you may wish to consider providing the client with forms or questionnaires to be completed prior to or in conjunction with the appointment. Some examples include, at the initial appointment, providing forms to be completed before next scheduled appointment; mailing the forms to the client before the first appointment and asking the client to bring the completed forms; or having the client complete the forms while waiting for the appointment.

In the inpatient setting, because of time constraints and limited patient contact, the use of forms or questionnaires may not be possible or efficient. Instead, the forms or questionnaires can be used to record nutrition assessment information collected orally from the patient.

Some suggestions for ways to maximize the information provided by the client include:

➤ take time to develop rapport and establish trust;
➤ be nonjudgmental in the way you ask questions and react to responses; there are no wrong answers;
➤ respect the client's emotional state, which may require waiting to obtain comprehensive assessment data.

Assessment Summary

Nutrition assessment serves an educational purpose for both the diabetes educator and the client because it can improve the client's awareness of health status, treatment options, and lifestyle factors that affect his or her health. Nutrition assessment also provides the diabetes educator with an opportunity to establish the tone of the relationship with the client. Ideally, the diabetes educator and client should develop a working partnership. The diabetes educator should ask not only for information, but also for the client's reactions, feelings, and thoughts about the information being discussed, which is a natural progression into the next step of the four-step model of diabetes medical nutrition therapy—goal setting.

Goal Setting

Definition

Goal setting is a crucial part of diabetes self-management training, as well as the process of lifestyle change. Diabetes management goals are clinical or metabolic outcomes of treatment intervention and may include clinical parameters, such as lipid levels, blood glucose levels, and body weight. Goals for diabetes medical nutrition therapy have been established[3] and are summarized in Chapter 3.

Lifestyle change goals are also an important aspect of the management and education plan. They are less clinically focused but are specifically individualized to the client's needs. The purpose of setting goals is to establish realistic target behaviors that can be used to evaluate their success in making positive lifestyle changes. Goals are established by mutual agreement between the diabetes educator and the client. This contributes to the likelihood that the client will "own" the goals and become committed to the self-care behaviors that will enable him or her to reach and maintain them. A form to assist the diabetes educator and client in goal setting is shown in Appendix 5.

Standardized goals for education and counseling have been established by many organizations representing educators involved in health care. For diabetes self-management training, the American Diabetes Association has established education goals.[4] These goals acknowledge that diabetes self-management training occurs at different stages and is a continuous process; thus, it is appropriate to develop both initial and continuing education goals.

Negotiating Goals

To negotiate goals, educators need to be sensitive to clients' needs for flexibility and structure. It is important to respond to requests for guidance, but also to encourage clients to develop a realistic degree of independence in self-care. Following are some examples of questions that can be asked to elicit valuable information about the client's goals and to help establish a lifestyle plan:

- What goals are most likely to help you develop a healthier lifestyle?
- What behavior would you like to change?
- What changes can you make in your current lifestyle?
- What obstacles do you see to making these changes?
- What benefits do you see as a result of these changes?
- What are you willing to do right now?

The way in which goals are set affects the tone of the relationship between the diabetes educator and the client because of the emphasis on negotiation and values. The nature of the relationship will have a strong influence on the outcome of treatment, making goal setting a critical step in the sequence of diabetes medical nutrition therapy leading to the intervention.

Goals are not permanent. As time passes, the client's health, lifestyle, and attitudes can be expected to change, necessitating a renegotiation of goals. Thus, the diabetes educator should view goal setting as a continuous process. The ongoing relationship with the client provides the diabetes educator with a means of assisting him or her to see new alternatives and to renegotiate goals.

The case study included at the end of this chapter includes two resource forms from *Facilitating Lifestyle Change*, the Eating Behavior Diary and the Lifestyle Change Plan, which can be used to assist the diabetes educator and client in goal setting (specific to clinical outcomes, lifestyle change, and/or education). The Eating Behavior Diary is an assessment tool designed to provide the client with experience in monitoring eating behaviors. It focuses on the client becoming more aware of factors that influence eating (for example, social situations and feelings). The Lifestyle Change Plan is a tool to assist in setting goals for evaluating and ultimately improving problem lifestyle behaviors.

Intervention

Definition

Intervention refers to the diabetes educator's activities that facilitate or support the client's nutrition self-management plan. Effective nutrition intervention requires the diabetes educator to function as both an information provider and a counselor. As a counselor, a diabetes educator can help the client understand what having diabetes means personally and support the client in an effort to cope responsibly with the disease. Often, in the counselor role, diabetes educators think their responsibility is to motivate the client; however, this is a false premise. The diabetes educator's role is to serve as guide to help clients discover how they are motivated and to help them use their motivation so that they can bring about positive changes in eating behavior. The role of information provider is more in keeping with the traditional information-centered approach to diabetes management. The role of counselor is in keeping with the more client-focused trends in health care. Both are part of an essential balance that expands the role of the diabetes educator and contributes to quality health care.

Components of Nutrition Intervention

Nutrition intervention specifically refers to the *basic* and *in-depth education stages* of the nutrition intervention process. Basic education is providing primary information about nutrition and nutrient requirements, discussing the diabetes nutrition management guidelines, and introducing other survival skills information that may be important to the specific type of diabetes. In-depth education is selecting an appropriate meal-planning approach for achieving individually determined goals.

Nutrition Intervention Resources

Intervention includes the use of education resources for the development of meal-planning skills and strategies for behavior change. When choosing the type of intervention resources to use, take into consideration the following points:

- ➤ The client's ability and/or willingness to learn,
- ➤ The client's level of motivation to make the needed changes in his or her eating habits,
- ➤ The nutrition goals established by the client and the diabetes educator,
- ➤ The type and amount of insulin or oral glucose-lowering medication used (if any),
- ➤ The client's current activity level,
- ➤ The client's lifestyle (job or school schedule, current eating habits, favorite foods, religious/ethnic food beliefs, social and economic factors).

Nutrition Intervention Summary

Sometimes available education materials may not be appropriate for certain clients. Instead, you may want to develop your own materials or choose not to give any printed material. Another strategy may be to establish short-term eating behavior goals with a client, writing them out on paper, and simply using that as your education resource. It is important to choose from a variety of materials. Client backgrounds, lifestyles, needs, and interests differ vastly, and as a result, their educational needs differ considerably. The goal is to individualize the education and counseling session for each person with diabetes, rather than to use the same procedure or process of education for everyone.

Evaluation

Definition

Evaluation is a system of quality control for identifying what works and what does not. It refers to the activities of the diabetes educator and the client that enable them to determine the effectiveness of a plan, identify its strengths and weaknesses, and reinforce changes that need to be made. The educator evaluates whether the agreed-upon behavioral goals have been met and whether specific clinical outcomes (such as glycosylated hemoglobin, lipids, or weight) have improved. Adjustments in either goals or educational interventions should be negotiated jointly.

Types of Evaluation

Evaluation specific to client care involves process, outcome, and impact evaluation. A process evaluation involves a description of the specific activities carried out in developing a diabetes medical nutrition therapy plan with a client (eg, types of assessment(s) conducted and their results, description of individual nutrition/lifestyle goals, type of intervention and/or resources that were recommended, and plan for follow-up visits). In clinical settings this process is often referred to as "charting" or documenting in the medical record. Outcome evaluation is an assessment of the achievement of intermediate goals (eg, medical, behavioral, and psychosocial). *Table 12.3* outlines specific client outcome measures that can be considered when evaluating outcomes. Impact evaluation is an assessment of the achievement of ultimate goals (eg, prevention or delay of chronic complications of diabetes).

A process evaluation of client care activities is important primarily for the purposes of documentation. This is necessary for developing standards and improving quality of care, as well as for purposes of hospital accreditation, program recognition, and staff certification.

Outcome and impact evaluations are conducted for the purpose of measuring and evaluating the client's health care experience and are designed to help the client, providers, and payers make more rational and informed health care–related decisions.[9]

Practice guidelines are a series of steps or sets of criteria that are linked to expected outcomes. It is expected that implementing practice guidelines will minimize the current diverse approaches to care, control costs, and also result in a decrease in long-term mortality/morbidity rates.[10] Practice guidelines have now been developed for diabetes medical nutrition therapy for persons with both type I and type II diabetes (see Chapter 3).[7,11] The real benefit of practice guidelines is greater consistency of care based on the most current and scientifically supported information.

Resources

Facilitating Lifestyle Change includes two forms that can be used for evaluation: the Lifestyle Change: Food and Physical Activity Record and the Lifestyle Change: Summary Record.

The Food and Physical Activity Record form provides space for up to 3 days of records of food intake, nutrient information (eg, exchanges, grams of fat or carbohydrate), physical activity, and other information (eg, blood glucose results for persons with diabetes). It is recommended as a temporary tool for clients who may need to monitor their nutrient intake and/or physical activity to improve problem lifestyle behaviors, evaluate patterns, and solve problems.

The Summary Record form provides space to record up to 30 days of information, such as nutrient intake, physical activity, blood glucose results, medication, weight, and emotional and social support issues. This form is designated for longer-term record-keeping and is useful in tracking progress and evaluating the effects of changes in eating and physical activity. For example, a person with diabetes taking insulin might use the form to record nutrient information (eg, carbohydrate grams), amount of physical activity, and blood glucose results, which would be useful in making decisions about insulin adjustments or changes in meal timing or the type or amount of food eaten.

The case study at the end of this chapter incorporates all of these resource forms and shows how they may be completed.

Table 12.3
Client Outcome Measures

Medical Factors

Medical history*
Present health status*
> ➤ Glucose control*
> ➤ Complications

Health resource utilization*
> ➤ As indicator of need
> ➤ As indicator of prevention

Risk factors*
> ➤ Hypoglycemia unawareness
> ➤ Smoking

Behavioral Factors

Diabetes knowledge and skills*
> ➤ BG relationships and dynamics*

Health behavior and goals/intentions*
> ➤ BG monitoring*
> ➤ Medication*
> ➤ Diet*
> ➤ Exercise*
> ➤ Prevention/management of complications*
> ➤ Pregnancy management*

Psychosocial Factors

Social support systems*
> ➤ Family
> ➤ Peer
> ➤ Health care professional

Health beliefs and attitudes*
Psychosocial adjustment*
> ➤ Quality of life
> ➤ Psychological well-being

Contextual factors
> ➤ Barriers to learning*
> ➤ Socioeconomic factors*
> ➤ Cultural influences*

*Measure required by ADA Recognition Program (*Meeting the Standards: A Manual for Completing the American Diabetes Association Application for Recognition*, 4th ed (Alexandria, Va: American Diabetes Association, 1995).

Reprinted with permission from M Peyrot, Evaluation of patient education programs: how to do it and how to use it, *Diabetes Spectrum*, 1996;9(2):86–93.

Evaluation Summary

Evaluation in diabetes medical nutrition therapy is a continuous and cyclical process. It is not just a one-time step conducted after the assessment, goal setting, and intervention steps. For clients to learn and maintain new behaviors, the entire four-step model of diabetes medical nutrition therapy must be reinforced. Over time, clients need to be reassessed, new or revised goals need to be established, and new or revised interventions should be tried. Many diabetes educators call this cyclical process *follow-up*.

Follow-up refers to ongoing visits and should be both immediate and long-term. After the second or third visit, it should be possible to determine whether the client is making progress toward his or her goals. If no progress is evident, the client and the educator need to reassess and, perhaps, revise the plan for intervention. Evaluation is a component of all the steps involved in diabetes medical nutrition therapy and occurs continuously, rather than just at the time of follow-up. In the long term, clients need to understand that diabetes is a chronic disease and that they should return to their nutrition educator at least annually for follow-up.

Summary

The sequence for diabetes medical nutrition therapy includes assessment, goal setting, intervention, evaluation/follow-up. Each of the steps in diabetes medical nutrition therapy is necessary to promote success in facilitating lifestyle change. It is also important to recognize that each step in the process of nutrition therapy is cyclical, and that completing the process involves more than a short-term encounter with a client.

Implementing the process of diabetes medical nutrition therapy also requires documentation for communication to members of the diabetes care team. Documentation is essential for reimbursement and should include the identified nutrition problems, goals established and accomplished, the type of nutrition intervention, and an evaluation of the diabetes nutrition self-management plan. Documentation is needed to show that diabetes medical nutrition therapy and diabetes self-management training are part of quality treatment, are cost-effective, and are manageable. Data documenting effectiveness can be used to justify coverage and reimbursement for these services.

The recommended time frames for conducting the steps involved in the process of diabetes medical nutrition therapy are outlined in *Table 12.4*. These time frames represent the *minimum* time it would take to complete an initial assessment, the *minimum* number of visits and time it would take to provide basic nutrtion intervention, and the *minimum* number of visits recommended for follow-up. However, for clients with more extensive or complex lifestyle change/treatment plans, an increase in frequency and/or duration of visits is often necessary.

Table 12.4
Time Frames for Diabetes Medical Nutrition Therapy

Adapted with permission from MA Powers, Accessing nutrition care, in *Therapy for Diabetes Mellitus and Related Disorders*, 2nd ed (Alexandria, Va: American Diabetes Association; 1994), p 104.

Initial Workup Assessment
1–2 hours; 1–2 appointments
Nutrition Self-Management Training
Minimum of 2 visits consisting of 15–60 minutes Daily/weekly phone calls with self-monitoring records
Follow-up
As needed for lifestyle and life-cycle changes Minimum of every 3–6 months for children, every 6–12 months for adults

Case Study
(from *Facilitating Lifestyle Change: A Resource Manual*)

Summary of Client Data (See Lifestyle Questionnaire)

Delores is a 45-year-old woman with type II diabetes. She is referred to a diabetes outpatient clinic for diabetes medical nutrition therapy. The family practice physician states in his referring letter that Delores has a long history of "dietary noncompliance" and that if this course of nutrition intervention does not achieve the desired results, insulin therapy will be initiated.

Demographic Information

Height: 5 ft 5 in
Weight: 223 lb (currently at maximum adult weight)
Reasonable body weight: 180 lb

Nutrition Assessment
Physical Information

A review of her food record reveals that Delores is a frequent snacker, often including 4 or 5 snacks in her daily eating pattern. Upon questioning, Delores says she snacks when she is lonely, bored, or stressed. Although she is using some special products, such as diet carbonated beverages, sugar-free ice cream, low-fat dairy products, and low-calorie frozen entrees, Delores frequently makes high-fat, high-calorie snack choices (eg, cheese and peanut butter crackers, potato chips with dip, and cookies). Her high calorie and total fat intake, low fiber intake, and infrequent consumption of fruits and vegetables are problem areas. Estimated calorie intake = 3,170.

Nutrition History (usual food intake): See Food Record Form

Her current level of physical activity is low and consists primarily of housework once a week. She is interested in a walking program, but doesn't like to exercise alone.

Exercise Schedule

Delores also has hyperlipidemia. A lipid profile was recently completed with the following results: total cholesterol = 218 mg/dL; HDL cholesterol = 27 mg/dL; LDL cholesterol = 148 mg/dL; and triglycerides = 278 mg/dL.

Other Medical Problems

Delores was diagnosed with type II diabetes approximately 6 years ago. She is currently being managed on the maximum dose of a second-generation oral glucose-lowering medication. She monitors her fasting blood glucose level. A review of her glucose log book brought to the clinic visit reveals fasting glucose levels ranging from 100 mg/dL to 258 mg/dL. Recent laboratory values sent with the physician referral letter indicate a glycosolated hemoglobin level of 13.2%.

Diabetes Information

High school graduate.

Education/Knowledge

Delores lives alone and does her own food shopping and preparation. She eats away from home at lunch and eats out once or twice a week for dinner,

Psychosocial/ Economic

111

usually at a fast-food restaurant. Delores states she is interested in losing weight and doesn't care how long it takes "if I don't have to go on insulin!"

Rationale for Selecting *Facilitating Lifestyle Change: A Resource Manual*

A primary concern for Delores is having to start taking insulin. She has received nutrition intervention in the past and 2 years ago she lost 15 pounds by "avoiding sweets and sticking to a 1,200-Calorie exchange diet" and walking 5 days a week, but has gained it all back over the past year. She knows how important it is for her to lose weight, but doesn't know how to lose it and keep it off. She is interested in learning to manage her weight, increase her level of physical activity, and improve her glucose control. Using the resources contained in *Facilitating Lifestyle Change* will help the dietitian and Delores to become more aware of the specific problems associated with eating, to develop goals and a specific plan of action for accomplishing the individualized goals, and to track and evaluate the progress by using the monitoring forms.

Nutrition/Behavior Change Goals

During the goal-setting session and by completing the Action Plan portion of the Lifestyle Change Plan, Delores decided that she would address the problem of snacking, increase fruit and vegetable consumption, and begin comprehensive monitoring for diabetes self-management using the following tactics:

➤ Eat 5–7 servings of vegetables and fruits each day,
➤ Eat low-fat crackers, pretzels, popcorn, or cookies for snacks,
➤ Explore alternative evening activities to decrease time spent alone,
➤ Use monitoring forms to record glucose levels, food intake, and nutrient information,
➤ Test blood glucose results daily, but at random times during the day.

Education Plan

First Visit

Delores was asked to complete the Lifestyle Questionnaire in the waiting room before her appointment (see the end of this case study). The dietitian reviewed the questionnaire with Delores during the appointment and asked her to monitor her eating behavior by using the Eating Behavior Diary form. She was asked to bring 3–5 days of records at her return clinic visit in 1 week to establish goals and determine initial nutrition intervention.

Second Visit

The Eating Behavior Diary forms were reviewed with Delores. Delores said that major issues for her are snacking too much and eating in response to being alone. The Lifestyle Change Plan was used with Delores to identify eating behaviors to change, establish goals, and develop an action plan for accomplishing her goals. Delores decided that her priorities for behavior change are to address the problem of snacking and limited intake of fruits and vegetables. Delores's specific goals and action plans are described in the completed and attached Lifestyle Change Plan. Delores was asked to sign the Lifestyle Change Plan as a form of written agreement to work on these goals until her follow-up visit in 1 month.

Delores was provided with information on increasing intake of fruits and vegetables and with a handout from the National Cancer Institute on the Five-A-Day Program. Ideas for healthy snacks were also discussed.

She was given several copies of the Lifestyle Change: Food and Physical Activity Record and a copy of the Lifestyle Change: Summary Record to use in recording information about blood glucose monitoring results, nutrient information (ie, total servings of fruit and vegetables), and physical activity, as well as instructions on how to complete the form.

An appointment was made for Delores to return for a clinic visit with the dietitian in 1 month. Delores agreed to bring in 3-4 complete Lifestyle Change: Food and Physical Activity Records.

Third Visit

A review of Delores's Lifestyle Change: Food and Physical Activity Record attached to this case study shows a big improvement with fat intake and consumption of fruits and vegetables. She introduced new products into her daily eating pattern (eg, low-fat crackers and frozen yogurt), primarily at snack time. Delores was able to increase her fruit and vegetable intake to 5-7 servings/day. Her weight decreased by 2 pounds. Delores discussed her snacking problems with her cousin. They decided to join a volleyball team together at the local City Park and Recreation Intramural Program to increase their physical activity and social support levels. A return clinic appointment was made for Delores in 1 month.

Further Follow-up

Continued to see Delores on a monthly basis until she met initial goals. Reviewed monitoring forms at each visit and continued to revise goals and action plans as necessary.

Diabetes Medical Nutrition Therapy

Lifestyle Questionnaire

Name: *Delores*   Date: *April, 1995*

Do You Want to Change Your Lifestyle?

The time you take to provide this information will help your health care team work better for you. Thank you for taking an important step to manage your health.

- Have you made any changes in your lifestyle that you feel good about?   (X) Yes ( ) No
  If yes, what changes have you made? ....
  ....

- If you and your nutritionist discover changes you could make in your lifestyle to improve your health (e.g., eating, exercise, or self-monitoring plan), would you be open to the changes?
  (X) Yes ( ) No

    If yes, who will support and encourage you as you make these changes? *Friends at work*
    ....

    If no, what would keep you from making these changes? ....
    ....

- What information would you like from the nutritionist?

  ( ) Meal planning   (X) Weight management
  ( ) Eating out   (X) Exercise
  ( ) Food label reading/supermarket shopping   ( ) Record keeping
  ( ) Eating less fat   ( ) Other ( )

- What changes would you like to make?

  ( ) Improve my eating habits   ( ) Get more information
  ( ) Improve my activity level   (X) Feel better about my health
  (X) Improve my blood glucose control   (X) Learn how to manage my weight
  (X) Lower my blood pressure   (X) Improve my energy level
  ( ) Improve my cholesterol, triglyceride levels   ( ) Control food cravings
  ( ) Learn how to prevent high or low blood
      glucose levels
  ( ) Other ( )

114

Process of Diabetes Medical Nutrition Therapy

Lifestyle Questionnaire

Name *Delores* **Date** *April, 1995*

Nutrition History

- Have you ever wanted to make changes in what you eat? (X) Yes ( ) No
  If yes, what advice have you been given? *Lose weight, avoid sweets, eat more fruits and vegetables*

- Are you following any type of meal plan, such as exchange lists, calorie counting, carbohydrate counting, low cholesterol, low fat, or low sodium? ( ) Yes (X) No
  If yes, please describe. *Not currently; have followed 1200-calorie exchange list diet.*

  If yes, how much of the time are you able to follow your meal plan?
  ( ) Rarely ( ) Sometimes ( ) Often ( ) Usually

- How many people live in your household? *just myself* Ages _____

- Who usually does the cooking? *me* The shopping? *me*

- How many times each week do you eat away from home? *6-7*
  a. Which meals are usually eaten away from home? *lunch*
  b. In which type of restaurant do you usually eat or carry out? (mark **F** for Frequently, **O** for Occasionally, **N** for Never)
     - (F) Fast food (hamburger, chicken, seafood, pizza, subs, tacos)
     - (O) Buffets/All-you-can-eat
     - (O) Sit-down restaurant (Types: *steakhouse*)
     - (O) Sweets/Dessert Shops

- Do you drink alcohol? (*no*) Beer (*no*) Wine (*no*) Liquor
  How often? _____ How much? _____

- Do you take vitamins, minerals, herbs, or any other food or nutritional supplement? ( ) Yes (X) No
  If yes, please list. _____

- Do you regularly skip meals? ( ) Yes (X) No
  If yes, list which meals you skip most often and why. _____

- Do you have "trigger" foods that often cause you to overeat? (X) Yes ( ) No
  If yes, please list. *sweets, especially chocolate*

- Have you ever been on an extreme diet (such as fasting) or a fad diet? ( ) Yes (X) No
  If yes, please describe. _____

- Do you eat for other reasons than hunger? (X) Yes ( ) No
  If yes, please describe. *boredom, loneliness*

115

Lifestyle Questionnaire

Name: Delores **Date:** April, 1995

Food Record

- This food record can help you and your nutritionist better understand how food affects your health.

- Please write down everything you eat and drink from the time you wake up to the time you go to bed. Include meals, snacks, and drinks. If you eat or drink anything when you wake up, that should be added to the list.

Time	Type of Food / Beverage	Amount
7:30 a.m.	cornflakes	1 cup
	skim milk	1/2 cup
10:00 a.m.	peanut butter/cheese crackers	1 package
	diet cola	1 can
noon	tossed salad (lettuce, tomato, carrots, red cabbage, onions)	large
	salad dressing—ranch	2 Tbsp.
	cottage cheese—low-fat (2%)	1 cup
	diet cola	1 can
3:00 p.m.	Twinkies	3
	Slurpee	1 medium
5:30 p.m.	potato chips	4 oz
	onion dip	1/2 container
7:00 p.m.	Lean Cuisine—chicken entree	1
	diet cola	1 can
9:30 p.m.	oatmeal-raisin cookie	4
10:00 p.m.	sugar-free ice cream	4 scoops

Process of Diabetes Medical Nutrition Therapy

Lifestyle Questionnaire

Name: Delores   Date: April, 1995

Weight History

- Height (5'5")   Present weight (223 lbs)   Usual weight (over 200)

- Has your weight changed any over the past year?   (X) Yes ( ) No

    If yes, please describe how. *I gained back the 15 pounds I lost 2 years ago*

    How do you feel about your weight now? *I need to lose weight. I don't want to take insulin shots!*

- What has been your weight range as an adult? (180–223 lbs)

- What would you consider to be a healthy weight for you? (180 lbs)

    Would you feel comfortable at that weight?   (X) Yes ( ) No

- Have you ever tried to change your weight before?   (X) Yes ( ) No

    If yes, what have you tried? *- avoided sweets; "stuck to" 1200-calorie exchange diet.*
    - ate more fruits and vegetables; walked 5 days a week (with cousin—for 1 year)

    Have you been successful? *no*

- Are you interested in working to change your weight?

    (X) Yes, right now
    ( ) Yes, but I can't right now
    ( ) No, but I will think it over
    ( ) No, not now
    ( ) No, I'm not interested

117

Diabetes Medical Nutrition Therapy

Lifestyle Questionnaire

Name *Delores* **Date** *April, 1995*

Physical Activity History

- What type of activities do you do regularly and how much time each week do you spend doing them? Examples include walking, dancing, golf, tennis, biking, aerobics, and swimming.

Activity	Times per Week	Minutes per Activity
none	*none*	*none*

- Do you like to do these activities alone or with others? ....

- Do you perform other physical activities of daily living, such as housework, gardening, or climbing stairs? If yes, list type and amount. *housework, once a week for 2 hours*

- Are you interested in becoming more physically active?

  (X) Yes, right now
  ( ) Yes, but I can't right now
  ( ) No, but I will think it over
  ( ) No, not now
  ( ) No, I'm not interested

  If yes, what type of physical activity could you see yourself doing regularly?
  walking, played volleyball in high school

  If no, why? ....

Process of Diabetes Medical Nutrition Therapy

Lifestyle Questionnaire

Name (*Delores*)   **Date** (*April, 1995*)

Stress History

- Have you had a significant change in life events (such as marriage, divorce, death of a family member, new home, or change in employment) over the past year? ( ) Yes (X) No
   If yes, please describe. ....

- How does stress affect you physically or emotionally (e.g., headaches, neckaches, sleeping difficulties, eating too much or too little, fear, depression)? *overeat when stressed*

- How do you deal with stress (e.g., meditation, exercise, avoidance)? *avoidance*

Record Keeping

	Yes	No	How Often
Do you keep food records?	( )	(X)	
Do you keep blood glucose records?	(X)	( )	*daily*
Do you keep exercise records?	( )	(X)	
Do you keep any other kind of records? (for example, blood pressure)	( )	(X)	

Type ....

- Who benefits from your record keeping?

  (X) Self
  ( ) Family
  (X) Doctor
  ( ) Other (..................)

119

Diabetes Medical Nutrition Therapy

Eating Behavior Diary

Time	Location or Place	Food/Beverage Consumed Amount/Description	Degree of Hunger[1]	Social Situation[2]	Comments[3]
7:30 a.m.	home— kitchen	cornflakes with Equal—1 cup skim milk—1/2 cup	1	home— alone	
10:00 a.m.	work—desk	peanut butter/cheese crackers—1 package diet cola—1 can	2	work—break with friends	— busy at work trying to catch up.
noon	work—desk (brought lunch from home)	1 sandwich—ham & Swiss cheese, mustard, lettuce, whole-wheat bread nonfat fruited yogurt—1 cup diet cola—1 can	2	ate alone at desk	
3:00 p.m.	work—desk	M & M's—1 package diet cola	2	vending machine across hall	— feel stressed at work!
7:00 p.m.	home—in front of TV	cheeseburger—2 french fries—large chocolate milkshake—large	3	worked late, stopped for fast food	— very hungry and tired!
9:00 p.m.	home—in front of TV	low-fat devil's food cake cookie—1 box diet cola	3	home— watching TV	— bored, depressed

What did I learn about my eating habits?   — I snack too much!
                                            — I eat in response to my emotions.

1 Use rating scale of: 1 = not hungry, 2 = moderately hungry, 3 = very hungry
2 Who were you with? What were you doing?
3 Include feelings (e.g., sad, bored, angry), thoughts (e.g., eating out with friends), concerns (e.g., stressed out at work)

Name: Delores
Day/Date: Monday, 04/95

Process of Diabetes Medical Nutrition Therapy

Lifestyle Change Plan

Behavior	Goal(s) (what to do)	Action Plan (how to do it)	
Eating	– eat healthier snacks	– eat 5-7 servings of vegetables & fruits/day – eat low-fat crackers, pretzels, popcorn, cookies for snacks – increase social support by exploring alternative evening activities	– feel better about myself – lower triglyceride levels – lose weight
Physical Activity			
Record Keeping	– keep records of glucose, food intake, and fruits and vegetables eaten	– keep food and physical activity records 3 times/week for 1 month – continue blood glucose testing but at random times throughout the day	– improve my blood glucose levels
Other			
My reward for making a lifestyle change		buy a pair of walking shoes to begin walking program.	

For the period from 5/95 to 6/95 , I Delores agree to the above goals and plan to change my behavior(s).

Day/Date Monday, 04/95

Name Delores

Lifestyle Change
Food and Physical Activity Record

Time	Food Eaten — Day: Monday	Nutr. Info. F	Nutr. Info. V
7:30	1 cup cornflakes 1 cup skim milk 1 banana	1	
10:00	15 LF cheese crackers diet cola		
12:00	1 cup LF cottage cheese 1 tomato carrots and celery 1 onion bagel orange	1	1 1
3:00	16 oz tomato juice 15 pretzel sticks		1
6:00	Lean Cuisine chicken entree tossed salad w/ 1 T LF dressing 2 slices French bread 1 T diet margarine		1
9:00	1 cup LF vanilla yogurt 1/2 cup fresh strawberries 2 T chocolate syrup	1	
Nutrient Totals		**3**	**4**

Time	Food Eaten — Day: Wednesday	Nutr. Info. F	Nutr. Info. V
7:40	1 cup cornflakes 1 cup skim milk 1 banana	1	
10:00	15 LF cheese crackers diet cola		
12:15	1 cup LF yogurt turkey sandwich w/ 2 slices rye bread, mustard, lettuce, tomato grapes	1	1
3:30	6 oz orange juice 3 LF devil's food cookies	1	
6:30	1 piece lasagna 2 slices French bread 1 T diet margarine fresh pineapple	1	1
9:30	1 cup LF chocolate yogurt		
Nutrient Totals		**4**	**2**

Time	Food Eaten — Day: Friday	Nutr. Info. F	Nutr. Info. V
7:15	1 cup cornflakes 1 cup skim milk 1 banana	1	
9:45	1/2 bagel diet cola		
12:00	chef salad w/ 1/2 cup tuna, lettuce, tomato, cucumber, pepper 10 crackers 1 apple	1	2
3:15	5 jelly beans 16 oz tomato juice 15 pretzels		1
6:30	1 grilled chicken breast sandwich w/ lettuce, tomato corn on the cob watermelon	1	1 1
10:00	1 cup LF vanilla yogurt 2 T chocolate syrup		
Nutrient Totals		**3**	**5**

Physical Activity — Type / Amt.

Other Information — glucose: 179 mg/dl (7:20 am)   215 mg/dl (2:15 pm)   182 mg/dl (9:00 pm)

Comments: I liked the low-fat crackers & pretzels—even the low-fat yogurt!

Instructions: F = fruit servings, V = veg. servings, LF = low-fat

Name: Delores
Start Date: 04/1/95

122

References

1. Fels Tinker L, Heins JM, Holler HJ. Commentary and translation: 1994 nutrition recommendations for diabetes. *J Am Diet Assoc.* 1994;94:838–839.
2. Arnold MS, Stepien CJ, Hess GE, Hiss RG. Guidelines vs practice in the delivery of diabetes nutrition care. *J Am Diet Assoc.* 1993;93:34–39.
3. American Diabetes Association. Nutrition recommendations and principles for people with diabetes mellitus. *Diabetes Care.* 1994;17:519–522.
4. Brink S, Siminerio L, eds. *Diabetes Education Goals.* Alexandria, Va: American Diabetes Association; 1995.
5. Prochaska JO, DiClemente CC, Norcross JC. In search of how people change: applications to addictive behaviors. *Am Psychol.* 1992;47:1102–1114.
6. Prochaska JO, Ruggiero L, eds. Readiness for change. *Diabetes Spectrum.* 1993;6:22–60.
7. Leontos C, Splett PL. Nutrition practice guidelines for type I diabetes mellitus: development and field testing. *Diabetes Spectrum.* 1996;9(2):128–130.
8. Peyrot M. Evaluation of patient education programs: how to do it and how to use it. *Diabetes Spectrum.* 1996;9(2):86–93.
9. Ellwood PM. Outcomes management: a technology for patient experience. *N Engl J Med.* 1988;318:1549–1556.
10. Monk A. Linking practice guidelines to outcomes. *On the Cutting Edge.* 1995;16:10–12.
11. Monk A, Barry B, McClain K, Weaver T, Cooper N, Franz MJ. Practice guidelines for medical nutrition therapy provided by dietitians for people with non-insulin-dependent diabetes mellitus. *J Am Diet Assoc.* 1995;95:999–1006.

Resource

Facilitating Lifestyle Change: A Resource Manual can be purchased through The American Dietetic Association at 1-800-877-1600, ext 5000, and the American Diabetes Association at 1-800-ADA-ORDER. The cost of the publication is $23.50 for nonmembers and $19.95 for members.

For Further Reading

American Association for Diabetes Educators. Psychosocial issues. In: *A Core Curriculum for Diabetes Educators.* 2nd ed. Chicago, Ill: American Association of Diabetes Educators; 1993:27–108.

Franz M, Monk A, Barry B, McClain K, Weaver T, Cooper N, Upham P, Bergenstal R, Mazze R. Effectiveness of medical nutrition therapy provided by dietitians in the management of non-insulin-dependent diabetes mellitus: a randomized, controlled clinical trial. *J Am Diet Assoc.* 1995;95:1009–1017.

Halford BH. Nutrition assessment. In: Powers MA, ed. *Handbook of Diabetes Medical Nutrition Therapy.* 2nd ed. Gaithersburg, Md: Aspen Publications, Inc; 1996:61–76.

Prochaska JO, DiClemente CC, Norcross JC. In search of how people change: applications to addictive behaviors. *Am Psychol.* 1992;47:1102–1114.

Wheeler ML, Kulkarni K, eds. The art of nutrition: multiple aspects of medical nutrition therapy. *Diabetes Spectrum.* 1996;9(2):97–98.

Part 3
Basic Nutrition Intervention

Introduction to Basic Nutrition Intervention 13

As the name implies, *basic nutrition education* should focus primarily on providing information about basic nutrition and diabetes nutrition guidelines. The approaches discussed in Chapters 14, 15, and 16 are limited to resources that can be used to teach basic nutrition and diabetes nutrition guidelines and, as such, can be referred to as *guideline approaches.*

Basic nutrition education involves the following three areas:

1. *Basic nutrition guidelines* provide the client with an understanding of the basic principles of nutrition and guidance in selecting an adequately balanced eating plan for optimal health.
2. *Diabetes nutrition guidelines* provide the client with an understanding of the connection between nutrition and diabetes. They give the client direction in making appropriate food choices for managing diabetes.
3. *"Beginning" changes in eating habits* identify changes in food consumption, purchase, and preparation, and establish nutrition goals (eg, use of low-fat milk in place of whole milk).

Basic nutrition education includes providing information and goal setting. The goal of nutrition education is to promote long-term behavior change. This can best be accomplished by working with the client to change a few eating behaviors at a time. It is imperative to be realistic and to listen to the concerns of the client when negotiating changes in eating behavior.

However, basic diabetes nutrition guidelines do not include the commonly used nutrition prescription or simplified educational approach referred to as *no concentrated sweets.* This term misinforms both clients and health care professionals, leading them to believe that the primary nutrition goal should be avoidance of simple sugars. This belief contradicts the current diabetes nutrition recommendations.[1] In addition, most clients' primary problem is an eating pattern too high in total calories and fat. The use of a "no concentrated sweets" diet is often an attempt to provide a simplified form of education to clients. A more acceptable strategy would be to use and teach the diabetes nutrition guidelines that are much broader in focus. The dietitian may want to consider using a "regular" or "low-fat" diet as a more appropriate nutrition prescription in the inpatient setting.[2] Although a "regular" diet may not be "heart healthy," it can be used as a teaching tool for the dietitian and client in an inpatient setting. The self-selection by the client using a "regular" menu can assist the dietitian in determining the "starting place" of the client and can help in establishing individualized goals.

Time Frame

It is difficult to identify a time frame for providing basic nutrition education. The educator's time in providing the information depends on the amount of education needed and the client's readiness to learn. The time frame also is determined by the client's willingness and readiness to change his or her eating habits. The diabetes educator may be able to provide basic nutrition education in one or two sessions, but for some clients an unlimited number of sessions may be necessary.

Other Issues That Should Be Addressed

Clients with diabetes who are treated with insulin should receive other information in addition to basic nutrition education during the initial contact with the diabetes educator. Important points that should be discussed include the following:

➤ Eating meals and snacks in consistent amounts and at appropriate times to coincide with exogenous insulin patterns,
➤ Sick-day management guidelines,
➤ Treatment guidelines for hypoglycemia.

The recommendation concerning amounts of food and times of meals should be individualized to the client's current lifestyle, eating pattern, and insulin schedule. This recommendation should not be taken to mean that all clients using insulin need to follow a structured meal plan. Implementing this recommendation can be accomplished successfully for some clients by teaching the diabetes nutrition guidelines and making simple adjustments to current eating patterns.

Obese clients with type II diabetes should also receive information in addition to basic nutrition education during the initial visit with the diabetes educator. Because weight loss may be a goal for overweight clients with type II diabetes, attention should be focused on eating awareness rather than simply suggesting a low-calorie meal plan. This can be achieved in some of the following ways:

➤ Promote self-monitoring through use of food behavior records, which are designed to increase awareness of total food consumption and stimuli that promote overeating (see Chapter 12 about the various types of record-keeping forms).
➤ Discuss the connection between portion size and calories.
➤ Review the calorie and fat content of foods.
➤ Discuss exercise recommendations for weight management and glucose control.

Food behavior records should be used initially to identify problem areas and to develop tactics for changing eating behaviors. For many overweight clients, using a behavioral approach may be more effective in promoting long-term weight loss than the more traditional approach of prescribing a low-calorie meal plan and teaching a structured system of meal planning.

There are many creative ways to teach portion control and calorie and fat content of foods, including food labels, restaurant menus, cooking demonstrations, and grocery store tours. The development of a support group for overweight clients with type II diabetes can also be effective in many ambulatory care clinic settings. An important factor is keeping clients connected so they can receive continued support and reinforcement for a difficult and complex problem.

Educational Resources

To provide basic nutrition education for clients, the following resources can be used:

- ➤ Basic Nutrition—*Dietary Guidelines for Americans; Guide to Good Eating; Food Guide Pyramid* (see Chapter 14)
- ➤ Diabetes Nutrition—*First Step in Diabetes Meal Planning; Healthy Food Choices; Healthy Eating; Single-Topic Diabetes Resources* (see Chapters 15 and 16)

References

1. American Diabetes Association. Nutrition recommendations and principles for people with diabetes mellitus. *Diabetes Care.* 1994;17:519–522.
2. Schafer B, McLaughlin S. How to use the 1994 diabetes nutrition recommendations in health care institutions: a task force looks at translation. *Diabetes Spectrum.* 1996;9(2): 118–119.

Basic Nutrition Guidelines 14

Dietary Guidelines for Americans

Definition

Dietary Guidelines for Americans is a basic nutrition guide aimed at all Americans for the purpose of health promotion and the prevention of chronic diseases. The seven guidelines are:

1. Eat a variety of foods.
2. Balance the food you eat with physical activity—maintain or improve your weight.
3. Choose a diet with plenty of grain products, vegetables, and fruits.
4. Choose a diet low in fat, saturated fat, and cholesterol.
5. Choose a diet moderate in sugars.
6. Choose a diet moderate in salt and sodium.
7. If you drink alcoholic beverages, do so in moderation.

Dietary Guidelines for Americans is intended to give healthy people guidance in choosing a more nutritionally balanced eating plan. The emphasis is on an approach that is simple, easy to understand, and adaptable to individual needs.

Historical Background

The current, fourth edition was developed and distributed by the US Department of Agriculture and Department of Health and Human Services (USDA-HHS) in 1995. It was adapted from "Dietary Goals for the US," developed as a result of hearings of the US Senate Select Committee on Nutrition and Human Needs in 1977. The first, second, and third editions of the guidelines were released in 1980, 1985, and 1990, respectively.

Method of Use

There are many methods for using the *Dietary Guidelines for Americans*. Below is one for use with clients with diabetes:

1. Obtain nutrition history or have the client keep a food record for a minimum of 3 days.
2. Assess the nutritional adequacy of the history or food records (see Chapter 12 and Appendix 3).
3. Review the *Dietary Guidelines for Americans* brochure.
4. Using the history or food records, highlight recommended food choices from the *Dietary Guidelines for Americans.*
5. Using the history or food records, highlight food choices that need to be changed.

Table 14.1
Suggestion for Using Dietary Guidelines

Guideline 4: Choose a diet low in fat, saturated fat, and cholesterol	
High-Fat Food Choices from Sample Food Record	*Suggested Low-Fat Alternatives*
Bacon	Turkey or Canadian bacon
Butter	Margarine (with liquid oil as first ingredient)
Lunch meat	Turkey, deli roast beef
Fried meat	Broiled, baked, or grilled meat

6. Provide suggestions for only one area of the *Dietary Guidelines for Americans* to be changed during the visit. The other areas identified for change can be worked on during future visits. The client will work on this area until the next visit (see the example in *Table 14.1*).

Intended Population for Use

Dietary Guidelines for Americans provides general guidelines to help clients identify eating habits that should be changed. Emphasis is on helping clients understand the general principles of good nutrition. *Dietary Guidelines for Americans* can be used for clients with either type I or type II diabetes and is especially useful when there is a need to keep the message simple. This approach is appropriate for clients who are unable or choose not to employ complex concepts such as exchanges, grams, or calories.

Clinical Setting

Dietary Guidelines for Americans can be used for nutrition education in both inpatient and ambulatory care settings. The approach is appropriate for group and individual nutrition self-management training sessions.

Length of Time to Teach

The amount of time to teach this approach can vary, depending on the needs of the client. For a client who has limited knowledge of basic nutrition and has many food habits to change, the use of *Dietary Guidelines for Americans* may require two to four sessions consisting of 30 minutes each. If a client has some basic nutrition knowledge, fewer sessions may be needed.

Advantages/ Disadvantages

The major advantage of using the *Dietary Guidelines for Americans* is its simplicity, which is helpful for clients who have difficulty coping with complex issues. Another advantage to using this approach is the ability to individualize the education to specific areas of improvement without providing large amounts of information.

The major disadvantage may be the lack of a structured approach to meal planning for some clients. The *Dietary Guidelines for Americans* may be less effective than other nutrition resources in achieving the degree of glucose control desired.

Guide to Good Eating

Definition

The *Guide to Good Eating* categorizes foods according to their major nutrient composition. Each of the food groups (milk, meat, vegetable, fruit, and grain) is characterized by certain leader nutrients; for example, the leader nutrients for each of the five food groups are calcium, iron, vitamin A, vitamin C, and fiber, respectively. Foods of low nutrient density, those containing calories primarily from sugar or fat, are placed in the "others" category.

Serving sizes of various foods within a food group are approximately equivalent in leader nutrients but not necessarily equivalent in caloric value. A minimum number of daily servings from each group is recommended for each age group to achieve approximately 80% of the daily requirement of nine leader nutrients. It is assumed that if a variety of foods is chosen from each of the food groups, the daily requirement for all nutrients will be met.

The intent of the *Guide to Good Eating* is to give guidance in choosing nutritionally adequate daily food intakes. The emphasis is on providing an approach that is simple and easy to understand. The *Guide to Good Eating* emphasizes the minimum nutrients required for health.

Historical Background

The Basic Four Food Groups were developed in 1954 by the USDA, replacing the earlier Basic Seven, and were intended to translate the quantitative nutrient-based Recommended Dietary Allowance (RDA) information into practical terms for the average person. The Basic Four Food Groups guide has been the most widely used food grouping system in the United States by a number of organizations. The National Dairy Council (NDC) adapted the *Guide to Good Eating* several times to reflect the recommendations of the USDA and changes in the RDA and to incorporate newer knowledge about the nutrient content of foods. The NDC recently released its revised *Guide to Good Eating* as a tool to complement the *Food Guide Pyramid* (which was introduced in 1992 and is discussed later in this chapter) by emphasizing the nutrition concepts that are given less emphasis by the *Food Guide Pyramid*.

Method of Use

There are many methods for using the *Guide to Good Eating*. Below is one for use with clients with diabetes:

1. Obtain nutrition history or have the client keep a food record for a minimum of 3 days.
2. Assess the usual food intake by using the minimum number of servings from each of the basic food groups included in the *Guide to Good Eating*.
3. Review the *Guide to Good Eating*; identify adequate intake of food groups and inadequate intake of food groups.
4. Discuss strategies to improve the intake of a food group.
5. Discuss portion sizes of suggested foods.
6. Use the *Guide to Good Eating* as a tool to assess future food records.

Intended Population for Use

The *Guide to Good Eating* can be used as a follow-up tool after the introduction of *Dietary Guidelines for Americans*. It can also be used in place of exchange lists or counting approaches (calories, fat, carbohydrate), since it provides some general guidelines for recommended servings per day and suggested portions. For many clients this may provide the only structure necessary for making changes in their eating habits, while others may need to progress to other meal-planning approaches.

This approach may be used for clients with either type I or type II diabetes and is simple, yet practical. Again, this material may serve as the basis for diabetes nutrition education.

Clinical Setting

As with *Dietary Guidelines for Americans*, the *Guide to Good Eating* can be used in both inpatient and ambulatory care settings. The approach is appropriate for group or individual nutrition self-management training sessions.

Length of Time to Teach

Introduction of the concept of food grouping and portion sizes through use of the *Guide to Good Eating* may require 30 minutes to 1 hour. For clients already familiar with the concept, the session may be 15 to 30 minutes in duration. A follow-up visit to further expand the use of the *Guide to Good Eating* in menu planning would be encouraged, as well as plans for future nutrition self-management training.

Advantages/ Disadvantages

The major advantage of the *Guide to Good Eating* is the ability to provide some guidance regarding types and amounts of foods to use. The information is very simple and easy to utilize. Another advantage is the emphasis on normal nutrition versus the concept of a modified eating plan.

The major disadvantage of this approach is that it is less structured and may be less effective than other meal-planning approaches in obtaining the desired blood glucose control.

Food Guide Pyramid

Definition

The *Food Guide Pyramid* is an illustration of foods to eat according to the *Dietary Guidelines for Americans*. A general guide for choosing a well-balanced eating plan, the *Food Guide Pyramid* recommends eating a variety of foods to obtain the necessary nutrients. It also outlines how to obtain the needed calories to maintain a healthy weight.

The *Food Guide Pyramid* promotes the idea of using more starches (grains, fruits, vegetables), which form the base. Less emphasis is placed on foods that are high in fat and sugar (meats, dairy products), which is illustrated by the decreasing size of the pyramid. This educational piece represents visually the recommendations of the *Dietary Guidelines for Americans*. It also includes the concept of food grouping from the *Guide to Good Eating*.

Historical Background

The *Food Guide Pyramid* was developed by the US Department of Agriculture and the Food Marketing Institute in early 1990. It was reviewed by various nutrition-related organizations, modifications were made, and it was made available for distribution in 1992.

Method of Use

There are many ways to use the *Food Guide Pyramid*. Below is one for clients with diabetes:

1. Obtain nutrition history or have the client keep a food record for a minimum of 3 days.
2. Assess the usual food intake by using the number of servings from each food category of the *Food Guide Pyramid* (Figure 14.1).
3. Review the *Food Guide Pyramid* and discuss how the client's usual food intake compares with the recommendations (nutrient content and number of servings).

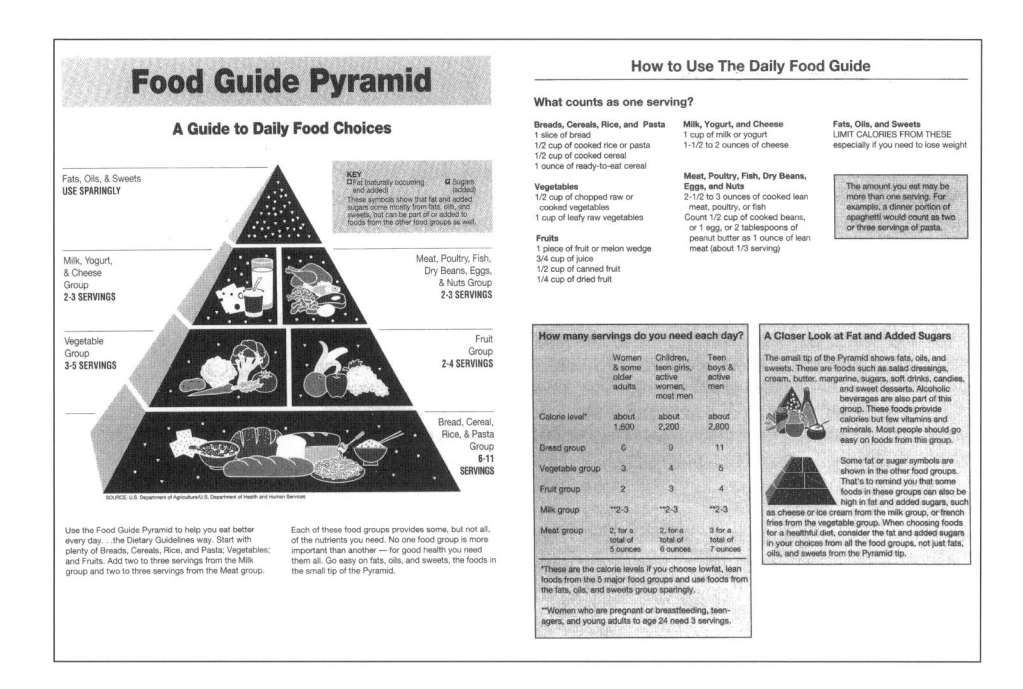

Figure 14.1
Food Guide Pyramid

Source: *The Food Guide Pyramid*, Home and Garden Bulletin Number 252, Human Nutrition Information Service, US Department of Agriculture, August 1992.

4. Identify ways to improve the nutrient composition of current eating habits and establish goals for eating behavior changes.
5. Review the sections of the *Food Guide Pyramid* entitled "How many servings do you need each day?" and "What counts as one serving?"
6. Have client continue to keep food records and assess future food intake.

The *Food Guide Pyramid* can be used as an introduction to basic nutrition or can be used for follow-up education after the introduction of *Dietary Guidelines for Americans*. As with the *Guide to Good Eating*, it can be used in place of exchange lists or counting approaches. It is appropriate for clients with either type I or type II diabetes. For some clients, this may be the only tool needed to change eating behaviors; however, others may need more structured approaches to meal planning.

Intended Population for Use

Dietary Guidelines for Americans, 1995 edition. For ordering information, contact the Superintendent of Documents, US Government Printing Office, Washington, DC 20401, 202/783-3238. Single copies: $ .50; 25% discount for bulk orders.

Food Guide Pyramid. To order a copy of the 30-page booklet about the *Food Guide Pyramid*, send a $1.00 check or money order made out to the Superintendent of Documents to: Consumer Information Center, Department 159-Y, Pueblo, CO 81009. To obtain a copy of the *Food Guide Pyramid* educational resource, contact the Superintendent of Documents, US Government Printing Office, Washington, DC 20401, 202/783-3238. Single copies: $1.00; 25% discount for bulk orders.

Guide to Good Eating. For information about the *Guide to Good Eating*, 1992 edition, contact your local Dairy Council office or National Dairy Council, 6300 N River Road, Rosemont, IL 60018-4233.

Ordering Information for Resources Described

Diabetes Nutrition Guidelines 15

For many years diabetes educators have needed a basic, simple, self-contained nutrition education resource that could be distributed to clients with diabetes. This need, combined with the development of the USDA/USDHHS *Food Guide Pyramid*, has resulted in this new diabetes nutrition resource.

The First Step in Diabetes Meal Planning

Definition

The First Step in Diabetes Meal Planning was jointly published by The American Dietetic Association and the American Diabetes Association in 1995. It is a trifold brochure opening to an 11 × 18–inch poster of the diabetes food guide pyramid. The first foldout *(Figure 15.1)* provides basic diabetes meal planning guidelines, including a "Here's How You Do It" section and "Changes You Can Make" section. The second foldout shows the diabetes food guide pyramid, which uses the exchange lists food groupings. The base (Grains/Beans/Starchy Vegetables) has the largest number of servings daily. Moving toward the top of the pyramid, Vegetables and Fruits categories are next, followed by the Milk category and the Meat & Others category. The tip represents Fats, Sweets, & Alcohol. The pyramid page also includes behavior change tips for each group, as well as general food examples and serving sizes.

Historical Background

The 1994 American Diabetes Association nutrition recommendations for diabetes (endorsed by The American Dietetic Association) emphasized the need to individualize nutrition management.[1,2] These recommendations made it clear that a number of resources needed to be updated or developed. After reviewing existing resources and surveying dietitians and other diabetes educators, the Diabetes Nutrition Education Resources Steering Committee, representing both The American Dietetic Association and the American Diabetes Association, identified as one priority the development of a basic diabetes nutrition education resource adapting the *Food Guide Pyramid*.

A volunteer dietitian writing group developed the initial draft of *The First Step in Diabetes Meal Planning* with the aid of professional editors. Next, the product was technically reviewed by dietitians and other health care professionals. Finally, the product was field-tested by dietitians throughout the United States with clients representing a variety of cultural and ethnic groups and educational levels.

The diabetes pyramid is based upon the *Food Guide Pyramid*, first used as the official food guide for the United States in 1992[3] (see Chapter 14 for more details). Conceptually, it is a graphic representation of the *Dietary Guidelines for Americans*[4] illustrating the concepts of variety, moderation, and balance.

Figure 15.1

The First Step in Diabetes Meal Planning

Healthy Eating Is the First Step in Taking Care of Your Diabetes

You can make a difference in your blood glucose control through your food choices.

You do not need special or diet foods.

The food that is good for you is good for your whole family.

Here's How You Do It

Eat a wide variety of foods every day.

Eat high-fiber foods, such as fruits, vegetables, grains, and beans, to fill you up.

Use less added fat, sugar, and salt.

Changes You Can Make

Eat meals and snacks at regular times every day.

Eat about the same amount of food each day.

Try new foods.

Try not to skip meals.

If you want to lose weight, cut down on your portion size. If you skip a meal, you may eat too much at your next meal.

Developed by:
Brenda A. Broussard, RD, MPH, MBA
Eva Brzezinski, MS, RD
Nancy Cooper, RD, CDE
Carolyn Leontos, MS, RD, CDE
Madelyn Wheeler, MS, RD, CDE

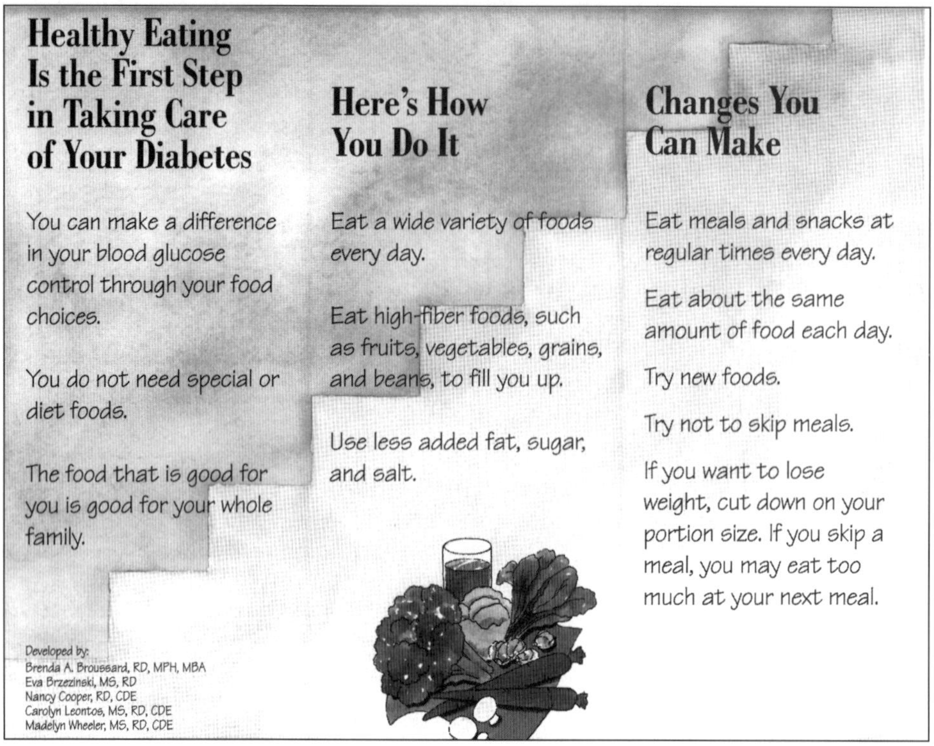

Source: *The First Step in Diabetes Meal Planning* (Alexandria, Va: American Diabetes Association, Inc, and The American Dietetic Association; 1995).

In contrast to previous food guides, it represents the total diet, addressing overnutrition as well as undernutrition.[5] The diabetes food pyramid, the first to focus specifically on a chronic illness, is similar to the *Food Guide Pyramid* but incorporates concepts from the 1994 American Diabetes Association nutrition recommendations, as well as grouping basic foods in a way similar to the *Exchange Lists for Meal Planning* (for example, cheese is placed in the Meat & Others category; nuts are in the Fats, Sweets & Alcohol category).

Method of Use

The First Step in Diabetes Meal Planning may be provided (mailed or handed) to clients with newly diagnosed diabetes with little or no explanation. It serves as a starting education resource in meal planning until the client can see a dietitian. Field-testing indicated that users can select a food-related behavior change after reading the pamphlet on their own without any additional discussion.

This resource may be the only meal-planning tool that diabetes educators use for some clients with diabetes. After reviewing the first foldout section, a client should be able to set a behavioral goal (eg, eat less fat). The pyramid itself could be used to support the client's efforts to achieve the behavioral goal. Or, after reviewing the pyramid, the client could use it as a daily check-off sheet to evaluate the nutritional quality of his or her daily food intake. The food pyramid could also be used to help the client develop simple menus.

Intended Population for Use

The intended audience is clients with newly diagnosed diabetes who may not have immediate access to diabetes medical nutrition therapy from a dietitian. It can also be used for education of clients with long-standing diabetes (type I or II) who need some simple guidelines or tips for planning meals.

Clinical Setting

The resource can be used in a physician's office, clinics, hospitals, home care agencies, or long-term care facilities. It can be used for self-education, individual nutrition self-management training sessions, or in a group class.

Length of Time to Teach

The resource is essentially a self-teaching education tool. If used by diabetes educators, the teaching time may be 10 to 30 minutes, depending on the assessed needs and goals of the client.

Advantages/Disadvantages

A major advantage of *The First Step in Diabetes Meal Planning* is that it is self-explanatory, so clients can start making changes in food habits before seeing a dietitian. It is simple to understand and is written at about a sixth-grade reading level. Because the concept of the *Food Guide Pyramid* can be understood visually, it has wide appeal for clients who need or desire a basic and simplified form of nutritional guidance. The concept of this piece is based on a nationally known resource that has been widely publicized. The resource has generic serving sizes for each of the six components of the pyramid. Also, it is useful in planning a generally more healthful way of eating.

A disadvantage of the resource is that it does not provide specific serving sizes for a wider range of foods. The resource does not control a specific nutrient, such as carbohydrate, calories, or fat. Also, the print size may be difficult for some for clients with visual impairments to read.

Healthy Food Choices (Guideline Section)

Definition

Healthy Food Choices is a pamphlet that promotes healthful eating practices. It is divided into two sections:

► Guidelines for making healthy food choices, discussed in this chapter *(Figure 15.2)*,
► Simplified exchange lists to be used as an introduction to the full exchange system (discussed in more detail in Chapter 18).

The guidelines help clients make healthy food selections without weighing and measuring foods; using exchanges; or counting calories and grams of fat or carbohydrate. Specific guidelines are included for those who want to decrease fat, salt, and sugar intake and increase fiber intake.

Historical Background

Healthy Food Choices, a joint publication of The American Dietetic Association and the American Diabetes Association, was designed and published concurrently with the 1986 revised exchange lists to enhance the concept that not all clients need to use the *Exchange Lists for Meal Planning*. *Healthy Food Choices* was intended to provide an introduction to diabetes meal planning with an emphasis on healthful eating practices. The client who desired to advance to the exchange system could use the simplified lists as the initial step.

Method of Use

Healthy Food Choices is useful during the initial level of education in diabetes meal planning. Many clients may remain at the initial level of education for quite some time or may never advance to the in-depth/continuing education

Figure 15.2

Healthy Food Choices (Guidelines)

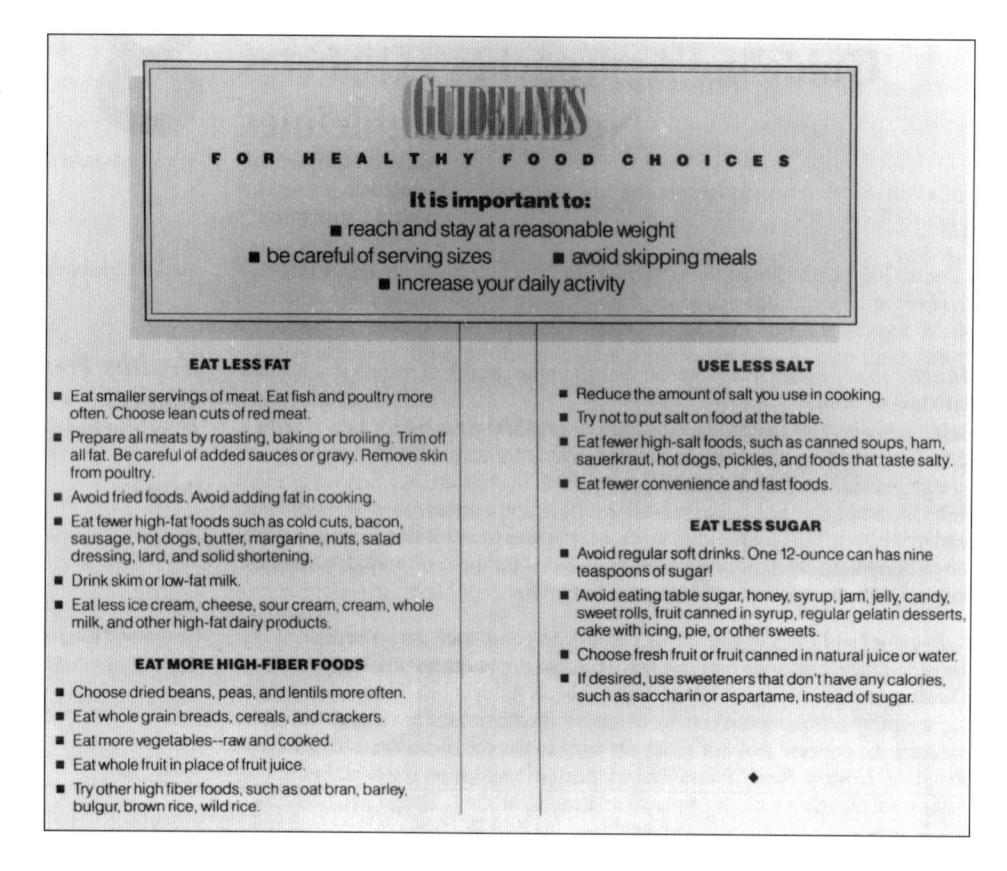

GUIDELINES FOR HEALTHY FOOD CHOICES

It is important to:
- reach and stay at a reasonable weight
- be careful of serving sizes
- avoid skipping meals
- increase your daily activity

EAT LESS FAT
- Eat smaller servings of meat. Eat fish and poultry more often. Choose lean cuts of red meat.
- Prepare all meats by roasting, baking or broiling. Trim off all fat. Be careful of added sauces or gravy. Remove skin from poultry.
- Avoid fried foods. Avoid adding fat in cooking.
- Eat fewer high-fat foods such as cold cuts, bacon, sausage, hot dogs, butter, margarine, nuts, salad dressing, lard, and solid shortening.
- Drink skim or low-fat milk.
- Eat less ice cream, cheese, sour cream, cream, whole milk, and other high-fat dairy products.

EAT MORE HIGH-FIBER FOODS
- Choose dried beans, peas, and lentils more often.
- Eat whole grain breads, cereals, and crackers.
- Eat more vegetables--raw and cooked.
- Eat whole fruit in place of fruit juice.
- Try other high fiber foods, such as oat bran, barley, bulgur, brown rice, wild rice.

USE LESS SALT
- Reduce the amount of salt you use in cooking.
- Try not to put salt on food at the table.
- Eat fewer high-salt foods, such as canned soups, ham, sauerkraut, hot dogs, pickles, and foods that taste salty.
- Eat fewer convenience and fast foods.

EAT LESS SUGAR
- Avoid regular soft drinks. One 12-ounce can has nine teaspoons of sugar!
- Avoid eating table sugar, honey, syrup, jam, jelly, candy, sweet rolls, fruit canned in syrup, regular gelatin desserts, cake with icing, pie, or other sweets.
- Choose fresh fruit or fruit canned in natural juice or water.
- If desired, use sweeteners that don't have any calories, such as saccharin or aspartame, instead of sugar.

Source: *Healthy Food Choices* (Alexandria, Va: American Diabetes Association, Inc, and The American Dietetic Association; 1986).

---

level. The diabetes educator should not try to cover all the information too quickly; instead, he or she should provide encouragement and guidance while relying on the client's questions and progress as indicators of readiness for advancement.

Both sections (the guidelines page and the simplified exchange list page, which folds out into a poster) can be used in a variety of ways. The diabetes educator should involve the client in making the initial decision about eating change(s) on which to focus. This teaching strategy emphasizes that the client can and should contribute to decision making about his or her health care and demonstrates that the educator respects his or her opinions.

The following five teaching situations show how the guidelines page can be used.

Example 1: You have inadequate time for a comprehensive nutrition assessment and a client with type II diabetes says he or she will not return for a nutrition appointment. Review the guidelines in the top box and explain that you could help him or her identify a reasonable weight and the best times to eat. State that a reasonable body weight often involves a weight loss of only 10–20 lb. Circle the four other specific eating points (relating to fat, fiber, salt, and sugar), adding that you are sure the client is already making healthy food choices, but you would not know which ones unless you had time for a nutrition therapy appointment. Then ask if he or she would like to reconsider an appointment. If not, tell the client to feel free to call if questions arise or if he or she decides to return for an appointment. Document the session and notify the primary care provider of the intervention.

Example 2: You have inadequate time for a comprehensive nutrition assessment, but the client agrees to return next week for further instruction. Review the four guidelines at the top of the page. Ask the client to review all of the specific points before the next appointment and to put a check by all that he or she currently follows. Also, ask the client to select the one or two points that he or she is not currently doing and would like help in achieving.

Example 3: After a nutrition assessment, review the first four guidelines and have the client write in his or her reasonable weight next to them. Next, ask the client to review the four specific eating points and to put a check by all those the client currently observes. This step is critical to remind the client that positive eating behaviors already exist. You may assist in this step by adding information gained in the nutrition history. Then ask the client to select one or two eating behaviors he or she feels can be worked on until the next nutrition therapy appointment. You may wish to add, in the space at the bottom of the page, specific changes that relate to information obtained in the nutrition history, eg, eat fruit for breakfast, eat five crackers before exercise class, eat meals and snacks at specific times as listed.

Example 4: After a nutrition assessment, you determine that the client's first short-term goal is to modify his or her fat intake. You discuss this and agree that modifying fat intake is the priority. Then review the six points under "eat less fat." Again, identify what the client is already doing and agree on one or two additional steps he or she should take toward eating less fat. Consider utilizing the *Single-Topic Diabetes Resources* to supplement the session.

Example 5: After a nutrition assessment, you realize the client's primary goal should be to refrain from skipping meals and to eat at regular times. You discuss this and the client agrees. Highlight the guideline "avoid skipping meals" and write in the meal and snack times the client agrees to follow. Mention that the client should review the other points on the page, but they are not as critical at this time as eating at regular times.

When the pamphlet is used for basic guidelines, as in these five examples, the diabetes educator should refer to the poster of the food choices so the client is not confused as to what to do with the second section. The diabetes educator may want to review it in detail with some clients, even if it will not be used. Other clients will need only a brief mention that it is a more structured meal plan and that it is not necessary for them at this time.

Intended Population for Use

Healthy Food Choices is appropriate for most clients because it offers an overview of diabetes medical nutrition therapy within the framework of basic eating guidelines and the simplified exchange system. The intended population is broad based; all age groups, with the exception of infants, can use the material. Because diabetes is not mentioned in the pamphlet, it is appropriate for use by any client who desires to improve his or her eating habits; it also emphasizes that the eating habits of clients with diabetes are similar to those of individuals without diabetes. It can be used by clients with either type I or type II diabetes. The amount of structure and the rate of progression depends on the needs of each client and his or her desire and ability to make changes in eating habits.

Clinical Setting This nutrition education resource can be used in a variety of clinical settings. The guidelines section (Section 1) is appropriate in the inpatient setting to teach diabetes nutrition guidelines and beginning ideas about meal planning. It is also appropriate in the outpatient and community setting to teach guidelines and to use as a simplified educational tool for teaching meal planning (Section 2).

Length of Time to Teach This nutrition education resource is very straightforward. The guidelines can be reviewed in one session (15 to 60 minutes). The time will depend on whether a nutrition assessment is completed, whether the basics of diabetes need to be presented, and on other self-management training needs the client may have. As with any nutrition self-management training, the client and the diabetes educator should discuss individualized goals pertinent to changes in meal planning. In that regard, this resource can be used for numerous teaching sessions.

Advantages/ Disadvantages The pamphlet is easy to use, concise, and is at a moderate reading level (sixth grade on SMOG readability test). It introduces two approaches to nutrition education—diabetes nutrition guidelines and a simplified exchange list, which uses the term *choices* instead of *exchanges* and simplifies portion sizes within exchange groups (eg, ½ cup of any fruit juice and 1 fresh medium fruit).

The primary disadvantage is that the two nutrition education approaches are included in the same pamphlet. This could lead to potential misuse in that both approaches might be introduced at the same time when it is appropriate to teach a single approach. The diabetes educator needs to conduct a comprehensive nutrition assessment to make the best decision about how to introduce nutrition and meal planning. Gradual change is often the key to incorporating changes into lifelong eating habits.

Healthy Eating

Definition *Healthy Eating* is a low-literacy booklet with illustrated food lists divided in two categories, "Good for You" and "Not as Good for You" *(Figure 15.3)*. General information on the role of meal planning in diabetes management is also covered.

This booklet is considered appropriate for adults with low reading skills. It is organized in a logical sequence and uses short sentences, short paragraphs, and as few scientific words and concepts as possible. *Healthy Eating* is written in a conversational tone, and the content of the material is emphasized by boldface type, subheadings, enumeration, or illustrations. The readability of *Healthy Eating* has been assessed using the Spache readability formula as between the second- and third-grade levels.

Historical Background *Healthy Eating*, developed to teach clients with low-literacy levels, was published in 1988 by the International Diabetes Center. The booklet was designed and field-tested for its intended populations. *Healthy Eating* is also a chapter in *Diabetes Care Made Easy: A Simple Step-by-Step Guide for Controlling Your Diabetes*. It includes a meal plan in which a sample menu can be written.

Diabetes Nutrition Guidelines

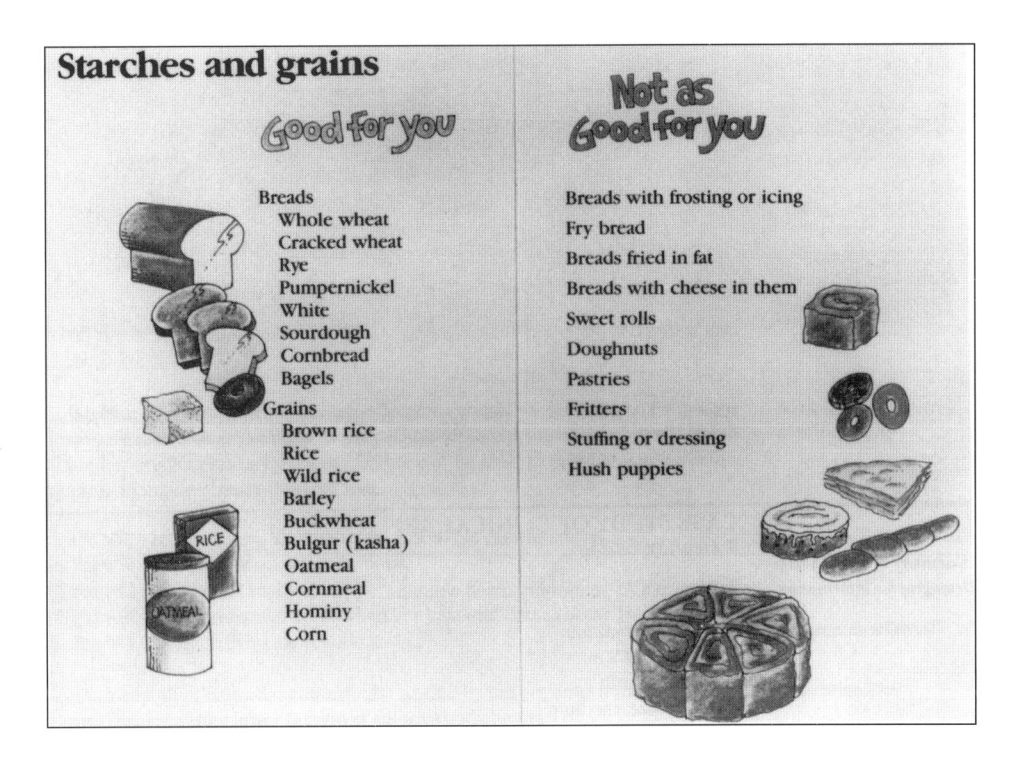

Figure 15.3
Healthy Eating Food Lists

Starches and grains

Good for you
- Breads
  - Whole wheat
  - Cracked wheat
  - Rye
  - Pumpernickel
  - White
  - Sourdough
  - Cornbread
  - Bagels
- Grains
  - Brown rice
  - Rice
  - Wild rice
  - Barley
  - Buckwheat
  - Bulgur (kasha)
  - Oatmeal
  - Cornmeal
  - Hominy
  - Corn

Not as Good for you
- Breads with frosting or icing
- Fry bread
- Breads fried in fat
- Breads with cheese in them
- Sweet rolls
- Doughnuts
- Pastries
- Fritters
- Stuffing or dressing
- Hush puppies

Reprinted with permission from *Healthy Eating*, ©1988 International Diabetes Center, Minneapolis, Minnesota. All rights reserved.

Method of Use

Below is one method for using this nutrition resource for clients with diabetes:

1. Review the diabetes nutrition guidelines, which can help the client make beneficial changes in eating habits *(Figure 15.4)*.
2. Ask the client to verbalize a few changes he or she would make in usual food intake based on the diabetes nutrition guidelines just discussed.
3. Especially for clients taking insulin, fill in suggested times for meals and snacks on the blank clocks included for each meal.
4. Explain the need to be accurate in measuring portion sizes; demonstrate how to measure foods.*
5. Explain food groups and the list of foods under the categories "Good for You" and "Not as Good for You" (see Figure 15.3).

Intended Population for Use

Use of this booklet is not limited to clients with low-level reading skills. It is appropriate and would be helpful for any adult with diabetes who would benefit from simplified materials, for the elderly, or for clients who need easily understood materials for initial education. It is not intended for use with children. Information in the booklet should be individualized based on each client's knowledge, interest, and ability to make changes in his or her eating pattern.

Clinical Setting

The booklet can be used in an inpatient or ambulatory care setting. It should be used during the educational sessions so that when the client is at home, he or she can relate the information to the text and pictures in the booklet. It can be used in one-on-one or small-group learning situations.

---

* This step may not be necessary for some clients, especially older adults with type II diabetes.

Figure 15.4
Healthy Eating Nutrition Guidelines

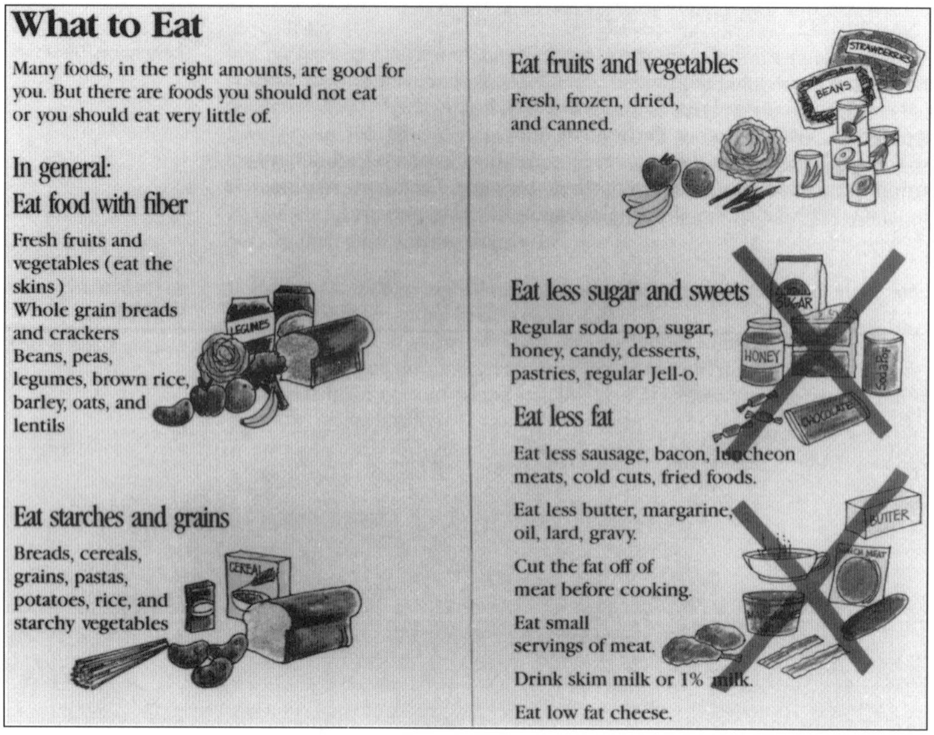

Reprinted with permission from *Healthy Eating,* ©1988 International Diabetes Center, Minneapolis, Minnesota. All rights reserved.

What to Eat

Many foods, in the right amounts, are good for you. But there are foods you should not eat or you should eat very little of.

In general: Eat food with fiber
Fresh fruits and vegetables (eat the skins)
Whole grain breads and crackers
Beans, peas, legumes, brown rice, barley, oats, and lentils

Eat starches and grains
Breads, cereals, grains, pastas, potatoes, rice, and starchy vegetables

Eat fruits and vegetables
Fresh, frozen, dried, and canned.

Eat less sugar and sweets
Regular soda pop, sugar, honey, candy, desserts, pastries, regular Jell-o.

Eat less fat
Eat less sausage, bacon, luncheon meats, cold cuts, fried foods.
Eat less butter, margarine, oil, lard, gravy.
Cut the fat off of meat before cooking.
Eat small servings of meat.
Drink skim milk or 1% milk.
Eat low fat cheese.

Length of Time to Teach

Shorter and more frequent sessions are important for clients with limited reading skills. Teaching one concept at each session, such as returning and keeping blood glucose as normal as possible, cutting back on fat, or regular meals, is helpful. At each session, clients should commit themselves to making at least one change in eating behavior (eg, eating three meals per day). At the follow-up visit, time must be allowed so that the clients can report on how they did with those commitments.

During the sessions only essential concepts should be taught—"need-to-know" rather than "nice-to-know." Information should be presented in a variety of ways and related to familiar examples. Vocabulary may also need to be taught. Visual aids are extremely useful. Clients should be asked to restate the information or learned behavior, or to demonstrate the new skill.

Advantages/Disadvantages

The booklet is colorful, written in a positive and conversational manner, and uses short sentences and short words. Paragraphs are limited to a single message and important points are repeated and reviewed. Type is simple and bold, and size is appropriate. Visuals illustrate the text.

Despite these features, *Healthy Eating* may be too advanced for clients who cannot read. It does not provide structured information about meal planning. For clients who need or desire this information, supplemental materials should be provided.

References

1. The American Diabetes Association. Nutrition recommendations and principles for people with diabetes mellitus (position statement). *Diabetes Care.* 1994;17:519–522.
2. Franz MJ, Horton ES, Bantle JP, Beebe CA, Brunzell JD, Coulston AM, Henry RR, Hoogwerf BJ, Stacpoole PW. Nutrition principles for the management of diabetes and related complications (technical review). *Diabetes Care.* 1994;17:490–518.

3. *Food Guide Pyramid: A Guide to Daily Food Choices.* Washington, DC: US Department of Agriculture, Human Nutrition Information Service; 1992. Home and Garden Bulletin No. 252.
4. *Nutrition and Your Health: Dietary Guidelines for Americans.* 4th ed. Washington, DC: US Departments of Agriculture and Health and Human Services; 1995. Home and Garden Bulletin No. 232.
5. Achterberg C, McDonnell E, Bagby R. How to put the Food Guide Pyramid into practice. *J Am Diet Assoc.* 1994;94:1030–1035.

Ordering Information for Resources Described

The First Step in Diabetes Meal Planning, 1995 (package of 25) is available from The American Dietetic Association (1-800-877-1600, ext 5000) and the American Diabetes Association (1-800-ADA-ORDER).

Healthy Eating (pack of 1 dozen) is available from Chronimed Publishing, PO Box 59032, Minneapolis, MN 55459-9686, 1-800-848-2793. Also available are Simplified Learning Series (8-book review pack), *Diabetes Care Made Easy* (low-literacy, English, and Spanish).

Healthy Food Choices pamphlet is available from The American Dietetic Association. For ordering information, call 1-800-877-1600, ext 5000.

Additional Resources and Ordering Information

Warshaw H. *Diabetes Meal Planning Made Easy: Put the Diabetes Food Pyramid to Work.* Alexandria, Va: American Diabetes Association/Contemporary Books; 1996. This book provides:
➤ expanded information for the client who wants to use the Diabetes Food Pyramid for meal planning,
➤ healthy eating tips and tactics for someone interested in eating healthier.

The book discusses current goals for diabetes management, principles of diabetes medical nutrition therapy, and ways these recommendations dovetail with the diabetes food pyramid (introduced in *The First Step to Diabetes Meal Planning*).

Part One provides a chapter on each food group, including fats, sweets, and alcohol. Each chapter includes nutrition and diabetes information, the number of servings to eat based on several calorie levels, extensive food lists with pertinent nutrition information, and quick and easy ways to achieve specific nutrition goals.

Part Two demonstrates how to apply the pyramid to make healthy food choices and plan meals and snacks. Chapters provide practical information about fast food, convenience food, portion control, preplanning, food labeling, foods with fat and sugar replacers, and restaurant eating.

Client scenarios throughout the book illustrate the process of behavioral change to achieve diabetes nutrition goals.

Available at any bookstore or by contacting the American Diabetes Association, 1-800-ADA-ORDER.

For Further Reading

Brezinski E. The first step in diabetes meal planning: simple and basic. *On the Cutting Edge.* 1996;17(2):11.

Broussard BA, ed. Diabetes nutrition education: reaching clients with low-literacy skills. *On the Cutting Edge.* 1993;14:1–24.

Daly A. Nutrition management. In: Lebovitz HE, ed. *Therapy for Diabetes Mellitus and Related Disorders.* 2nd ed. Alexandria, Va: American Diabetes Association; 1994:95–101.

Nitzke SN, Voichick J. Overview of reading and literacy research and applications in nutrition education. *J Nutr Educ.* 1992;24:261–266.

Pastors JG. Meal planning approaches for nutritional management of diabetes. In: Powers MA, ed. *Handbook of Diabetes Medical Nutrition Therapy.* Gaithersburg, Md: Aspen Publishers, Inc; 1996:207–226.

Powers MA. Accessing nutrition care. In: Lebovitz HE, ed. *Therapy for Diabetes Mellitus and Related Disorders.* 2nd ed. Alexandria, Va: American Diabetes Association; 1994:102–106.

16
Single-Topic Diabetes Resources

Definition

Single-Topic Diabetes Resources is a set of reproducible client handouts that contain basic information about diabetes nutrition topics commonly taught by dietitians or other diabetes educators. The 50-page booklet and pocket contain:

➤ General information about the purpose, design, and format of the client and professional resources,
➤ 21 single-topic client reproducible handouts (*Table 16.1* lists all the topics),
➤ 21 professional guides, which correspond to each client handout and provide specific information on and additional ideas for teaching each topic.

Table 16.1
Single-Topic Diabetes Resources: Contents

Category	Title
Nutrition and Food	*Alcohol, Diabetes, and You*
	Cooking, Baking, and Diabetes
	Diabetes: Sugars and Sweets
	Eating Out: From Burgers to Burritos
	Healthy Eating for Diabetes Before You See an RD
	Low-Calorie Sweeteners and Diabetes
	Portions: How Much Is Enough?
	Protein: Less Is Enough
	Shop Smart
	Understanding Fats
General Diabetes	*Diabetes Medicines (Pills and Insulin)*
	Disordered Eating and Diabetes
	Diabetes and Low Blood Glucose
	Exercise and Diabetes: On the Move
	Eat Healthy to Prevent Diabetes Complications
	When You Just Can't Eat
Diabetes and the Lifecycle	*Children with Diabetes (birth to 5 years)*
	Children with Diabetes (6–11 years)
	Diabetes Just During Pregnancy
	Food, Diabetes, and the Older Person
	Teens, Food, and Making Choices

Both the client and professional resources integrate the four-pronged approach to diabetes medical nutrition therapy: assessment, goal setting, intervention, and evaluation. The handouts are interactive and allow the educator to individualize the content and teaching process. They can be used alone or with other meal-planning approaches as supplemental information.

Historical Background

In 1993 a steering committee of The American Dietetic Association and American Diabetes Association was appointed to identify nutrition-related diabetes resources that needed updating, as well as new products for development. A resource identified for development was an educational tool that would enable educators to teach one diabetes-related nutrition topic at a single visit for purposes of simplification and individualization. To develop these single-topic resources, writing groups were formed consisting of volunteer dietitians with relevant expertise in each particular topic area. Each of the resources went through technical review and field-testing before publication.

Method of Use

Client Handouts

Each client handout contains the following sections (Appendix 6 contains 2 sample handouts):

➤ "What About You?" (self-assessment) asks clients three to six easy-to-answer questions about their own behaviors and knowledge. Completion of this section gives both the educator and the client insight into the client's current behaviors and knowledge. The educator can individualize learning, behavioral objectives, intervention strategies, or educational content based on these responses.
➤ "Why Learn About (specific topic)?" presents rationales for how this knowledge benefits diabetes self-management. For example, the rationale from "Alcohol, Diabetes, and You" is "Alcohol has calories. You need to know how to fit alcohol into your food plan, especially if you want to lose weight."
➤ "What Will You Learn?" presents three to five learning objectives. For example, from "Eat Healthy to Prevent Diabetes Complications" a client could expect to learn "how good food choices can help you control blood glucose to prevent/delay diabetes complications."

The content of these three sections should be individualized to the client. The educator can add or delete self-assessment questions, rationales, and learning objectives by simply writing them in or scratching them out. The professional guides suggest more ways to individualize the handouts and additional content to cover.

Each single-topic handout includes content information about the specific topic. The educator can review this basic information with the client before moving on to the final sections on the worksheet:

➤ "Set Your Sights" is the goal-setting section. Here the client and educator work together to develop behavioral goals that apply the content to the client's needs. Two to three goals are listed for consideration. Space is provided for the educator and client to develop and write in individualized goals. The number of goals should be small to give the client a sense that these are achievable. Additional goals can be set in future teaching sessions. For example, from "Portions: How Much Is Enough?": "This week I will measure food portions when I eat at home. First I will write down the size of mugs, glasses, bowls, and plates I will use to measure foods and beverages."

➤ "Keep Track" is the monitoring section. It helps the client monitor one small area of diabetes self-management. It helps the educator evaluate whether or not the client can apply the new knowledge, change behavior, and improve his or her diabetes self-management.

➤ "Here's the Challenge; What's Your Solution?" is the problem-solving section. The client's ability to solve problems helps the educator evaluate learning. Each handout contains two to three topic-specific problems. Additional space is provided for the educator to add another situation for problem solving. For example, from "Protein: Less Is Enough": "You buy sirloin steak to make dinner for four people. You want each person to eat 3 to 4 ounces of cooked meat. How much will you buy?"

The sections of *Single-Topic Diabetes Resources* that require input can be used as the basis for homework assignments. Listed below are examples of how homework assignments can be made based on the type of clinical setting:

➤ *Inpatient Setting.* Have the client work on the "Set Your Sights" section by developing a list of personal goals and return the next day to review and negotiate realistic and achievable goals.

➤ *Ambulatory Care Setting.* Recommend that your client complete the "Keep Track" monitoring section for an agreed-upon period. At the next follow-up visit, review monitoring records with the client to evaluate his or her success and challenges, develop plans, and identify new solutions.

➤ *Group Class Setting.* Ask clients to form small groups and have them complete the "Here's the Challenge; What's Your Solution?" section. Review the responses with the entire class and allow each class participant to share additional ideas.

Professional Guide

A professional guide is included for each of the 21 client handouts in this resource. The guides help the educator identify ideas for gathering assessment data, suggest creative ways to increase interaction between the educator and client, provide additional learning objectives, and identify additional client and professional resources. *Table 16.2* gives additional tips on using the client handouts.

The format of each professional guide is as follows:

➤ *How to assess need for and timing of content.* This section lists ways to collect information and data to determine if and when a client needs education on this topic.

➤ *How to help client set learning and behavioral objectives.* This section helps the educator use assessment information to establish individualized learning objectives and behavioral goals.

Table 16.2

Tips for Use of *Single-Topic Diabetes Resources* Client Handouts

> ➤ Think about grouping certain topics together that might be used in one session, eg, "Diabetes Medicines" with "Diabetes and Low Blood Glucose," or "Eating Healthy to Prevent Complications" with "Protein: Less Is Enough." A cross-reference guide is included in the professional guide to help the educator note the related client handouts.
>
> ➤ Provide information about a topic for which a client needs information (eg, "Alcohol, Diabetes, and You") or in which the educator feels the client needs more support (eg, "Disordered Eating and Diabetes").
>
> ➤ Show clients a list of the topics as an incentive to return for more follow-up.
>
> ➤ Show clients a list of the topics and have them choose ones they find interesting.
>
> ➤ Laminate the 21 reproducible masters to preserve them. Laminating can be done at most copy shops. Keep the masters separate from the copies to avoid losing the originals.
>
> ➤ Copy them on different colored paper based on their three major topic categories (see Table 16.1).
>
> ➤ Place your name, business or diabetes program logo, phone number and/or e-mail address in the "courtesy of" box. Order a stamp or print some labels with this information.
>
> ➤ Provide clients with a three-ring binder or folder to keep the handouts together.

➤ *How to make the handout interactive.* The client handouts are designed to maximize interaction between the client and educator. The client learns more if he or she is involved with the process and the education meets the client's specific learning and lifestyle needs. "What About You?", "Set Your Sights," and two other topic-specific sections increase the client's involvement in the educational process.

➤ *Client resources.* Several client resources are listed in each professional guide. These resources are familiar to many educators and easy to find. Many, but not all, are published by the American Diabetes Association and The American Dietetic Association and/or the Diabetes Care and Education dietetic practice group.

➤ *Professional resources.* Two to four easy-to-find professional resources are listed in each guide to provide the educator with more information about that specific content area. These are not exhaustive lists.

Intended Population

Single-Topic Diabetes Resources is tailored to meet the varying educational needs of people with diabetes. A handout can be used as the sole educational tool in a nutrition self-management training session or as a supplement to other information. Handouts can also be used in diabetes education classes or in individual nutrition self-management training sessions. Educators can enlarge the forms on a photocopy machine for clients who need larger print.

Single-Topic Diabetes Resources can be used to achieve individual behavioral goals without using other diabetes meal-planning resources or to expand on or supplement other diabetes meal-planning resources.

Here are two examples of uses of *Single-Topic Diabetes Resources*:

Example 1: A client prefers to cook foods at home instead of eating in restaurants or purchasing convenience foods. The client is unwilling to substitute lower-fat ingredients. For this client, the educator might establish goals related to trying new food preparation methods that use less fat. Two client handouts can be used together—"Cooking, Baking, and Diabetes" and "Understanding Fats."

Example 2: A 13-year-old client has been followed routinely for 5 years in the diabetes clinic and has been utilizing an exchange list meal plan. During an appointment, the teen expresses concern over recent excess late-night snacking, which is causing high blood glucose. You might use the client handout "Teens, Food, and Making Choices" to help the client explore his or her options for late-night snacking.

Clinical Setting

Single-Topic Diabetes Resources can be used in a variety of diabetes education settings, including:

➤ diabetes education center,
➤ hospital nutrition department (outpatient and inpatient),
➤ physician's office that employs a dietitian or diabetes educator,
➤ dietitian's private practice,
➤ home health agency,
➤ long-term care facility.

For example, the client handout "Food, Diabetes, and the Older Person" could be used by the home health educator or dietitian during a home health visit. This handout might lead to the introduction of *The First Step in Diabetes Meal Planning*, which includes the diabetes food pyramid, at the next visit. In another example, "When You Just Can't Eat" could be used in an outpatient clinic to teach rules for sick days and whom and when to call for help. Or Shop Smart could be used in a diabetes education class on supermarket shopping and/or reading food labels.

Length of Time to Teach

The teaching time required for *Single-Topic Diabetes Resources* depends on whether this method is used as a stand-alone meal-planning resource or used along with another meal-planning resource. A single topic can be covered in a minimum of a 30–60-minute session. Since this resource is designed to be interactive and track progress over time, a follow-up appointment is important to review the "Keep Track" section.

Advantages/ Disadvantages

A major advantage of *Single-Topic Diabetes Resources* is the integration of the four-step model of diabetes medical nutrition therapy—assessment, goal setting, intervention, and evaluation—into the layout and design of the resource. The handouts are interactive and allow the educator to individualize the content and teaching process. Another advantage is that the resources can be used alone or in combination with other meal-planning resources.

A disadvantage of *Single-Topic Diabetes Resources* is the inability of the resource to include all content available for each topic. Due to space limitations, only basic information is included in the resource.

Ordering Information for Resource Described

Single-Topic Diabetes Resources, published by the American Diabetes Association and The American Dietetic Association, 1996, is available from the American Diabetes Association, 1-800-ADA-ORDER, or The American Dietetic Association, 1-800-877-1600, ext 5000.

Part 4

In-depth Nutrition Intervention

Introduction to In-depth Nutrition Intervention

17

In-depth nutrition education can be defined as information that provides more structure to the process of meal planning and/or information on specific nutrient (eg, fat or carbohydrate) or calorie content to assist with meal planning. During the in-depth nutrition education stage, the dietitian works with the client to develop an individualized plan of eating. The resources discussed in Chapters 18 to 21 are more structured; they require the use of menus, food exchanges, grams, or calories to develop an individualized meal plan; and as such can be referred to as *meal-planning approaches.*

Meal-planning approaches have been placed into three subcategories, based on their similarities:

1. *Menu approaches* were designed to provide a simplified method for clients to plan their daily food intake. They provide daily menus that a client can follow in a rote manner.
2. *Exchange list approaches* provide structure since they are nutrient-based, involve the use of a meal plan, and require the client to understand grouping food by exchanges.
3. *Counting approaches* also provide structure by identifying a specific procedure. The calorie- and/or fat-counting approaches allow more flexibility with food choices and meal planning than the exchange list approaches. Carbohydrate counting is a more precise meal-planning method for matching food and insulin.

The meal-planning approaches discussed in Chapters 18 to 21 are more complex and should be taught by a diabetes educator who is a registered dietitian with advanced training and knowledge in clinical nutrition and diabetes.

Advancing to the In-depth Stage of Nutrition Intervention

Many people do well with guideline information and do not need more structured information about meal planning. This decision is based on more than intellect or literacy level. Many well-educated clients may need or want only basic information. They may not have time to use a more in-depth system of meal planning, or they may not need it to adopt an eating plan that meets their treatment goals. Conversely, clients who are not able to comprehend a more in-depth approach to meal planning may need to remain at the basic stage of nutrition education indefinitely. This does not mean that they need only one nutrition self-management training session or that any follow-up sessions should be just a review of information. The challenge is to present new information using techniques individualized to their particular needs. The information should empower them to make gradual but permanent changes in their lifestyles and eating behaviors.

In-depth Nutrition Educational Resources

The three subcategories of meal-planning approaches and their educational resources include:

- Menu approaches—individualized menus; *Month of Meals 1, 2, 3, 4, and 5* (see Chapter 18),
- Exchange list approaches—*Healthy Food Choices*; *Exchange Lists for Meal Planning* (see Chapter 19),
- Counting approaches—carbohydrate counting (Levels 1, 2, and 3); calorie counting; fat gram counting (see Chapters 20 and 21).

Menus 18

The menu is the basis of all meal-planning approaches. It is the written description of what actually can and should be eaten. Ideally, the dietitian will incorporate some degree of menu planning into whatever nutrition education approach is chosen. At least one sample menu should be written out to illustrate how meals can be designed to fit the client's individual nutrition care plan.

This chapter will describe two types of menu planning that may be useful in counseling the client:

- ➤ Individualized menus, which show how menus can be written with the client to meet the objectives of the nutrition prescription,
- ➤ Menu planning based on the set of publications titled *Month of Meals* by the American Diabetes Association.

The use of preprinted menus, another menu-planning approach, is traditionally discouraged because they are not individualized. However, there may be situations in which preprinted menus could be developed specifically for a certain population, and therefore could be more individualized to the eating style of that group. They can be useful for the dietitian when time is limited and there will be an opportunity at a later time to follow up with a more customized approach. The menu in *Table 18.1* shows an example of how a menu can be preprinted yet provide the opportunity for some choice. For even more flexibility without sacrificing menu structure, refer to *Table 18.2* to see how menu planning can be combined with the exchange list system to help provide additional guidance to clients who need assistance in meal planning.

Individualized Menus

Definition

For the purposes of this discussion, the term *individualized menus* is defined as a method of meal planning whereby the dietitian works with the client to prepare menus that specify the foods and appropriate quantities that should be eaten over a period of days. The written menus reflect whatever restrictions are called for in the nutrition prescription. There are no rules that govern this approach, and its main purpose is to help simplify meal planning. The menus can either be very specific or involve some food choices. The client is not expected to follow the menus forever, but will gradually learn, with the help of the dietitian, how to select foods and what are appropriate portion sizes.

Table 18.1
Specific Preprinted Menu

1,500-Calorie Meal Plan

Dietitian: _____ Phone: _____

√ = select as desired

MEAL	SAMPLE MENU
Breakfast	
1 milk	1 c skim milk *or* 1 c low-fat yogurt
1 fruit	small banana *or* ½ grapefruit *or* 2 tbsp raisins
2 starch	2 slices toast *or* 1½ c cold flake cereal *or* 1 2-oz bagel *or* 1 c hot cereal
1 meat	1 egg *or* 1 oz low-fat cheese
1 fat	1 tsp margarine *or* 1 tbsp cream cheese
Lunch	
√ vegetable	Green salad with fat-free salad dressing; 4 oz vegetable juice
1 fruit	1 pear *or* 1 orange *or* 1 apple
2 starch	2 slices bread *or* 1 roll (2-oz size) *or* 10 melba toast rectangles
2 meat	2 oz lean beef, poultry, or fish *or* ½ c tuna *or* ½ c cottage cheese
1 fat	1 tsp mayonnaise *or* 1 tsp margarine
Dinner	
√ vegetable	Green salad with fat-free salad dressing; 1 c green vegetables (eg, broccoli, asparagus)
1 fruit	½ c applesauce *or* 1 c cubed melon
3 starch	1 large potato *or* 1½ c corn *or* 1½ c pasta *or* 1 c rice
2 meat	2 oz lean meat, poultry, or fish
2 fat	2 tsp oil *or* 2 tsp margarine
Evening Snack	
1 starch	¾ c cold cereal *or* 1 Dutch pretzel *or* 3 graham cracker squares
½ milk	4 oz skim milk

Historical Background

Individualized menus have been used most often by dietitians as a supplement to meal planning, rather than as an independent meal-planning approach. The effectiveness of individualized menus is difficult to document or to compare with other approaches as a singular meal-planning approach. Individualized menus are tailored to the needs of each client and are not standardized; therefore, a great deal of variation among clients should be expected.

Method of Use

One way to start developing individual menus is to have the client record what is usually eaten and categorize the usual food consumed into exchange list servings. The dietitian uses the typical food intake to create the meal plan and sample menu by making necessary changes. This approach to menu planning emphasizes to clients that they are not following a special diet, but are just making some changes in the way they usually eat to improve blood glucose control.

The following is a step-by-step description of how to utilize individual menus with clients.

1. Whenever possible, have the client keep a 3- to 7-day food diary. This will be a valuable tool to design individualized menus.
2. Complete a routine nutrition assessment to best understand the client's usual eating habits, food preferences, and other factors that may influence food choices.
3. Identify specific foods or meals the client agrees to eat for a period of days. For example, he or she may agree to have cereal, milk, and fruit for one breakfast and bread, yogurt, and fruit for another breakfast.
4. Determine the times each meal (and snack) will be eaten. Coordinate meal and snack times with insulin action, when appropriate.
5. Keeping in mind the nutrition prescription, specify the amount of each food that can be eaten. Although the client is not taught exchanges, it may be helpful to use the exchange system for quickly determining appropriate quantities of each food. For example, the dietitian may be designing a breakfast that is approximately 300 kcal. In the foods selected by the client in step 3, this would translate into 1 starch, 1 milk, and 1 fruit.
6. The total number of menus developed will depend on the dietitian, the client, the time available, the number of days until the next visit, and the client's usual eating habits.

The dietitian can write an individualized menu to be very specific. It can also be written to allow for some choices, as illustrated in *Table 18.2*. A second breakfast menu may be written so the client may alternate menus every other day. These may be referred to as *odd-day menus* and *even-day menus*. For example, the breakfast from meal plan 1 is eaten Monday, Wednesday, Friday, and so forth.

Adherence to this approach can be monitored in several ways. Clients can keep daily food records or, more simply, check off or scratch through food items on their daily menu sheet to illustrate what they actually ate. The menu sheet will need to be copied for the number of times the client will be recording. Obviously, a good, trusting relationship is required between the client and the dietitian to encourage open and honest recording.

Intended Population for Use

Individualized menus can be designed to fit almost any type of client in any kind of situation. They may be suitable for clients with type I or type II diabetes. They are probably most appropriate for those who have either little experience or interest in meal planning and who have fairly routine eating habits. The design can be simple or complex and therefore can be planned to meet any educational background.

Other clients who might find this approach useful include those who:

- have had little experience with meal planning and do not currently have a healthful eating plan;
- want to be told what to eat and when to eat; and
- have difficulty making or limiting food choices.

Clinical Setting

Because of its flexibility, this menu approach can be used in any setting, at any time. The design, implementation, and success of individualized menus will depend on the amount of time available and degree of client participation.

Table 18.2
Flexible Preprinted Menu

	Sample Menu	Food Choices
*Breakfast Time*____		
___Starch		1 slice bread, 2 slices diet bread, ½ English muffin, ½ cup hot cereal, ¾ cup cold cereal, 2 pancakes (4" size), ½ bagel
___Fruit		1 cup berries, small banana, 1 cup melon, ½ cup fruit juice, ½ cup canned fruit, 1 orange, 3 dried prunes, 2 Tbsp raisins
___Milk		1 cup nonfat or low-fat milk, ¾ cup plain yogurt, 1 cup low-fat yogurt, 2 packs sugar-free hot chocolate
___Meat		1 egg, ¼ cup egg substitute, ¼ cup cottage cheese, 1 ounce low-fat cheese, 1 Tbsp peanut butter, 1 oz lean ham
___Fat		1 tsp margarine, 1 Tbsp diet margarine, 1 slice bacon, 1 Tbsp cream, 1 Tbsp cream cheese, 1 tsp oil
*Snack Time*____		
*Lunch Time*____		
___Starch		1 slice bread, 2 slices diet bread, ½ hamburger or hot dog bun, ½ cup corn, ⅔ cup lima beans, ½ cup spaghetti or noodles, ⅓ cup rice, 4–6 crackers, 1 cup soup, 3 graham cracker squares
___Fruit		½ cup fruit juice, ½ cup canned fruit, 1 cup berries, small banana, 15 grapes, 1 small orange or apple, 2 Tbsp raisins
___Milk		1 cup nonfat or low-fat milk, ¾ cup plain yogurt, 1 cup low-fat yogurt
___Vegetables		½ cup cooked or 1 cup raw asparagus, green beans, beets, broccoli, cabbage, carrots, spinach, tomatoes
___Fat		1 tsp margarine, 1 Tbsp diet margarine, 1 Tbsp salad dressing, 2 Tbsp diet salad dressing, 1 tsp vegetable oil, 1 Tbsp cream cheese

Length of Time to Teach

As this is a very straightforward approach, it can be taught in one session (usually 45 minutes to 1 hour). However, follow-up sessions may be needed for further meal planning and nutrition self-management training.

Advantages/ Disadvantages

The simplicity of this approach is its major advantage. Clients who have fairly routine eating habits and who eat at consistent times and in consistent places are likely to do better than clients who have no routine. However, this method is also good for clients who follow no routines because it encourages some structure and discipline while allowing the client the freedom of choosing what to include in the menus.

The primary disadvantage of this approach is the structure; some clients may find individualized menus too restrictive or monotonous in regard to food choices. Additionally, it can be very time consuming for the dietitian to develop individualized menus.

Table 18.2
(continued)

	Sample Menu	Food Choices
Snack Time____		
Dinner Time____		
___Starch		1 slice bread, 2 slices diet bread, ½ hamburger or hot dog bun, ½ cup corn, ½ cup peas, ½ cup spaghetti or noodles, ⅓ cup rice, ½ cup mashed potatoes, 3 graham cracker squares
___Fruit		½ cup fruit juice, ½ cup canned fruit, 1 cup berries, small banana, 15 grapes, 1 small orange or apple, 2 Tbsp raisins
___Milk		1 cup nonfat or low-fat milk, ¾ cup plain yogurt, 1 cup low-fat yogurt
___Vegetables		½ cup cooked or 1 cup raw asparagus, green beans, beets, broccoli, cabbage, carrots, spinach, tomatoes
___Meat		1 oz beef, chicken, turkey, or pork, 1 egg, ¼ cup tuna or salmon, 1 oz low-fat cheese, 1 Tbsp peanut butter
___Fat		1 tsp margarine, 1 Tbsp diet margarine, 1 Tbsp salad dressing, 2 Tbsp diet salad dressing, 1 tsp vegetable oil, 1 Tbsp cream cheese
Snack Time____		

Combination Foods:
Casseroles and hot dishes   1 cup   2 starch, 2 meat, 1 fat
Plain cheese pizza   ⅛ of 14"   1 starch, 1 meat, 1 vegetable, 1 fat
Macaroni and cheese   ½ cup   1½ starch, 2 fats
Taco   1   1 starch, 2 meat, 1 fat

Goals for Good Eating:
I agree to _____

_____

Month of Meals

Definition

Month of Meals 1, Month of Meals 2, Month of Meals 3, Month of Meals 4, and *Month of Meals 5* are five separate books that teach the menu-planning approach. Each book contains 28 days of complete menus for breakfast, lunch, dinner, and snacks to provide a balanced, healthful eating plan. Menus are written for a basic meal plan of 1,500 kcal daily, including three meals plus two 60-kcal snacks or one 125-kcal snack. Lists of 125-kcal and 170-kcal snacks are also provided to be used in an 1,800-kcal meal pattern. Instructions are provided for how to adjust the calorie level upward or downward, with sample patterns for 1,800 kcal or 1,200 kcal in all five books and 2,100 kcal in *Month of Meals 5.*

Menus are designed to follow guidelines for good nutrition and the exchange lists for meal planning. Menus provide 45% to 50% of calories from carbohydrate, 20% from protein, and about 30% from fat. Since each breakfast, lunch, and dinner contains approximately the same number of calories (350, 450, and 550, respectively), the client is encouraged to mix and match meals (which can be done, since the pages are cut into thirds) to suit his or her own tastes. Whenever a special recipe is described, the actual recipe ingredients and preparation directions are included. Many menus incorporate recipes reprinted from American Diabetes Association cookbooks or *Diabetes Forecast*, while others are original or from other sources.

While certain elements are consistent in all five volumes, each volume has unique features. Thus, the volumes can be used individually or as a set. All five volumes include a review of diabetes nutrition guidelines, as well as the food groups in the *Exchange Lists for Meal Planning;* "how-to" features are available in each volume. *Month of Meals 1* includes a special occasions section. *Month of Meals 2* adds more ethnic foods and quick-to-fix items and meals, with a special chapter on dining out. *Month of Meals 3* continues the emphasis on time-saving meals, incorporating convenience foods and microwave recipes. Special sections cover food labeling, fast foods, fiber, meal planning during illness, and picnics and barbecues. *Month of Meals 4* contains menus emphasizing old-time family favorites like pot roast and meat loaf. Recipes for one or two people are featured and hints for turning family-size meals into healthy leftovers are included. *Month of Meals 5* features all meatless meals and snacks for people choosing a vegetarian diet. Recipes call for whole-grain foods whenever possible. This book describes new and old favorites of vegetarian fare, common vegetarian staples, and tips for cooking with nuts, seeds, whole grains, and legumes.

Historical Background

The five *Month of Meals* books were developed by dietitians in the Council on Nutritional Science and Metabolism of the American Diabetes Association and staff members of the American Diabetes Association National Service Center in 1989, 1990, 1992, 1993, and 1994, respectively. The publications were developed in response to frequent requests for menus by people with diabetes. Five volumes have been created.

Method of Use

1. The dietitian should point out the prescribed meal pattern in the front of the book. The specific calorie level (ie, 1,200, 1,500, 1,800) and desired number of snacks must be negotiated with the client *(Figure 18.1)*.
2. The dietitian encourages the client to select 2 or 3 days of breakfasts, lunches, dinners, and snacks to sample initially. Clients can then arrange menus in any desired order, since meal patterns are consistent in all menus *(Figure 18.2)*.
3. Any menu can be exchanged with another menu for the same meal, as desired.
4. Some clients may choose to use menu cycles shorter than 1 month (eg, 1 week) to promote familiarity, while others may prefer a longer menu cycle for wider variety.
5. Clients using *Month of Meals* along with another meal-planning approach may wish to start by selecting a few recipes to try.

Intended Population for Use

Month of Meals is a highly flexible teaching tool. It can be used to teach clients with type I or type II diabetes, since consistent calorie levels are included in meal plans. This approach is adaptable for lean or obese clients,

Figure 18.1

Month of Meals:
Setting Calorie Levels

HOW TO USE THIS BOOK

Sample Meal Plan #1
Here's how to adjust the Basic Meal Plan (1500 calories) for about a 1200-calorie diet.

Meal		Calories
Breakfast		350
Plus or minus -1 Starch/Bread serving(s)		-80
	Subtotal	270
Lunch		450
Plus or minus -1 Fruit serving(s)		-60
	Subtotal	390
Dinner		550
Plus or minus -1 Fat serving(s)		-45
	Subtotal	505
	TOTAL DAILY CALORIES	1165

Sample Meal Plan #2
Here's how to adjust the Basic Meal Plan (1500 calories) for about a 2200-calorie diet.

Meal		Calories
Breakfast		350
Plus or minus +1 Starch/Bread serving(s)		+80
	Subtotal	430
Lunch		450
Plus or minus +1 Fruit serving(s)		+60
Plus or minus +1 Fat serving(s)		+45
	Subtotal	555
Dinner		550
Plus or minus +1 Starch/Bread serving(s)		+80
+1 Med-Fat Meat servings(s)		+75
+1 Fat serving(s)		+45
	Subtotal	750
Snacks (Morning, Afternoon, and/or Evening)		420
+1 Fruit serving(s)		+60
	Subtotal	480
	TOTAL DAILY CALORIES	2215

Reprinted with permission from *Month of Meals, 1–5: A Menu Planner* (Alexandria, Va: American Diabetes Association, Inc; 1989–1994).

offering potential for weight loss as well as glucose control. *Month of Meals* can be used for all age groups, but it is the best tool for clients with the common plea "Please—just show me what I should eat." In particular, the beauty of this tool is that it can be used with clients who do not understand or are frustrated by the exchange system. Nevertheless, clients who are familiar with the exchange system or a guideline approach will find this to be a useful tool as well. Some prior nutrition self-management training in one of these

Figure 18.2
Month of Meals:
Menu Selection

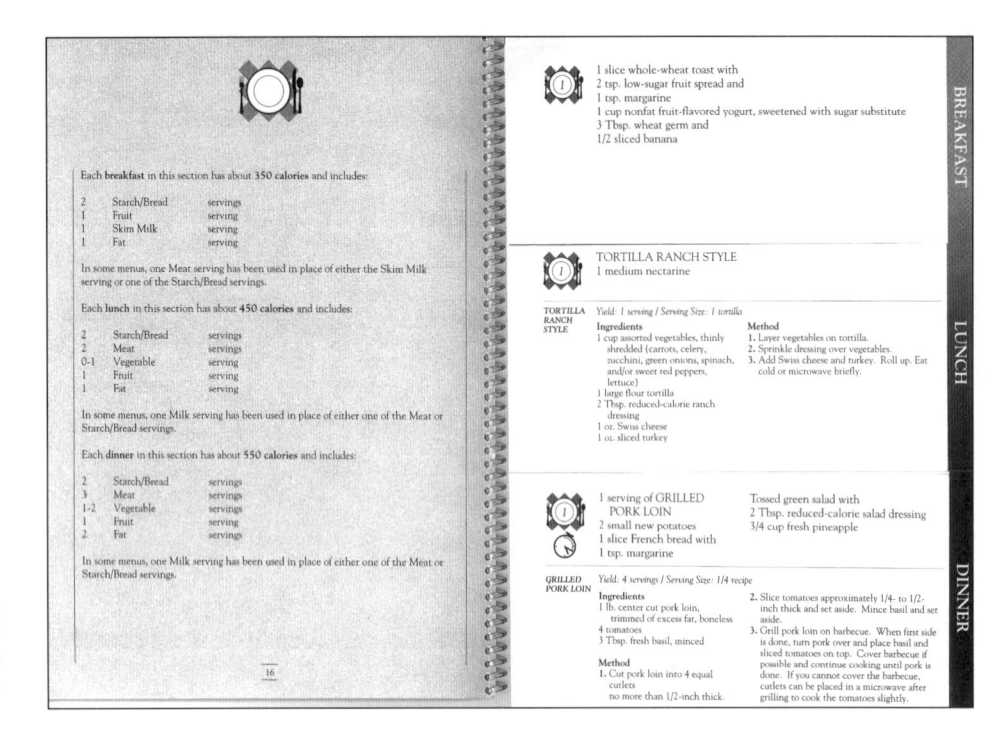

Reprinted with permission from *Month of Meals, 1: A Menu Planner* (Alexandria, Va: American Diabetes Association, Inc; 1989).

methods would be useful, although the books can also stand alone, since each volume covers basic guidelines and a discussion of the food groups.

Other clients who might find this approach advantageous include those who have had little experience with meal planning and do not make healthy food choices, those who want to be told what to do and what to eat, and overweight clients who have difficulty making or limiting food choices.

Clinical Setting

Month of Meals is especially appropriate for use in ambulatory care settings, since the primary focus is on meal preparation in the home setting. Adequate supermarket shopping and meal-planning skills (eg, how to use leftovers) are helpful when using *Month of Meals*.

Length of Time to Teach

The length of time to teach *Month of Meals* depends upon the knowledge and skill level of the client. At least one visit with a follow-up session is recommended.

Advantages/ Disadvantages

As with individualized menus, the simplicity of this approach is the major advantage. Clients who have fairly routine eating habits and who eat at consistent times and in consistent places are likely to do better than clients who have no routine. Another advantage is that clients do not require any prior knowledge or experience with any meal-planning approach and can follow the menus easily. Also, this option provides structure with food choices and amounts.

The primary disadvantage of this approach is the structure; some clients may find individualized menus too restrictive or monotonous in regard to food choices.

Summary

Several menu approaches to meal planning are available for nutrition self-management training. Menu approaches can be used as short-term methods until additional in-depth education can be accomplished, or they may be used as the primary method to teach clients with diabetes what can and should be eaten. Menu-planning approaches offer flexibility and a simple alternative, useful for many clients.

Ordering Information for Resources Described

Month of Meals 1: A Menu Planner. Alexandria, Va: American Diabetes Association, Inc; 1989.
Month of Meals 2: A Menu Planner. Alexandria, Va: American Diabetes Association, Inc; 1990.
Month of Meals 3: A Menu Planner. Alexandria, Va: American Diabetes Association, Inc; 1992.
Month of Meals 4: A Menu Planner. Alexandria, Va: American Diabetes Association, Inc; 1993.
Month of Meals 5: A Menu Planner. Alexandria, Va: American Diabetes Association, Inc; 1994.

All these publications can be obtained by calling the American Diabetes Association, 1-800-ADA-ORDER.

For Further Reading

Pastors JG. Alternatives to the exchange system for teaching meal planning to persons with diabetes. *Diabetes Educator.* 1992;1:57–62.

Pastors JG. Expanding meal planning options. In: Powers MA, ed. *Handbook of Diabetes Medical Nutrition Therapy.* Gaithersburg, Md: Aspen Publishers, Inc; 1996: 207–226.

Exchanges 19

Exchange Lists for Meal Planning

Definition

Exchange Lists for Meal Planning categorizes foods into three main groups: Carbohydrate, Meat and Meat Substitutes, and Fat. Foods are further subdivided in these three groups into specific exchange lists. An exchange list contains a listing of measured or weighed foods of approximately the same nutritional value; therefore, foods on each list can be substituted or "exchanged" with other foods on the same list. With each food list, one exchange is appropriately equal to another in calories, carbohydrate, protein, and fat.

The Carbohydrate group contains the starch, fruit, milk, other carbohydrates, and vegetable lists. Foods from the starch list, fruit list, milk list, and other carbohydrates list can be interchanged in the meal plan, since each of the lists contains foods that contain 60–90 Calories and 12–15 grams of carbohydrate.

The Meat and Meat Substitutes group contains food sources of protein and fat. This group is divided into four lists: very lean meats, lean meats, medium-fat meats, and high-fat meats. The lists have foods containing 35, 55, 75, and 100 Calories and 1, 3, 5, and 8 grams of fat, respectively.

The Fat group contains the monounsaturated fats, polyunsaturated fats, and saturated fats lists. Each food source contains an average of 45 Calories and 5 grams of fat.

The exchange lists also identify foods that contribute significant amounts of sodium. A sodium symbol is shown next to foods that contain 400 mg or more of sodium per exchange serving.

Historical Background

The concept of "exchange" or "substitution" of different foods that are acceptable for use by clients with diabetes was developed by The American Dietetic Association, the American Diabetes Association, and the US Public Health Service in 1950. Prior to its development, meal-planning resources in the United States were chaotic, with no agreement on education and meal planning among the major organizations involved with diabetes and nutrition. The goal was to develop an educational tool that would provide uniformity in meal planning and allow a wider variety of foods to be included.

The exchange lists were revised for the first time in 1976. The goals at that time were to be more accurate in the caloric content of listed foods and to emphasize fat modification and the need for individualized meal plans to be used with the exchange lists.

The exchange lists were revised again in 1986. The goals of this revision were to develop a simplified meal planning resource to be used when appropriate for the initial phase of education (see the sections in this chapter on

Healthy Food Choices), to ensure that both educational resources would better reflect the principles of nutrition, and to develop a database of the foods listed in the booklet. The database supported a revision in the nutrient values assigned to some exchanges (eg, fruit from 10 g to 15 g carbohydrate, with subsequent increase in calories from 40 to 60 per exchange serving).[1]

1995 *Exchange Lists for Meal Planning*

In 1995 the exchange lists were again updated. The goals of the 1995 revision were:

➤ to update the lists of foods and the database, primarily to add fat-modified foods, vegetarian food items, and fast foods;
➤ to group carbohydrate food sources to provide more flexibility in food choices that have a major impact on blood glucose levels; and
➤ to allow for more accurate calculation of exchanges from nutrient information on labels, recipes, and prepared foods.[2]

The criteria to determine which foods should be included were taken from Pennington's 1992 identification of core foods in the US food supply.[3] In addition, newer food products, such as fat-modified foods, and other common foods, such as ethnic and vegetarian foods, were added. The 1994 American Diabetes Association Diabetes Nutrition Recommendations[4] also served as the basis for the 1995 update of the exchange lists.

The updated booklet provides nutrition tips and selection tips for each exchange list. In addition, several changes were made to the meal plan form in the back of the booklet. A blank was added to list the number of Carbohydrate exchanges for each meal. If desired, the number of Carbohydrate exchanges can be subdivided into the number of exchanges for starch, fruit, and milk. Blanks are provided for the number of Meat and Meat Substitutes exchanges and Fat exchanges. After both of these groups are blanks that can be used, if desired, to indicate the type of meat (very lean, lean, medium-fat, or high-fat) or fat (monounsaturated, polyunsaturated, or saturated) that is preferred by the client.[2] A check mark (√) has been added before Vegetables on the Meal Plan page of the booklet. Its purpose is to encourage regular consumption of vegetables at the midday and evening meals. One to two servings of vegetables are recommended at each meal and will have a minimal impact on blood glucose levels. If a client consumes three or more servings per meal, they should be counted as one carbohydrate choice (1 starch or 1 fruit or 1 milk).

The most significant revision to the exchange list is the order and grouping of the lists. The Carbohydrate group is listed together in the front of the booklet. The "other carbohydrates" list expands food choices containing carbohydrate (sucrose) and fat (eg, pie, cake, ice cream). Foods on the other carbohydrates list usually provide 1 to 2 carbohydrate and 1 to 2 fat exchanges, and may be interchanged with an item on the starch, fruit, or milk lists and the fat list, if appropriate.[2] The vegetable list is included in the carbohydrate list; vegetables can be considered a free food unless three or more servings are eaten at one time.

The Meat and Meat Substitutes group includes a new list, very lean meat, which contains 7 g protein and 0–1 g fat. This new list enhances the emphasis on eating less fat for clients with diabetes. However, the type of meat that clients typically eat (lean or medium-fat meats) is used to calculate the meal plan. There is no need for clients to add or subtract fat exchanges when choosing meats from any of the other meat lists.

The Fat group has been subdivided into three fat lists: monounsaturated fats, polyunsaturated fats, and saturated fats. This change should assist clients in identifying monounsaturated fats and saturated fats in their meal plans.

Method of Use

The following outline provides a logical sequence for using the *Exchange Lists for Meal Planning*:

1. Complete the nutrition assessment (see Chapter 12).
   a. Estimate reasonable body weight (see Appendix 2, Table 3).
   b. Estimate caloric requirements (see Appendix 2, Table 4).
   c. Obtain a nutrition history (see Appendix 3, Table 1) to guide the development of the meal plan.
2. Evaluate nutrition history.
   a. Categorize usual food intake into exchange amounts and divide the exchanges among meals/snacks, staying as close to the current eating pattern as possible (see *Table 19.1*, which shows a sample nutrition history in which a typical day's intake is converted into exchange list values). A handheld computer that calculates nutrients and exchanges can be used to save time.
   b. Fill in grams of carbohydrate, protein, and fat according to total number of exchanges per day (see Table 19.1).
   c. Total the grams of carbohydrate, protein, and fat and the calories for the day. Determine percentages of carbohydrate, protein, and fat in the diet.
   d. Review the usual food intake and consider the following factors for developing an individualized meal plan:
      i. calorie intake versus calorie requirements,
      ii. distribution of food intake, meal size, and spacing of meals (see step 4),
      iii. integration of insulin therapy into the meal plan for insulin users.
3. Establish goals for client (see Appendix 5). The possible changes that the client is willing and able to make to improve food choices and distribution of food should be discussed.
4. Individualize a meal plan for the client that he or she can follow (see *Table 19.2*, which refers to an individualized meal plan based on the sample nutrition history from Table 19.1). The dietitian then calculates a meal plan for initial treatment keeping the following points in mind:
   a. The distribution of meals and snacks depends on lifestyle and activity patterns, diabetes medications, nutrition assessment data, and the established goals. With increasing use of more flexible insulin regimes, it is usually not necessary to divide the meal plan or the carbohydrate content into various fractions throughout the day. With consistent food intake from day to day, insulin therapy can usually be adjusted to match customary food intake.
   b. The dietitian guides the client to coordinate medication regimen and target blood glucose values, usual activity pattern, and food intake. Self-monitoring of blood glucose (SMBG) is used to evaluate the effectiveness of the meal plan (see Chapter 6).

Diabetes Medical Nutrition Therapy

Table 19.1

Converting Nutrition History Into Exchange List Values

Nutrition History

Breakfast:
- 1 c orange juice
- 2 slices toast with peanut butter
- 1 c dry cereal
- 1 c 2% milk
- Coffee

Lunch:
- Sandwich—2 slices bread, 3 slices lunch meat, mayonnaise, butter
- Potato chips—1 bag
- Cola

Afternoon snack:
- 12 oz can cranberry juice cocktail

Dinner:
- 1–1½ c casserole
- Tossed salad with dressing
- 1–2 slices bread with mayonnaise
- 1–2 c 2% milk

Bedtime snack:
- 1 c ice cream or 2-4 cookies

Recommended calorie intake based on assessment and goal setting: 1,400–1,600 kcal

Food Group	Meal	Snack	Meal	Snack	Meal	Snack	Total (Day)	CHO (g)	Protein (g)	Fat (g)	Calories
Starch	3		5		5	4	17	255	51	—	1,360
Fruit	2		3				5	75	—	—	300
Milk*	1		0		1		2	24	16	10	240
Veg					1		1	5			25
Meat & Sub†	1		3		3		7	—	49	35	525
Fat	0		6		4	6	16			80	720
TOTALS								359	116	125	
								×4 = 1,436	×4 = 464	×9 = 1,125	
								% of cal 45	% of cal 15	% of cal 35	
										TOTAL CALORIES	**3,170**

*Milk, 2%, used for calculation.
†Meat, medium-fat, used for calculation.

c. Refer to *Table 19.3*[5] for additional helpful hints for calculating meal plans.

d. Refer to *Table 19.4*[5] for exchange lists guidelines for recipe calculations.

5. Ask the client to complete several days of food records or menus so that the appropriateness of the initial meal plan and understanding of

Table 19.2
Individualized Meal Plan

Meal Plan for: _____			Grams	%kcal
		Carbohydrate	174	45%
Dietitian: _____		Protein	82	21%
		Fat	58	32%
		Calories	1,600	

Meal	Number of Exchanges/Choices		
Breakfast	__4__	Carbohydrate group	
	__2__	Starch	
	__1__	Fruit	
	__1__	Milk	__2%__
	__1__	Meat group	__high-fat__
	__0__	Fat group	
Snack	_____	_____	
	_____	_____	
Lunch	__2__	Carbohydrate group	
	__2__	Starch	
	__0__	Fruit	
	__0__	Milk	
	__√__	Vegetables	
	__2__	Meat group	__medium-fat__
	__1–2__	Fat group	
Snack	__1__	Carbohydrate group: 1 Fruit or 1 Starch or 1 Milk	
Dinner	__4__	Carbohydrate group	
	__2__	Starch	
	__1__	Fruit	
	__1__	Milk	__2%__
	__√__	Vegetables	
	__3__	Meat group	__medium-fat__
	__2__	Fat group	
HS Snack	__1__	Carbohydrate group: 1 Fruit or 1 Starch or 1 Milk	

the meal pattern and the exchange-list approach can be evaluated at a follow-up visit. Revise the meal plan and/or approach as necessary.
6. Communicate the meal plan and goals to the members of the diabetes care team.

Intended Population for Use

Exchange lists can be used for clients with type I or type II diabetes. Exchange lists can be used to emphasize the need for consistency in the timing of food intake and to identify the amount of food to be eaten at meals and snacks while providing for needed variety and flexibility. For clients with type II diabetes, they can be used to teach the caloric and fat values of foods, along with the carbohydrate content. Clients who request or need structured meal-planning guidance and are able to comprehend complex details may be best suited to using the exchange lists.

Table 19.3
Helpful Hints for Calculating Exchange Lists Meal Plans[5]

- Calorie level estimates in calculated meal plans should be rounded off to the nearest 50 or 100 Calories because calculations of food intake based on the exchange system are not accurate enough to allow more precision. Clients may consume 50–60 Calories from free foods. Since self-reports of food intake generally underestimate calories, values should be rounded up rather than down. Recommending a wide variety of foods is important so that a client is not always at the high or low end of calorie and macronutrient values, which could affect expected clinical outcomes.

- Some foods have been placed in one particular list, but they may fit just as appropriately in another list. For example, foods in the starch, fruit, and milk lists of the Carbohydrate group each contain similar carbohydrate and calorie content and may be interchanged. If fruits or starches are regularly substituted for milk, calcium intake may be decreased and, for children, protein intake may be significantly reduced. Conversely, regularly choosing milk instead of fruits or starches may result in inadequate fiber intake and an unanticipated increase in protein intake. Foods from the other carbohydrate list of the Carbohydrate group, the combination foods list, and the fast foods list are also interchangeable with the starch, fruit, and milk lists. Consequently, the same precautions regarding calcium, fiber, and protein apply. In addition, most of the dessert-type foods on the other carbohydrate list are higher in sugars and fat, and need to be used within the context of a healthy meal plan. The dietitian needs to provide definite guidelines for interchanging foods.

- Beans, peas, and lentils are included in the starch list of the Carbohydrate group. The serving size (usually ½ cup) is counted as 1 starch and 1 very lean meat for vegetarian meal planning. Clients not practicing vegetarianism use these foods less frequently and often as side dishes rather than main dishes. In this case, the very lean meat exchange need not be counted and ⅓ cup is equivalent to 1 starch.

- The exchanges for the type of milk the client drinks should be used to calculate the meal plan. Skim and low-fat milks are recommended for adults and children (over 2 years of age), rather than whole milk.

- Vegetables are included in the Carbohydrate group and should be a part of the meal plan. However, since 3 servings of vegetables are the equivalent of 1 Carbohydrate choice, clients wanting only 1 or 2 servings per meal need not count the calories or macronutrients, unless they are tightly controlling calories and/or carbohydrate. This encourages consumption of vegetables and simplifies meal planning.

- The types of meat and meat substitutes typically consumed by the client should be used to calculate the meal plan. Lean meats or even medium-fat meats will probably be used most often. The very lean meats and high-fat meat lists will probably be used more for exchange calculations for recipes or the Nutrition Facts component of food labels. It is not recommended that clients add or subtract fat exchanges when using meat lists that are different from those ordinarily consumed.

- Foods in the starch exchange list contain, on average, slightly less than 1 g fat per serving. The dietitian should use 1 g fat in calculations to yield the appropriate calorie level for the exchange group. If the dietitian knows the client uses very few food choices that contain fat (see the database), then it is appropriate to use 0 g fat and adjust the calorie value of the exchange.

- For calculating protein amounts for diabetes renal meal plans, use the average value of 2.3 g protein per starch exchange or the average grams of protein for each subcategory on the starch list (see the database).

The exchange lists can also be used with intensified insulin regimens (see Chapter 7). Using exchange lists can provide an initial understanding of the carbohydrate content of foods. Clients can then advance to the carbohydrate-counting approach to meal planning to assist them in understanding pattern management and to develop carbohydrate/insulin ratios for fine-tuning glucose control (see Chapter 20).

Clinical Setting

Clients should receive education in the use of *Exchange Lists for Meal Planning* in an ambulatory care setting. This approach may not be conducive for teaching in an inpatient setting because of its complexity. A series of visits needs to be scheduled to assist the client and family members in learning how to use the exchange system effectively.

Length of Time to Teach

Nutrition self-management training should ideally be provided over a period of time. A minimum of two to three sessions is ideal for self-management training with the exchange lists, in the following order:

➤ The first session consists primarily of assessment, goal setting, and planning the educational intervention. Simplified meal guidelines can be given to assist the client in making food choices on a temporary basis.
➤ The second session involves introducing the exchange system and an individualized meal plan. Clients can also be asked to keep a food record or to plan several days of meals to be evaluated at the third session.
➤ The third session involves evaluation of the suitability of the meal plan and comprehension of the client in applying the exchange system. If the third session cannot occur, a phone call or letter to the client to assess comprehension should be considered.

A follow-up session should be scheduled in 3 to 4 weeks. Ongoing nutrition self-management training should occur every 6 months to 1 year, or more often if needed.

Advantages and Disadvantages

When used with appropriate clients, exchange lists offer two primary advantages. First, they provide a framework for grouping foods that takes into account their calorie, carbohydrate, protein, and fat content. Second, they emphasize important nutrition management concepts: calorie control, fat modification, awareness of the carbohydrate content of foods, and awareness of high-sodium foods.

Another advantage is that the exchange lists can be used to teach clients and health professionals the amount of carbohydrate, protein, fat, and calories contributed by foods. With an understanding of the nutrient composition of the exchange list groups, clients and professionals can use nutrient values from food labels and can incorporate a wider variety of foods into the meal plan.

The exchange lists are not appropriate for use if the client and/or family members cannot understand the concept of "exchanging" foods. Because the exchange lists booklet is written at a ninth- to tenth-grade reading level,

Table 19.4
Exchange List Guidelines for Recipe/Food Label Calculation[5]

- Do not use ¼ or ⅓ exchanges, ½ vegetable exchanges, or ½ meat exchanges. It is not realistic for clients to utilize such small fractional amounts in their meal plan. However, ½ exchanges of starches, fruits, or milk are more easily utilized because of the larger serving sizes and the interconversion of the Carbohydrate group.
- Use the smallest number of exchange lists possible. For example, use 1 starch exchange rather than ½ starch and ½ fruit.
- Even though the Carbohydrate group food lists may be interchanged, it is helpful to clients to have the chosen exchange list(s) match not only the product ingredients, but also the way the food is used. For example, try not to use a milk exchange unless the food product or recipe has an obvious milk source in it and the food is appropriate for a milk exchange.
- Use lean meat or medium-fat meat exchanges unless the product is obviously a very lean or high-fat meat. For recipes or products with meat and other sources of fat, the meat list chosen can vary depending upon the additional fat. For example, 2 lean meats plus 1 fat is the same as 2 medium-fat meats. Since high-fat meats are generally not used in meal plans, use other meat categories such as medium-fat meat plus fat exchanges. For example, 2 high-fat meat exchanges is the same as 2 medium-fat meats plus 1 fat.
- A free food contains up to 20 Calories and up to 5 g carbohydrate per serving.
- Use the following recommendations when calculating exchanges for food products or recipes:
  1. To round off carbohydrate exchanges for the starch, fruit, and milk lists,
     - 1–5 g: do not count
     - 6–10 g: ½ exchange
     - 11–20 g: 1 exchange
  2. To round off protein exchanges for the meat and meat substitutes list,
     - 0–3 g: do not count
     - 4–10 g: 1 exchange
  3. To round off fat exchanges for the fat list,
     - 0–2 g: do not count
     - 3 g: ½ exchange
     - 4–7 g: 1 exchange
- Matching macronutrients and calories per serving to exchange values:
  1. Match carbohydrate content to exchanges.
  2. Keep the calorie content close to the exchange calories per serving.
  3. The fat and protein content will usually fall within the range limits given.
- The other carbohydrate list includes dessert-type foods and foods that do not fit into the starch list (such as chips). In recipe analysis or food label exchange calculations, these foods can be designated as "x carbohydrate exchanges (and y fat exchanges, if appropriate)." For example, ⅙ of a two-crust fruit pie = 3 starch (or 3 carbohydrate) and 2 fat exchanges.
- While clients need not count 1–2 vegetable exchanges per meal, recipes or food label exchange information should include the vegetable category wherever appropriate.
- If a serving from a recipe or food contains greater than 50% of its fat content as a particular fatty acid, "fat, monounsaturated," "fat, polyunsaturated," or "fat, saturated" could be listed rather than a generic "fat" exchange.
- When calories don't equal the general factors of 4, 4, and 9 calories per gram for protein, total carbohydrate, and fat, there are several possible explanations:
  1. The fruit and fat lists contain, on average, a little less than 1 g protein per serving and the fat and meat and meat substitutes lists contain, on average, 1 g carbohydrate, whereas the exchange average values are zero.
  2. On a Nutrition Facts food label the grams of fiber are included in the total grams of carbohydrate. However, in calculating calories for food labels, the

Table 19.4
(continued)

grams of carbohydrate from *insoluble* fiber do not have to be included. On a practical basis, when determining starch exchanges or carbohydrate choices, the only time fiber grams need to be subtracted from the total carbohydrate is with cereals containing a high amount of insoluble fiber. These foods will generally contain 5 grams or more of insoluble fiber in a serving. For example, the carbohydrate for the cereals and grains portion of the starch list is higher than expected because the insoluble fiber was not subtracted from the total carbohydrate for the higher-fiber cereals in the database.

3. In a situation analogous to fiber, grams of sugar alcohol (polyols) are included in the total grams of carbohydrate on the Nutrition Facts panel of a food label; however, in deriving energy values for food-labeling purposes, they are calculated as having about half the calories (2 kcal/g) of most other carbohydrates (4 kcal/g). Specific sugar alcohol calorie values "allowed" by the Food and Drug Administration are hydrogenated starch hydrolysate (HSH): 3 kcal/g; isomalt: 2.0 kcal/g; lactitol: 2.0 kcal/g; maltitol: 3.0 kcal/g; mannitol: 1.6 kcal/g; sorbitol: 2.6 kcal/g; and xylitol: 2.4 kcal/g. This should not make a difference in recipe calculations unless there are 5 grams or more of sugar alcohol in a serving. If this is the case, subtraction of ½ of the grams of sugar alcohol from the grams of total carbohydrate should make calculation of the exchange(s) easier.

4. When alcohol is used in a recipe, it is initially assumed to have 7 kcal/g; however, the nutrient makeup is not carbohydrate, fat, or protein. When a small amount of alcohol is used in a recipe and heat is applied, it will usually reduce the alcohol content to a reasonable level, which will not upset the balance of the calories versus the macronutrient calories. To determine how many calories to consider for the alcohol remaining in a prepared food after heat is applied, use the percentage retention factors determined by the USDA.

5. For food-labeling purposes, calories are rounded off to the nearest 5 calories, and protein, fat, and carbohydrate are rounded to the nearest gram per serving size. These rounding errors may contribute to a significant difference if the label serving size is small (1 or 2 tablespoons) and the amount in a recipe is large (1 cup).

---

clients must be able to read at this level or understand the concept of "exchanging" foods.

Healthy Food Choices (Poster Section)

The foldout section of the *Healthy Food Choices* pamphlet is a poster that shows a simplified version of the exchange lists *(Figure 19.1)*. For simplicity, the term *food choices* is used in this pamphlet. An eating plan for 1,200 kcal is provided as a reference. The guidelines section of the pamphlet is discussed in Chapter 15.

Definition

Historical Background

Healthy Food Choices was developed by the committee that coordinated the revision of the exchange lists in 1986. It is a joint publication of The American Dietetic Association and the American Diabetes Association. The goal in designing this piece and publishing it concurrently with the revised exchange lists was to enhance the concept that not all clients need to use the *Exchange Lists for Meal Planning*. It was intended to provide an introduction to diabetes meal planning with an emphasis on healthful eating. The client who wishes to

Figure 19.1
Healthy Food Choices
Poster Section

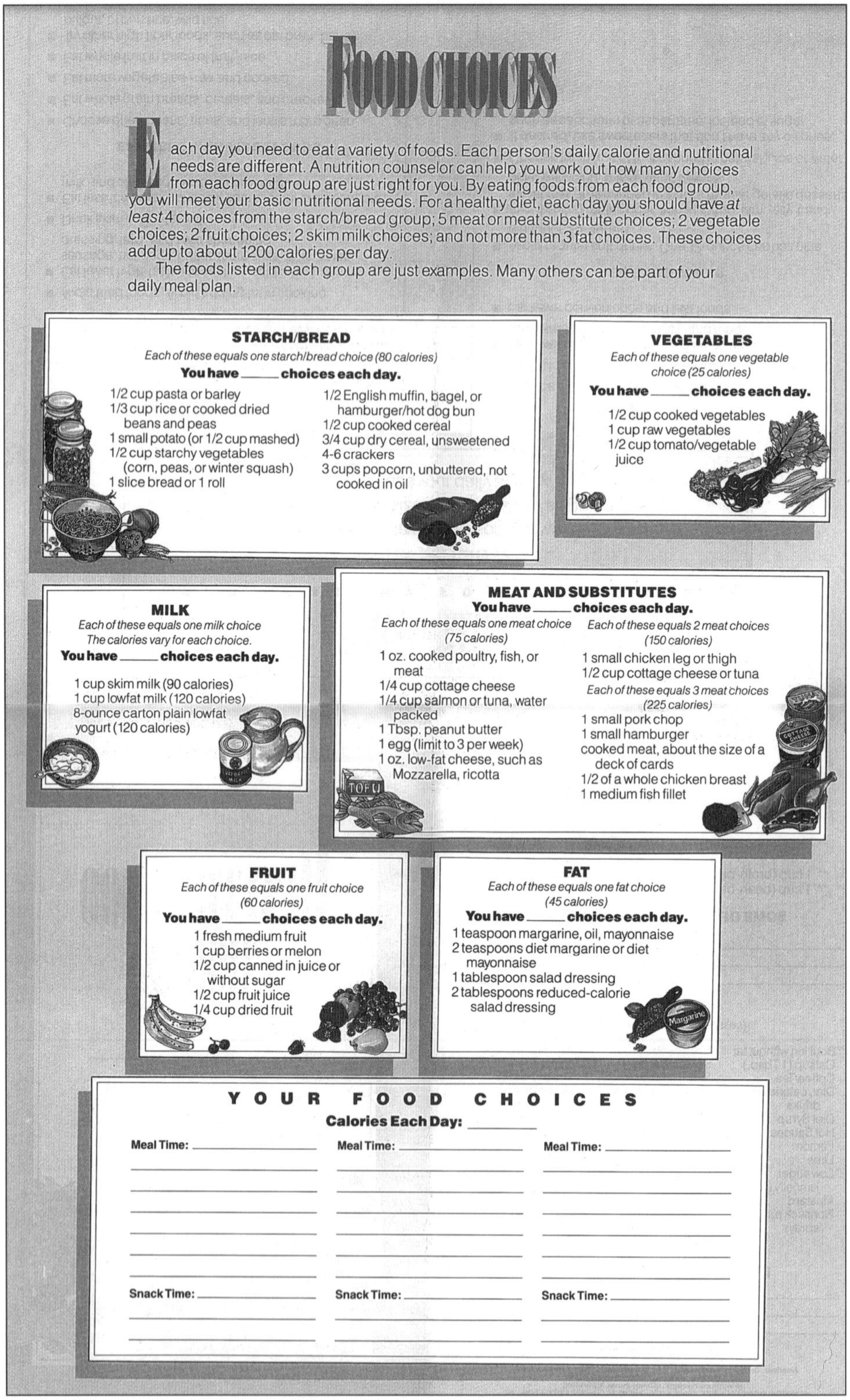

FOOD CHOICES

Each day you need to eat a variety of foods. Each person's daily calorie and nutritional needs are different. A nutrition counselor can help you work out how many choices from each food group are just right for you. By eating foods from each food group, you will meet your basic nutritional needs. For a healthy diet, each day you should have *at least* 4 choices from the starch/bread group; 5 meat or meat substitute choices; 2 vegetable choices; 2 fruit choices; 2 skim milk choices; and not more than 3 fat choices. These choices add up to about 1200 calories per day.

The foods listed in each group are just examples. Many others can be part of your daily meal plan.

STARCH/BREAD
Each of these equals one starch/bread choice (80 calories)
You have ____ choices each day.

- 1/2 cup pasta or barley
- 1/3 cup rice or cooked dried beans and peas
- 1 small potato (or 1/2 cup mashed)
- 1/2 cup starchy vegetables (corn, peas, or winter squash)
- 1 slice bread or 1 roll
- 1/2 English muffin, bagel, or hamburger/hot dog bun
- 1/2 cup cooked cereal
- 3/4 cup dry cereal, unsweetened
- 4-6 crackers
- 3 cups popcorn, unbuttered, not cooked in oil

VEGETABLES
Each of these equals one vegetable choice (25 calories)
You have ____ choices each day.

- 1/2 cup cooked vegetables
- 1 cup raw vegetables
- 1/2 cup tomato/vegetable juice

MILK
Each of these equals one milk choice
The calories vary for each choice.
You have ____ choices each day.

- 1 cup skim milk (90 calories)
- 1 cup lowfat milk (120 calories)
- 8-ounce carton plain lowfat yogurt (120 calories)

MEAT AND SUBSTITUTES
You have ____ choices each day.

Each of these equals one meat choice (75 calories)

- 1 oz. cooked poultry, fish, or meat
- 1/4 cup cottage cheese
- 1/4 cup salmon or tuna, water packed
- 1 Tbsp. peanut butter
- 1 egg (limit to 3 per week)
- 1 oz. low-fat cheese, such as Mozzarella, ricotta

Each of these equals 2 meat choices (150 calories)

- 1 small chicken leg or thigh
- 1/2 cup cottage cheese or tuna

Each of these equals 3 meat choices (225 calories)

- 1 small pork chop
- 1 small hamburger
- cooked meat, about the size of a deck of cards
- 1/2 of a whole chicken breast
- 1 medium fish fillet

FRUIT
Each of these equals one fruit choice (60 calories)
You have ____ choices each day.

- 1 fresh medium fruit
- 1 cup berries or melon
- 1/2 cup canned in juice or without sugar
- 1/2 cup fruit juice
- 1/4 cup dried fruit

FAT
Each of these equals one fat choice (45 calories)
You have ____ choices each day.

- 1 teaspoon margarine, oil, mayonnaise
- 2 teaspoons diet margarine or diet mayonnaise
- 1 tablespoon salad dressing
- 2 tablespoons reduced-calorie salad dressing

YOUR FOOD CHOICES
Calories Each Day: ____

Meal Time: ____	Meal Time: ____	Meal Time: ____
Snack Time: ____	Snack Time: ____	Snack Time: ____

Source: *Healthy Food Choices* (Alexandria, Va: American Diabetes Association; Chicago, Ill: The American Dietetic Association; 1986).

advance to the exchange system could use the simplified lists as the initial step. Two alternative approaches to meal planning, basic guidelines and simplified exchanges, are presented. These two approaches encourage individualization of the delivery of nutrition self-management training for clients.

Method of Use

Healthy Food Choices is primarily useful for the initial level of diabetes meal planning education. It can be used to provide either basic guidelines or a simplified exchange plan. It must be remembered that many clients may remain at the basic education level for quite some time or may never advance to the in-depth level. The dietitian provides encouragement and guidance while relying on the client's questions and progress as indicators of readiness for advancement. Supplemental reading materials on the various points addressed (eg, fat, sodium, fiber, food preparation) may be provided to provide more in-depth information. *Single-Topic Diabetes Resources* may be used for this purpose. The method of use outlined for *Exchange Lists for Meal Planning* can be used in developing the meal plan.

Intended Population for Use

Healthy Food Choices is appropriate for most clients because it offers an overview of diabetes medical nutrition therapy within the framework of basic eating guidelines and the simplified exchange system. The intended population is broad-based; all age groups can use the material. It is appropriate for use by any client with type I or type II diabetes who desires to improve his or her eating habits and blood glucose levels. The amount of structure and the rate of progression depends on the needs of each client and his or her desire and ability to make changes in eating habits.

Clinical Setting

The poster section is appropriate for use in an ambulatory care setting as a simple tool to teach meal planning.

Length of Time to Teach

This education resource can be reviewed in two or three sessions, depending on the client's goals. If the client is progressing from the guidelines section to developing a meal plan, a session will be needed to establish a simplified eating plan. During a follow-up session, the dietitian will need to review food records or sample menus to evaluate the client's understanding of the approach. This session will also allow for further refinement of the meal plan based on SMBG records. In some cases, during another follow-up session, the client could progress to learning the use of the *Exchange Lists for Meal Planning*.

Advantages and Disadvantages

The pamphlet is easy to use, concise, and at a moderate reading level (sixth grade on SMOG readability test). It introduces simplified exchange lists, which use choices instead of exchanges and simplified portion sizes within exchange groups (eg, ½ cup of any fruit juice and 1 medium fresh fruit).

The primary disadvantage with this educational resource is that the two approaches (guidelines and simplified exchange lists) are included in the same pamphlet. This could lead to potential misuse in that both approaches might be introduced at the same time when it is only appropriate to teach a single approach. The dietitian needs to conduct a comprehensive nutrition assessment to make the best decision about how to introduce nutrition guidelines and meal planning. Gradual change is often the key to incorporating changes into lifelong eating habits.

References

1. Franz MJ, Barr P, Holler H, Powers MA, Wheeler ML, Wylie-Rosett J. Exchange lists, revised 1986. *J Am Diet Assoc.* 1987;87:28.
2. Franz MJ. Exchange lists for meal planning: what you should know about the 1995 version. *On the Cutting Edge.* 1996;17(2):12–15.
3. Pennington JAT. Total diet studies: the identification of core foods in the United States food supply. *Food Additives and Contaminants.* 1992;9:253–264.
4. American Diabetes Association. Nutrition recommendations and principles for people with diabetes mellitus. *Diab Care.* 1994;17:519–522.
5. Wheeler ML, Franz M, Barrier P, Holler H, Cronmiller N, Delahanty L. Macronutrient and kilocalorie database for the 1995 Exchange Lists for Meal Planning: a rationale for clinical practice decisions. *J Am Diet Assoc.* 1996;96:1167–1171.

Ordering Information for Resources Described

Exchange Lists for Meal Planning. 1996. Available from The American Dietetic Association (1-800-877-1600, ext 5000) or the American Diabetes Association (1-800-ADA-ORDER).

Healthy Food Choices. 1988. Available from The American Dietetic Association (1-800-877-1600, ext 5000).

Additional Resources

Anderson JW. *HCF Exchanges: A Sensible Plan for Healthy Eating: The HCF Guide Book.* Lexington, Ky: HCF Nutrition Research Foundation, Inc; 1987. The High-Carbohydrate/High-Fiber (HCF) exchange lists follow a format similar to the *Exchange Lists for Meal Planning.* Each serving of food within an exchange group is approximately equal in calories, carbohydrate, protein, fat, and fiber content. In the HCF plan, foods are divided into eight exchange groups: Starches, Garden Vegetables, Fruits, Cereals, Beans, Milk, Proteins, and Fats. The Cereals and Beans exchange groups are unique to this meal-planning approach, which emphasizes intake of fiber from food sources, particularly those rich in water-soluble fiber, such as oat bran and beans.

Franz MJ. *Exchanges for All Occasions: How to Use the Exchange System for Healthy and Creative Food Choices.* Alexandria, Va: American Diabetes Association; 1993. This book can help anyone to effectively use the exchange system for meal planning. It includes exchanges for Italian, Asian, and Jewish foods; sample meal plans; and planning suggestions for just about any occasion.

For Further Reading

Franz MJ. *Exchange Lists for Meal Planning*: what you should know about the 1995 version. *On the Cutting Edge.* 1996;17(2):12–14.

Holler HJ. The exchange system: a comprehensive review. In: Powers MA, ed. *Handbook of Diabetes Medical Nutrition Therapy.* Gaithersburg, Md: Aspen Publishers, Inc; 1996:227–254.

Carbohydrate Counting 20

Carbohydrate counting is a meal-planning approach used for clients with diabetes. Scientific evidence and clinical observations have shown that carbohydrate found in foods is the primary nutrient affecting postprandial blood glucose levels, and thus insulin requirements.[1] Additionally, scientific evidence shows that carbohydrate sources, whether monosaccharides, disaccharides, or polysaccharides, basically affect blood glucose levels similarly when eaten in the same gram amounts.[2,3]

Definition

In its simplest form, carbohydrate counting can be used to help people with diabetes focus on the consistency of their food consumption. At an intermediate level, the focus will be on adjustment of food, medication, and activity, based on patterns from daily records. A more advanced level of carbohydrate counting allows clients on multiple daily injections (MDI) of insulin or continuous subcutaneous insulin infusion (CSII) of regular insulin in an insulin pump to determine ratios of insulin units to grams of carbohydrate. In order to use this advanced level of carbohydrate counting with clients with diabetes, it is essential to understand intensive insulin therapy (eg, how to make food and/or insulin adjustments based on blood glucose results). It may be helpful to review the discussion of intensive insulin therapy in Chapter 7 before reading this chapter.

The *Carbohydrate Counting* series was jointly developed and published by The American Dietetic Association and American Diabetes Association in 1995. It is organized into three levels as follows:

➤ *Carbohydrate Counting: Getting Started* (Level 1) is the basic booklet, which introduces the following concepts: how each of the macronutrients (carbohydrate, protein, and fat) affect blood glucose levels and overall nutrition; which foods contain carbohydrate; the importance of consistent amounts of carbohydrate; food portions that equal one carbohydrate choice (15 grams); references for determining the carbohydrate content of foods; and developing a beginning level meal plan.

➤ *Carbohydrate Counting: Moving On* (Level 2) is the intermediate booklet, which assumes an understanding of the basic level of knowledge and focuses on educating the client to understand the relationships between food, medication, and activity. This level also teaches initial steps for making adjustments in insulin based on additions and/or deletions to usual carbohydrate intake. Intermediate carbohydrate counting allows more practice in weighing and measuring foods. The roles of fat, protein, and fiber are discussed, as well as the use of combination foods and precautions about hypoglycemia and weight gain. Learning to use a variety of references, including food labels, exchange lists, and carbohydrate reference books, is stressed for skill development.

➤ *Carbohydrate Counting: Using Carbohydrate/Insulin Ratios* (Level 3) is the advanced booklet. It assumes an understanding of the intermediate level knowledge and concentrates on the client's individual responses to food, medication, and activity. This level introduces concepts that assist clients using MDI or CSII to match insulin to carbohydrate, using carbohydrate-to-insulin ratios. Clients selected to use Level 3 carbohydrate counting should have good blood glucose control, with a well-adjusted basal dose of insulin.

Historical Background

Carbohydrate counting as a meal-planning resource has been used at some centers in the United States since 1935 and in Europe for even longer.

Nevertheless, traditional dietetics curricula have not included this meal-planning approach because of its complexity and focus on carbohydrate with minimal consideration of protein, fat, and total calories. However, carbohydrate counting was one of the four approaches used successfully in the Diabetes Control and Complications Trial (DCCT). Since the DCCT, interest in carbohydrate counting has been renewed.

Method of Use

Carbohydrate Counting: Getting Started

Four steps are involved when teaching Level 1 carbohydrate counting:

1. Determining usual food intake;
2. Practicing how to determine amounts of carbohydrate in different portion sizes of carbohydrate foods (see *Table 20.1*);
3. Figuring usual carbohydrate intake at meals and snacks;
4. Completing a meal plan with agreed-upon carbohydrate goals (see *Table 20.2*).

During Step 2, the dietitian can simultaneously assess clients' knowledge and skills for counting carbohydrate. A written carbohydrate quiz and "hands-on" food labs are useful. After the initial appointment, clients may fax or mail food records to save time at the next visit. Follow-up visits for Level 1 carbohydrate counting may include an office visit or telephone consult. During Level 1, the client and the diabetes care team should discuss a goal or target range for blood glucose levels. Daily SMBG is recommended when using Level 1 carbohydrate counting.

As part of teaching the basics of carbohydrate counting, specific carbohydrate targets should be negotiated for each meal and snack. These should be based on usual carbohydrate intake and/or nutrition goals as set by the client and the dietitian. In some cases, the dietitian may need to define carbohydrate targets when information regarding usual intake is incomplete, unavailable, or unusable. Consumption of consistent amounts of carbohydrate within

Table 20.1
Tips for Using Level 1 Carbohydrate Counting

> ➤ Encourage clients to acquire a food scale. A scale, along with measuring cups and measuring spoons, is essential.
> ➤ Clarify that the serving size listed by gram weight on a food label is not the same as the number of grams of total carbohydrate per serving.
> ➤ Emphasize the serving size on the food label may not be the same as the portion consumed or the portion equal to one carbohydrate choice.
> ➤ Encourage clients to use a calculator.
> ➤ Review foods to be measured by weight (ounces) vs volume (cups) and the difference between a level and a heaping measuring cup/tablespoon.
> ➤ Teach techniques to assess portion size skills, including:
>   • having clients "guesstimate" before they actually measure and then compare their two answers;
>   • conducting a "food lab" demonstration with hands-on practice.
> ➤ Begin teaching portion size skills on combination foods, such as casseroles, pizza, and baked goods.

specified targets enables the diabetes care team to fine-tune the diabetes self-management plan. The dietitian should assess the client's ability to adhere to a consistent carbohydrate plan, and communicate this to the other diabetes care team members.

Clients need to be provided with a meal-planning form with individual carbohydrate goals, such as that shown in Table 20.2. Self-care information (ie, SMBG, food intake, timing, diabetes medications, and physical activity) will provide data to assess the effectiveness of this approach and document the need for adjustments and/or other information.

Carbohydrate Counting: Moving On

There are three steps for teaching pattern management in Level 2 carbohydrate counting:

1. Study records of food, medication, physical activity, and blood glucose levels;
2. Interpret blood glucose patterns;
3. Determine appropriate actions or strategies to achieve blood glucose goals.

During Level 2, the client begins to learn how to adjust food, activity, and medications to improve blood glucose control. Initially, the diabetes care team makes adjustments with explanations to the client. Over time, the client assumes increasing responsibility for making adjustments, with appropriate coaching.

Table 20.3 provides a sample food and blood glucose record. The procedure for using pattern management with these sample records is described below:

➤ *Step 1—Study the data.* Identify patterns in the data. Circle prelunch blood glucose over 120 mg/dL (premeal target range). List possible explanations for blood glucose being out of range. Circle breakfast meals with greater than 65 g carbohydrate.
➤ *Step 2—Interpret the data.* Blood glucose levels are too high before lunch. Client is eating the agreed-on amount of carbohydrate at breakfast (60–65 grams).

Table 20.2

Meal-Planning Form for Level 1 Carbohydrate Counting

Meal Plan for: _____	Daily Totals
Dietitian: _____	Carbohydrate _____ g
Phone: _____	Protein _____ g
	Fat _____ g
	Calories _____

Time	Carbohydrate Choice or Grams Carbohydrate	Menu Ideas	Menu Ideas
	___ Carbohydate choices or ___ grams Carbohydrate ___ oz Meat/Meat Substitutes ___ servings Fat ___ Carbohydrate choices/grams		
	___ Carbohydate choices or ___ grams Carbohydrate ___ oz Meat/Meat Substitutes ___ servings Fat ___ Carbohydrate choices/grams		
	___ Carbohydate choices or ___ grams Carbohydrate ___ oz Meat/Meat Substitutes ___ servings Fat ___ Carbohydrate choices/grams		

Source: *Carbohydrate Counting: Getting Started* (Alexandria, Va: American Diabetes Association, Inc, and Chicago, Ill: The American Dietetic Association; 1995).

▶ *Step 3—Determine possible actions or strategies.* Possible strategies include:

- Adjust activity: Add a morning walk.
- Adjust food: Reduce breakfast carbohydrate. Divide breakfast carbohydrate into a smaller breakfast and a midmorning snack.
- Adjust or add medication: Add oral glucose-lowering medication.

Client should discuss with the diabetes care team which of the above strategies are of the highest priority.

Carbohydrate Counting: Using Carbohydrate/Insulin Ratios

At this level the dietitian and the client work together to develop the carbohydrate/insulin ratio. This is accomplished by reviewing the last two weeks of records of the amount of carbohydrate eaten and the number of units of regular insulin used to meet the target blood glucose. Ideally, the client's food consumption and physical activity will be consistent for those two weeks. The carbohydrate/insulin ratio covers the usual amounts of protein and fat, as well as the carbohydrate in the meal.

There are two methods to determine an individual carbohydrate/insulin ratio: the *carbohydrate gram method* and the *carbohydrate choice method*. Both methods allow the client to see the differences in carbohydrate/insulin ratios

Table 20.3
Sample Food and Blood Glucose Records

Name: S. Smith			BG Target: premeal less than 120 mg/dL			
Type II Diabetes			Medical nutrition therapy only			
Breakfast Carbohydrate Goal: 60–65 g						

Breakfast

Day/Date	Time	BG	Food	Serving Size	Carbohydrate	Activity
Mon 6/10	8:00	112	corn cereal	1 cup	20 g	watchTV
			milk, skim	8 oz	12 g	
			orange juice	4 oz	15 g	
			bagel	½	15 g	
	12:00	(222)		Total	62 g	
Tues 6/11	8:00	98	rice cereal	1 cup	20 g	clean
			milk, skim	8 oz	12 g	
			grapefruit	½	15 g	
			toast	1 slice	15 g	
	12:30	(229)		Total	62 g	
Wed 6/12	7:30	70	toaster waffles	3	45 g	watchTV
			margarine	2 tsp	—	
			coffee with	8 oz		
			milk	1 oz	2 g	
			syrup, light	2 tbsp	15 g	
	12:15	(201)		Total	62 g	

Source: *Carbohydrate Counting: Moving On* (Alexandria, Va: American Diabetes Association, Inc, and Chicago, Ill: The American Dietetic Association, 1995).

from one meal to another. For example, some people find their ratio at dinner to be different from their ratio at breakfast. Many clients will have a lower carbohydrate/insulin ratio at breakfast than they have at dinner. For example, at breakfast the ratio may be 10/1, while at dinner the ratio is 15/1. This means that at breakfast 1 unit insulin covers 10 grams carbohydrate, while at dinner 1 unit covers 15 grams carbohydrate. Be aware that the lower the carbohydrate/insulin ratio, the more insulin is needed to cover food consumed.

Carbohydrate Gram Method

This method allows for greater precision in matching insulin to carbohydrate and is useful for people who are more sensitive to insulin, who are on smaller doses of insulin, and who are willing to count grams of carbohydrate rather than carbohydrate choices.

Using the carbohydrate gram method to calculate the carbohydrate/insulin ratio, use the following steps (see *Table 20.4* for an example):

1. Have the client record the carbohydrate grams consistently eaten at each meal based on blood glucose levels and food records.
2. Have the client record the regular insulin doses taken before meals that consistently meet target blood glucose levels.
3. To determine the carbohydrate grams per unit of insulin for each meal, divide the total grams of carbohydrate for each meal by the number of units of regular insulin.

Table 20.4
Example of Carbohydrate Gram Method

1. Total the grams (g) of CHO that you consistently eat at each meal, using figures from the exchange lists book, food labels, and carbohydrate value books:
   Breakfast (B) __45__ g   Lunch (L) __60__ g   Supper (S) __75__ g

2. Regular insulin meal dose prescribed:
   B __4__ units   L __5__ units   S __6__ units

3. Determine the g of CHO per **one** unit of insulin for each meal by dividing the total g of CHO for the meal by the number of units of regular meal dose insulin:

   $$\frac{\text{g CHO}}{\text{units of insulin meal dose}} \quad B\ \frac{45}{4u} = 11.2\ \text{g per one unit insulin} \quad L\ \frac{60}{5u} = 12\ \text{g per one unit insulin} \quad S\ \frac{75}{6u} = 12.5\ \text{g per one unit insulin}$$

4. Average g CHO per **one** unit of insulin:

   B __11.2__ g CHO per **one** unit insulin + L __12__ g CHO per **one** unit insulin + S __12.5__ g CHO per **one** unit insulin = __35.7__ Total **divide by 3** = __12__ average g CHO per **one** unit insulin

5. CHO/insulin ratio is __12__ g CHO per **one** unit insulin.

$$\frac{\text{grams CHO}}{\text{units regular insulin}} = \_\_\_\_\ \text{grams/unit}$$

Breakfast = ___ g/u   Lunch = ____ g/u   Dinner = ____ g/u

4. If the answers in Step 3 vary from each other by no more than 1 gram carbohydrate, add the answers together and divide by 3 to get the average grams carbohydrate per unit of insulin.
5. If the answers in Step 3 vary from each other by more than 1 gram carbohydrate and the client and diabetes care team agree that the basal insulin doses are well adjusted, then use your answers to Step 3 as your carbohydrate/insulin ratios for each meal.
6. To make insulin adjustments for more or less carbohydrate eaten, add up the total carbohydrate and divide by the appropriate carbohydrate/insulin ratio.

$$\frac{\text{Total grams CHO}}{\text{gram/unit ratio}} = \_\_\_\_\ \text{units regular insulin}$$

Carbohydrate Choice Method

If your client does not want to count actual grams of carbohydrate and is familiar with carbohydrate choices or exchanges, this method will be more appropriate. The premise of this method is that 1 carbohydrate choice or exchange = 15 grams carbohydrate. This method is based on information in the *Exchange Lists for Meal Planning*. Using the carbohydrate choice method to figure the carbohydrate/insulin ratio can be accomplished by following these steps (see *Table 20.5* for an example):

Table 20.5
Example of Carbohydrate Choice Method

1. Regular insulin meal dose prescribed:
   B __4__ units   L __5__ units   S __6__ units

2. Total number of CHO choices that you consistently eat at each meal, using the exchange lists book, food labels, and carbohydrate value books:
   Breakfast (B) _3_ CHO choices   Lunch (L) _4_ CHO choices   Supper (S) _5_ CHO choices

3. Determine the units of regular insulin per CHO choice for each meal by dividing the number of units of regular insulin by the number of CHO choices:

   $\dfrac{\text{units insulin}}{\text{CHO choices}}$ B $\dfrac{4}{3}$ = 1.3 units insulin per CHO choice   L $\dfrac{5}{4}$ = 1.25 units insulin per CHO choice   S $\dfrac{6}{5}$ = 1.2 units insulin per CHO choice

4. Average units of insulin per CHO choice:

   B _1.3_ units insulin per CHO choice + L _1.25_ units insulin per CHO choice + S _1.2_ units insulin per CHO choice = _3.75_ Total **divide by 3** = 1 (if MDI) 1.2 (if CSII)* average units insulin per CHO choice

5. CHO/insulin ratio is __1 or 1.2__ units insulin per CHO choice.

*Clients using an insulin pump can deliver insulin in tenths of a unit.

---

1. Have the client record the regular insulin doses taken before meals that consistently meet established target blood glucose levels based on the client's blood glucose and food records.
2. Have the client record the number of carbohydrate choices that are eaten consistently at each meal.
3. Determine the units of regular insulin per carbohydrate choice for each meal by dividing the number of units by the number of carbohydrate choices.

   $\dfrac{\text{units regular insulin}}{\text{carbohydrate choices}}$ = _____ units per CHO choice

   Breakfast = ___ units per CHO choice
   Lunch   = ___ units per CHO choice
   Dinner   = ___ units per CHO choice

   Carbohydrate/insulin ratio = ___ units per CHO choice

4. If the answers to Step 3 vary by more than 1 unit per CHO choice, have the client use more than one ratio.
5. To make insulin adjustments for more or fewer carbohydrate choices, add up the total carbohydrate choices and multiply by the client's ratio (unit/CHO choice).

   Total CHO choices ____ × ____ unit/CHO choice = ___ units regular

185

Comparison of Carbohydrate Gram and Carbohydrate Choice Methods

The carbohydrate gram method offers more precise insulin adjustments for the grams of carbohydrate that are eaten. To fine-tune the adjustments using this method, it is important for the client to weigh and measure foods and use food label information, along with carbohydrate reference books. Estimating carbohydrate to be eaten based on the *Exchange Lists for Meal Planning* or the carbohydrate choice method is simpler, but not as accurate. An essential factor is accurate weighing and measuring of foods to match the portion sizes in the exchange lists. *Table 20.6* demonstrates the difference between the two methods.

Other Considerations Related to Carbohydrate Counting

Weight Gain

Weight management is a concern for most people with diabetes. Clients with type II diabetes tend to be overweight and may improve glycemic control with modest weight loss.[4,5] Based on the results of the DCCT, people with type I diabetes who are on intensive insulin therapy are at increased risk for weight gain—approximately 10 pounds in the first year.[6,7]

Using carbohydrate counting increases the client's flexibility when dining out or desiring an occasional treat of a favorite candy or dessert. With that flexibility also comes the possibility of weight gain. Clients on insulin therapy may consume extra calories from additional carbohydrate while maintaining nearly normal blood glucose levels through adjustment of insulin doses. Clients may keep their carbohydrate intake consistent, but not pay attention to added protein and fat intake. Also, better glucose control reduces wasting calories through glycosuria and therefore can promote weight gain. Self-management training regarding food/blood glucose trade-offs and reminders that protein and fat calories do count are especially important when the enjoyment of meal-planning flexibility alters more regimented eating habits.

Hypoglycemia

In the DCCT, the risk of severe hypoglycemia was approximately three times greater during intensive therapy than during conventional therapy.[8] The client should be educated regarding:

- signs and symptoms of hypoglycemia (adrenergic and neuroglycopenic) and the fact that these symptoms are often more difficult to identify with tighter blood glucose control;
- appropriate hypoglycemia treatment;
- readily available carbohydrate source; and
- regular use of SMBG to reduce and manage the risk.

Overtreatment of hypoglycemia should be pointed out as a potential cause of subsequent hyperglycemia and weight gain. Frequency of hypoglycemia and inappropriate treatment both contribute to weight gain.[9,10] See Chapter 10 for detailed treatment guidelines for hypogylcemia.

Clients who increase insulin doses to cover extra carbohydrate in meals need to be especially vigilant about the possibility of hypoglycemia, especially at night. Alterations in insulin doses should not be attempted unless the client is educated in how to make these adjustments appropriately.

Erratic Schedules

The client who works swing shifts, travels often, or has erratic schedules can benefit remarkably from the use of intensive insulin therapy (ie, multiple

Table 20.6
Comparison of Carbohydrate Counting Methods

Food	Carbohydrate Gram (g) Method	Carbohydrate Choice Method
1½ cups cooked noodles	55 g	3
½ cup broccoli cooked†	5 g	0
1 small roll (1 oz)*	14 g	1
3 oz pork tenderloin	0 g	0
½ cup fruit cocktail†	15 g	1
2 tsp margarine	0 g	0
Totals	89 g	5 choices or 75 g

*Foods to weigh if label information not available.
†Foods to measure with measuring cup if using grams on food label or exchanges.

Source: *Carbohydrate Counting: Using Carbohydrate/Insulin Ratios* (Alexandria, Va: American Diabetes Association, Inc, and The American Dietetic Association; 1995).

daily injections or an insulin pump) and the flexibility provided by carbohydrate counting. Knowledge of the carbohydrate content of various foods will allow the client to use available foods (eg, vending machines, airline meals) to substitute appropriately for usual carbohydrate foods in the meal plan.

Nutrient-Related Factors Affecting Blood Glucose Levels

Fat Intake

A meal high in fat can slow gastric emptying and thereby blunt the postprandial rise in blood glucose levels.[11] To check the effect of high-fat meals, the dietitian may suggest that clients occasionally check blood glucose 3 to 4 hours postprandially. If a pattern of elevated blood glucose emerges, an adjustment of the long-acting insulin dose or the short-acting premeal insulin may be appropriate. If the client understands how fat may affect blood glucose, he or she will be able to plan for the slower absorption of food.

In assessing the impact of fat, it may be helpful to think about the client's eating pattern in one of the following ways: 1) usual diet is high in fat; 2) particular meals tend to be high in fat; or 3) occasional high-fat foods are consumed. For the client who typically consumes a high-fat diet, the dose of insulin or glucose-lowering medication may already accommodate that level of fat.

Protein Intake

Research is limited on the effects of protein ingestion on blood glucose levels. While it has been traditionally taught that 50% to 60% of protein is converted to glucose, there is research that suggests that protein has a limited effect on blood glucose levels.[11,12] A significant change in the protein content of a meal—for example, eating 10 oz of prime rib instead of a usual serving of 3 oz of cooked lean meat—can produce a delay in postprandial blood glucose levels and may require an insulin adjustment. It is not known whether this effect is due to the increased fat or protein content, and the effects of protein and fat on blood glucose levels need additional research. However, until such research is available, variations in blood glucose associated with variable fat and protein intake should be evaluated and addressed pragmatically, by modifying insulin and/or food intake to minimize glucose excursion. For the client who is consuming a high-protein meal, a recommendation can be made to do one of the following:

- increase insulin at the meal;
- take the usual amount of insulin, then take additional insulin following the meal; or
- take an insulin supplement 3 to 5 hours later when the extra protein is being absorbed and converted to glucose.

Then follow up with SMBG to check effectiveness of the above.

Fiber Intake

Soluble fiber delays the absorption of glucose, but the effect on postprandial glucose is not significant.[3,13,14] However, foods high in fiber are a healthy addition to a meal plan. Since fiber is not completely digested and absorbed, and is unavailable as glucose, a high-fiber meal would not provide as much available carbohydrate as a low-fiber meal of similar total carbohydrate content. One strategy for dealing with blood glucose variations associated with variable fiber intake is to subtract the grams of total dietary fiber from the total carbohydrate in determining the available carbohydrate. When there are 5 or more grams fiber per serving, subtract them from the total grams of carbohydrate to determine how much carbohydrate is available. For example, a breakfast cereal containing 28 grams carbohydrate per serving with 6 grams dietary fiber can be counted as 22 grams carbohydrate.

Intended Population for Use

Carbohydrate counting may be used in clients with all types of diabetes and from all age groups, including children, adolescents, and the elderly. Level 1 carbohydrate counting can be used in clients with type I diabetes, newly diagnosed or long-standing type II diabetes, and gestational diabetes mellitus (GDM). Clients who understand how to use the exchange system have a great start toward learning carbohydrate counting. However, carbohydrate counting may also be used as an initial approach, or as an alternative for people frustrated by other meal-planning systems.

Level 2 carbohydrate counting may be used in clients on medical nutrtition therapy only, oral glucose-lowering medications, and/or insulin. For clients not taking insulin, Level 2 carbohydrate counting is as in-depth as would be necessary.

Level 3 carbohydrate counting is designed for people who take insulin (MDI or an insulin pump) and choose to practice intensive diabetes self-management. Candidates for Level 3 carbohydrate counting ideally will have well-controlled blood glucose (ie, meeting target blood glucose range with current regimen) before starting. Further, clients should have demonstrated skill in insulin adjustment and insulin supplementation, and should have already been selected for intensive therapy based on their level of responsibility and motivation to be key players on the diabetes care team. Some clients may require a psychological assessment by a mental health professional involved with the diabetes care team. Clients must also have financial resources or adequate insurance coverage to manage the costs of additional visits to the diabetes care team.

Clinical Setting

Carbohydrate counting may be introduced in either the inpatient or ambulatory care setting. The ambulatory care setting offers the advantage of experiencing the effects of living in the "real world" while making adjustments to the new regimen. However, the inpatient setting offers the opportunity for frequent observation of response to insulin doses, and the ability to make adjustments or treat hypoglycemia promptly. Dietitians working in inpatient settings need carbohydrate counting skills to assist clients who use carbohydrate counting during their hospital stays. In the inpatient setting, the dietitian and the diabetes care team often have the opportunity to discuss food and insulin relationships on a meal-by-meal basis, thus ensuring that the client is documenting correctly and making appropriate observations, and possesses basic problem-solving skills.

Carbohydrate counting is recommended for use in settings where dietitians are available to do the teaching. Determining nutrition intervention priorities and choosing meal-planning approaches to match a client's needs are skills dietitians are best trained to perform. Other team members must work closely with dietitians to co-manage clients, assess client adherence with the particular plan recommended by the team dietitian, and know when to refer to or consult with the dietitian.

Level 1 carbohydrate counting is recommended for ambulatory care settings and hospitals where dietitians are available to do the education. Level 2 carbohydrate counting was developed for use by dietitians who have special training or experience in diabetes care and education, rather than dietitians who see clients with diabetes only occasionally. These dietitians are skilled in using blood glucose monitoring; interpreting blood glucose results; and discussing adjustments in food, activity, and medication. Level 3 carbohydrate counting was developed for dietitians who practice with a diabetes care team that is trained in intensive insulin therapy. The ambulatory care setting is most appropriate for establishing carbohydrate/insulin ratios.

Length of Time to Teach

Teaching clients to count carbohydrate requires multiple visits to allow time to gather, study, and interpret records. A carbohydrate counting checklist (*Table 20.7*) has been developed to give the dietitian a list of teaching activities to consider using.

Advantages/ Disadvantages

An advantage of *Carbohydrate Counting: Getting Started* (Level 1) is that it is focused on a single nutrient (carbohydrate) and may be less complex and offer more flexibility for some clients with diabetes than other methods of meal planning. *Carbohydrate Counting: Moving On* (Level 2) offers the same advantages but has additional potential for improving blood glucose control because of the focus on pattern management and adjustment of the carbohydrate level in response to blood glucose results. *Carbohydrate Counting: Using Carbohydrate/Insulin Ratios* (Level 3) has the same advantages as Levels 1 and 2, but has the greatest potential for fine-tuning blood glucose levels because of the ability to adjust both carbohydrate and insulin levels.

A disadvantage of all methods of carbohydrate counting may be undesirable weight gain because of the focus on carbohydrate and the inattention to total calories and fat. Carbohydrate counting may also result in the selection of fewer healthful food choices. All levels of carbohydrate counting require math skills. Levels 2 and 3 involve more advanced math skills and an addi-

Table 20.7
Carbohydrate Counting Checklist

Activities	Pre	LEVEL ONE	LEVEL TWO	LEVEL THREE
Patient contact	Pre	1 to 3	1 to 3	1 to 3
Contact intervals		1 to 4 weeks	1 to 2 weeks	1 to 2 weeks
Length of visit		30 to 90 minutes	30 to 60 minutes	30 to 60 minutes
Nutrition/diabetes history	X			
Why count carbo		X		
Starch vs sugar		X		
Effects of carbo		X	X	X
Effects of pro/fat		X	X	X
Good nutrition		X	X	X
Intro to carb choices		X		
Portion control		X	X	X
Food labels		X	X	X
Carbo resources			X	X
Set goals for carb*		X	X	X
Set goals for BG*		X	X	X
Keep food BG med records		X	X	
Assess readiness for next level*	X	X	X	
Review BG records*			X	X
Evaluate BG patterns*			X	X
Adjust plan*			X	X
Restaurant meals			X	X
Combo foods			X	X
Fiber			X	X
Choices vs grams		X	X	X
Estimate carb/insulin ratio				X
Use carb/insulin ratios				X
Snacking		X	X	X
Alcohol		X	X	X
Avoid wt gain		X	X	X

*Contact/activities can be done at visit, by phone or by fax.

tional time commitment for record keeping. Another disadvantage of carbohydrate counting is the added expense of SMBG for some individuals. Because Level 3 carbohydrate counting puts emphasis on tight blood glucose control, another disadvantage is the additional risk of hypoglycemia.

Summary

Since the DCCT, there is renewed interest in the United States in carbohydrate counting as a meal-planning approach for clients with diabetes. Carbohydrate counting can be used for all types of diabetes in clients of all age groups. Three levels of carbohydrate counting have been identified, based on increasing levels of complexity and skills required. All dietitians who practice clinical diabetes care should expand their skills in meal-planning approaches to include at least Level 1 carbohydrate counting. Since carbohydrate counting has not been widely used by dietitians, finding continuing education opportunities to increase professional knowledge and skills in using this approach will be helpful.

References

1. Nuttall FQ. Carbohydrate and dietary management of clients with insulin-requiring diabetes. *Diabetes Care.* 1993;16:1039–1042.
2. American Diabetes Association nutrition recommendations and principles for people with diabetes mellitus. *Diabetes Care.* 1994;17:519–522.
3. Franz MJ, Horton ES, Bantle JP, Beebe CA, Brunzell JD, Coulston AM, Henry RR, Hoogwerf BJ, Stacpoole PW. Nutrition principles for the management of diabetes and related complications (technical review). *Diabetes Care.* 1994;17:490–518.
4. Wing RR, Shoemaker M, Marcus MD, McDermott M, Gooding W. Variables associated with weight loss and improvements in glycemic control in type II diabetic patients in behavioral weight control programs. *Int J Obes.* 1990;14:495–503.
5. Watts NB, Spanheimer RG, DiGirolamo M. Gebhart SS, Musey VC, Siddiq K, Phillips LS. Prediction of glucose response to weight loss in patients with non-insulin-dependent diabetes mellitus. *Arch Intern Med.* 1990;150:803–806.
6. Diabetes Control and Complications Trial Research Group. The effect of intensive treatment of diabetes on the development and progression of long-term complications in insulin-dependent diabetes mellitus. *N Engl J Med.* 1993;329:977–986.
7. Diabetes Control and Complications Trial Research Group. Weight gain associated with intensive therapy in the Diabetes Control and Complication Trial. *Diabetes Care.* 1988;11(5):67–73.
8. Diabetes Control and Complications Trial Research Group. Epidemiology of severe hypoglycemia in the Diabetes Control and Complications Trial. *Am J Med.* 1991;90:450–459.
9. Cryer PE, Fisher JN, Shamoon H. Hypoglycemia (technical review). *Diabetes Care.* 1994;17:734–755.
10. Wheeler ML. Summary and comment on treatment of insulin reactions in diabetics in hypoglycemia: applications of current research. *Diabetes Spectrum.* 1988;1:307–308.
11. Peters AL, Davidson MB. Protein and fat effects on glucose response and insulin requirements in subjects with insulin-dependent diabetes mellitus. *Am J Clin Nutr.* 1993;58:555–560.
12. Nuttall FQ, Mooradien AD, Gannon MC. Effects of protein ingestion on the glucose and insulin response to standardized oral glucose load. *Diabetes Care.* 1984;7:465–470.
13. Nuttall, FQ. Perspectives in diabetes: dietary fiber in the management of diabetes. *Diabetes.* 1993;42:503–508.
14. Wursch, P. Dietary fiber and unabsorbed carbohydrates. In: Gracey M, Kretchmer N, Rossi E, eds. *Sugars in Nutrition.* Vol. 25. New York, NY: Raven; 1991:153–168.

Ordering Information for Resources Described

Carbohydrate Counting Series: Getting Started (Level 1), Moving On (Level 2), Using Carbohydrate/Insulin Ratios (Level 3) are available in packages of 10 each from The American Dietetic Association by calling 800/877-1600, ext 5000, or by calling the American Diabetes Association at 800/ADA-ORDER.

Additional Resources

Brackenridge BP, Frederickson L, Reed C. *Carbohydrate Counting: How to Zero in on Good Control.* Sylmar, Calif: MiniMed Technologies; 1995. 1-800-933-3322.
Exchange Lists for Meal Planning. Chicago, Ill: The American Dietetic Association and American Diabetes Association; 1995.
Krause B. *Calories and Carbohydrates,* 11th ed. New York: Penguin; 1995.
Netzer C. *The Complete Book of Food Counts.* New York: Dell Publishing; 1994.
Ruggles MF. *The Carbohydrate Counting Kit.* Booklet and camera-ready handouts, basic to intermediate levels of carbohydrate counting. $26.95 + $1.50 shipping and handling. Payable to Marie F Ruggles, MS, RD, 185 Cypress St, Floral Park, NY 11001.

For Further Reading

Brackenridge BP. Carbohydrate gram counting: a key to accurate mealtime boluses in intensive diabetes therapy. *Practical Diabetology.* 1992;11:22–28.
Choppin S, Jovanovic-Peterson L, Peterson CM. Matching food with insulin. *Diabetes Professional.* 1991(spring):1–14.

Daly A. A graduated approach to carbohydrate counting. *Practical Diabetology.* 1996;15(1): 19–23.

Daly A, Gillespie S, Kulkarni K. Tales from carboland. *Diabetes Forecast.* 1997;50(1):34–39.

Daly A, Gillespie S, Kulkarni K. Carbohydrate counting: vignettes from the trenches. *Diabetes Spectrum.* 1996;9(2):114–117.

Gillespie S. Meal planning approaches for management of intensive insulin therapy. In: Green Pastors J, Holler HJ, eds. *Meal Planning Approaches for Diabetes Management.* 2nd ed. Chicago, Ill: American Dietetic Association; 1994: 99–120.

Gregory RP, Davis DL. Use of carbohydrate counting for meal planning in type I diabetes. *Diabetes Educator.* 1994;20:406–409.

Rafkin-Mervis L. Carbo counting. *Diabetes Forecast.* 1995;48(2):30–37.

21 Calorie and Fat Counting

Calorie counting is a structured meal-planning approach that places major emphasis on the caloric density of food. This approach provides the client with a specific calorie limit to achieve weight loss. The client is given a calorie reference book to look up calorie values of foods, and completed food records along with calorie calculations are necessary.

As early as 1902, the relationship between energy intake and regulation of body weight can be found in the literature, and the use of calorie counting as a treatment for weight loss has been used since 1925.[1] Caloric restriction is associated with improved insulin sensitivity and glycemic control.[2] Although limited, studies have explored the benefit of using calorie counting in obese clients or examining the outcome differences between calorie counting and the exchange system. Wing and coworkers found that weight losses were greater using a calorie counting–lifestyle change approach than using an exchange-list approach during a 16-week intervention study in obese clients with type II diabetes.[3] Similar results were seen in an 8-week crossover German study when comparing exchange lists to calorie counting.[4] Fasting blood glucose and weight loss were slightly better in the calorie-counting group. Eighty-three percent of participants preferred the calorie counting method, citing simplicity and flexibility as major reasons for the preference.

No differences in weight, blood lipids, or glycemic control were seen in a longer study (18 months) of 70 participants with type II diabetes when comparing three sets of nutrition prescriptions (weight-management, high-carbohydrate, and lipid-lowering meal plans). Nutrition intervention, regardless of the prescription, was thought to be related to improvements in glycemic control and weight loss.[5] Nevertheless, participants found it difficult to meet recommended nutrient intakes in the long term. In obese clients without diabetes, lower attrition, improved compliance, and superior weight losses were seen with calorie-counting approaches more often than with traditional exchange lists.[6] It appears from these studies that calorie counting may provide an effective alternative for obese clients, with or without diabetes. Short-term studies indicate superior results and greater client preference with calorie-counting methods. Long-term issues with adherence, weight loss/maintenance, and permanent lifestyle change remain a challenge for the practitioner regardless of the method used.[7,8] However, tailoring the nutrition intervention to the client will facilitate initiation of change.[9,10]

Calorie Counting

Definition

Historical Background

Method of Use

The use of a food record form is the initial step for implementing calorie counting. The client is instructed to keep daily food records for 1 to 2 weeks. This step allows information to be collected that will help the client and the dietitian formulate individual nutrition goals and establish a calorie level that will achieve a negotiable weight loss. The client then is provided with a calorie book or list and asked to continue to keep food records, incorporating the established daily calorie goal. To also promote glycemic control, it is important to provide the client with blood glucose record forms and establish target glucose goals. Follow-up sessions provide an opportunity to review food records for assessing comprehension and to discuss individualized strategies for behavioral change.

Intended Population for Use

The calorie-counting approach is most appropriate for the obese client with type II diabetes who desires more accuracy in calculating calorie intake and who does not understand or want the structure of the exchange system. The calorie-counting method may be an appropriate alternative for clients who have experienced failure on other nutrition regimes. This method allows for flexibility in food choices and calorie intake so that a lapse does not lead to an "all-or-nothing" cognitive reaction.[11] Allowing the client to develop knowledge and eating management skills to deal with occasional slips, building healthy eating attitudes, and redefining foods into "choices" rather than "good" or "bad" is desirable, especially if long-term weight loss, glycemic control, and self-management skills are desired outcomes. The implementation and success of calorie counting will depend on the time available and the amount of participation from the client.[12,13] Additional follow-up with SMBG is necessary to evaluate the effectiveness of this approach in achieving improved glycemic control.

Clinical Setting

An ambulatory care situation provides the optimal setting for this approach, especially if the client continues self-management training for any length of time. However, the approach could be used in an inpatient setting if the client has adequate knowledge of nutrition. In this situation, ambulatory care follow-up would be desirable to further the educational process and provide support for lifestyle change and weight loss. This approach can be used in a group setting or for individual nutrition self-mangement training.

Length of Time to Teach

The teaching time required for this approach is at least one hour. However, follow-up sessions are recommended to suggest further changes in eating, evaluate or monitor food and SMBG records, and provide support for behavior change.

Advantages/Disadvantages

A major advantage of the calorie-counting approach is the expanded choice of foods and the flexibility in meal planning. Also, this approach promotes the concept of preplanning, through the technique of "banking" calories. Clients can develop skills to make choices through a process of accounting for and budgeting calories. For example, a special occasion dinner may cost 800 calories. The client accounts for this by limiting that day's calories or by "banking" extra calories for several days.

The biggest disadvantage with calorie counting is the inattention to glycemia and the focus on weight loss. Another disadvantage of calorie counting may be the amount of time involved in record keeping and calculation. A moderate degree of literacy is required. Calorie counting may also be more difficult to follow than less structured alternative approaches because it involves a restriction of calories. Calorie counting, by itself, does not produce a nutritionally balanced eating plan; combined with a guidelines approach, it does.

Fat Counting

Definition

Fat counting offers another approach to meal planning for overweight clients who are willing to keep food records. It is a simple self-monitoring approach that allows clients to have a considerable amount of flexibility and control over their food choices. A daily fat allowance is established, and the client counts the grams of fat he or she eats at each meal and snack. When explaining the concept, one could compare the daily fat allowance to a bank account. Instead of money, a limited number of fat grams is deposited into the client's account each day. These fat grams can be "spent" as desired until the account is empty.

Historical Background

Counting grams of fat evolved during the 1980s as a self-monitoring tool for clients following low-fat diets to reduce the risk of cancer. The system has been successfully used in several cancer prevention trials, in which clients learned to reduce fat intake to 15% to 25% of total calories. In developing the nutrition components of these trials, researchers realized the difficulties of establishing dietary guidelines based on percentage of calories from fat. Counting grams of fat was simpler, and the concept was easier for clients to grasp, since most Americans are familiar with counting calories or carbohydrates.[14,15]

Gradually, the concept has become more widely used in two other areas—cardiovascular disease and weight management. For weight management, fat counting helps clients learn how to reduce calorie intake by making low-fat food choices while still maintaining a sense of control over what they eat. They tend to react positively because they do not feel restricted or externally controlled. No clinical studies have been conducted to evaluate the effectiveness of this approach to managing diabetes. However, it is yet another alternative for clients with diabetes to consider. When combined with SMBG, it may be beneficial to some clients.

Method of Use

After determining the fat gram goal, the daily fat allowance is calculated in three steps:

1. Estimate daily calorie requirements.
2. Multiply daily calorie requirement by percentage of calories from fat (should be individualized based on treatment goals) to determine how many calories per day should come from fat.
3. To convert daily calories from fat into daily grams of fat, divide calories from fat by 9 (1 g fat = 9 calories).

Example:
1. Daily calorie requirement = 1,800
2. 30% fat (amount determined from treatment goals) × 1,800 calories = 540 calories per day from fat
3. 540 calories divided by 9 calories per gram = 60 g of fat per day

The client is taught to monitor daily fat intake by recording food consumption and noting the fat content of each food. There are many resources available to help clients identify the fat content of the foods they eat. Food labels now include this information, so it is important to teach clients how to understand nutrition labeling. Many fast-food restaurants have nutrient information pamphlets available and resources are available in most major bookstores.

In tailoring this approach for use with clients, it is also important to emphasize that the general nutritional guidelines for managing diabetes must still be observed. To promote glycemic control, it is important to provide the client with blood glucose record forms and establish target blood glucose goals. These include eating regular meals and snacks, emphasizing starch, and including sucrose in moderation as part of a mixed meal.

Intended Population for Use

The fat-counting approach is useful as a weight reduction tool for clients with type I and type II diabetes, particularly those who have become frustrated by previous unsuccessful attempts to lose weight. It is also appropriate for clients with elevated blood lipids and for those who have had difficulty with other meal-planning resources.

Clients introduced to this approach must be capable of reading food labels and books that provide information about the fat content of foods. They must also be willing and able to keep daily food records. For this reason, the system is not appropriate for children or for clients with limited reading skills.

Clinical Setting

Fat counting can be taught in an inpatient or ambulatory care setting. Ambulatory care follow-up would be desirable to further the educational process and provide support for lifestyle change and/or weight loss. This approach can be used in a group setting or individual nutrition self-management training.

Length of Time to Teach

The fat-counting approach can be explained in one teaching session, but follow-up is recommended. A minimum of one additional session should be scheduled after the client has had an opportunity to use the system. Most clients need additional instruction in estimating the fat content of unfamiliar foods, foods with many ingredients, and foods eaten away from home. As in all types of nutrition counseling, longer follow-up enhances compliance and success.

Advantages/ Disadvantages

Counting fat grams simplifies the process of nutrition monitoring and eliminates the difficulty of translating a portion of food into exchanges. But the flexibility and personal control the system offers may be its most important strength. Clients who use fat counting usually improve the overall quality of their food intake as well. As they become more aware of the fat content of various foods, they tend to select more fruits, vegetables, grains, and low-fat dairy products.

The primary disadvantage with fat counting is the inattention to glycemia and the focus on weight loss. Another disadvantage of fat counting is the obvious time commitment of record keeping, including recording food intake and determining the fat content of foods. In clients with diabetes, it is also important to consider the potential impact of a higher intake of carbohydrate. This may aggravate blood glucose and triglyceride levels, and overcompensation for reduced fat intake by ad lib eating of low-fat foods. Clients whose fat intake is initially very high are those who respond best.

References

1. Forbes JB. Energy intake and body weight: a reexamination of two "classic" studies. *J Clin Nutr.* 1984;39:349–350.
2. Wing RR, Blair EH, Bononi P, et al. Caloric restriction per se is a significant factor in improvements in glycemic control and insulin sensitivity during weight loss in obese NIDDM patients. *Diabetes Care.* 1994;17:30–36.
3. Wing RR, Nowalk MP, Epstein LH, et al. Calorie counting compared to exchange system diets in the treatment of overweight patients with type II diabetes. *Addict Behav.* 1986;11:163–168.
4. Keller U, Wakernagel C, Messer C, Riesen W. [Comparison of a calorie-defined diet with the conventional exchange diet in type 2 diabetes mellitus.] (German) Schweizerische Medizinische Wochenschrift. *Journal Suisse de Medecin.* 1991;121:1014–1019.
5. Mine RM, Mann JI, Chisholm AW, Williams SM. Long-term comparison of three dietary prescriptions in the treatment of NIDDM. *Diabetes Care.* 1994;17:74–80.
6. Ciaverella PA, Atkinson RL. Dietary therapy: exchange system vs calorie counting. *Diabetes.* 1983;32(suppl 1):6A.
7. Uusitupa M, Laitinen J, Siitonen O, et al. The maintenance of improved metabolic control after intensified diet therapy in recent type 2 diabetes. *Diabetes Res Clin Pract.* 1993;19:227–238.
8. Close EJ, Wiles PG, Lockton JA, et al. Diabetic diets and nutritional recommendations: what happens in real life? *Diabetic Med.* 1992;9:181–188.
9. Franz MJ, Horton ES Sr, Bantle JP, et al. Nutrition principles for the management of diabetes and related complications (review). *Diabetes Care.* 1994;17:490–518.
10. Franz MJ. Practice guidelines for nutrition care by dietetics practitioners for outpatients with non-insulin-dependent diabetes mellitus (consensus statement). *J Am Diet Assoc.* 1992;92:1136–1139.
11. Wilson GT. Relation of dieting and voluntary weight loss to psychological functioning and binge eating. *Ann Intern Med.* 1993;11(9):727–730.
12. Guare JC, Wing RR, Marcus MD, et al. Analysis of changes in eating behavior and weight loss in type II diabetic patients. *Diabetes Care.* 1989;12:500–503.
13. Wing RR. Behavioral strategies for weight reduction in obese type II diabetic patients. *Diabetes Care.* 1989;12:139–144.
14. Gorbach SL, Morrill-LaBrode A, Woods MN, Dwyer JT, Selles, WD, Henderson M, et al. Changes in food patterns during a low-fat dietary intervention in women. *J Am Diet Assoc.* 1990;90:802–809.
15. Buzzard IM, Asp EH, Chlebowski RT, Boyar AP, Jeffery, RW, Nixon DW, et al. Diet intervention methods to reduce fat intake: nutrient and food group composition of self-selected low-fat diets. *J Am Diet Assoc.* 1990;90:42–53.

Resources

Bellerson KJ. *The Complete and Up-to-Date Fat Book.* Garden City Park, NY: Avery Publishing Group; 1993.
Bellerson KJ. *The Shoppers Guide to Fat in Your Food.* Garden City Park, NY: Avery Publishing Group; 1994.
Carper J. *The All in One Calorie Counter.* 3rd ed. New York, NY: Bantam Books; 1994.
Dietary Treatment of Hypercholesterolemia: A Manual for Patients. Dallas, Tex: American Heart Association; 1988.
Krause B. *Calories and Carbohydrates.* 11th ed. New York, NY: Penguin Group; 1995.
LeGette B. *LeGette's Calorie Encyclopedia.* New York, NY: Time Warner; 1994.

National Dairy Council. *Calorie Catalog.* 4th ed. Rosemont, Ill: National Dairy Council; 1992.

Natow AB, Heslins JA. *The Supermarket Nutrition Counter.* New York, NY: Pocket Books; 1995.

Netzer C. *The Complete Book of Food Counts.* 3rd ed. New York, NY: Dell Publishing Company; 1994.

Roth H. *Harriet Roth's Fat Counter.* New York, NY: Signet Books; 1993.

Sonberg L. *The Quick and Easy Fat Gram and Calorie Counter.* New York, NY: Avon Books, 1992.

Step by Step: Eating to Lower Your High Blood Cholesterol. Washington, DC: National Institutes of Health, National Heart, Lung, and Blood Institute; 1994. NIH Publication No. 94-2920.

Ulene A. *The Nutribase Guide to Fat and Cholesterol in Your Food.* Garden City Park, NY: Avery Publishing Group; 1995.

Ulene A. *The Nutribase Guide to Fat and Fiber in Your Food.* Garden City Park, NY: Avery Publishing Group; 1995.

Part 5
Case Studies and Conclusion

Case Studies of Clinical Application

22

This chapter provides seven case studies that demonstrate the use of various meal-planning resources in different individual situations. These are only examples and are not intended to be strict guidelines for providing diabetes self-management training in nutrition. The case studies use the various resources discussed earlier in the book, and have been developed using the type II diabetes practice guidelines[1,2] (as discussed in Chapter 3) as the framework for providing diabetes medical nutrition therapy to a variety of different clients. Emphasis has been put on the importance of using nutrition assessment and goal setting to develop a diabetes self-management training plan that meets the unique needs of each client.

References

1. Monk A, Barry B, McClain K, Weaver T, Cooper N, Franz M. Practice guidelines for medical nutrition therapy provided by dietitians for persons with non-insulin-dependent diabetes mellitus. *J Am Diet Assoc.* 1995;95:999–1006.
2. *Nutrition Practice Guidelines for Type I and Type II Diabetes Mellitus.* Chicago, Ill: American Dietetic Association; 1996.

Case Study 1

Sarah is a 35-year-old Pima Indian woman of the Gila River Indian Community of Arizona.

Demographic Information

Client is referred by the Gila River Indian Community Health Clinic to the Gila River Diabetes Education Program for continued education for newly diagnosed type II diabetes.

Referral Data

Medical nutrition therapy only.

Diabetes Treatment Regimen

Random blood glucose: 250 mg/dL
Cholesterol: 160 mg/dL
LDL cholesterol: N/A
Blood pressure: 130/80

Glycosylated hemoglobin (HgbA$_{1c}$): 8.1%
HDL cholesterol: N/A
Triglycerides: 160 mg/dL
Microalbumin: N/A

Laboratory Values

Unremarkable.

Medical History

201

Diabetes Medical Nutrition Therapy

Diabetes History Sarah has a strong family history of diabetes and obesity; her mother died of complications of diabetes at the age of 55, and her older sister and maternal aunts have diabetes. She is fearful of her diagnosis; she thought she would develop diabetes, but not so soon. Her older sister has been able to manage her diabetes without the use of medication.

Medications That Affect Therapy None.

Exercise Guidelines Client has no exercise limitations, and has medical clearance to increase physical activity.

Medical Treatment Goals for Client Target blood glucose levels: fasting: 80–140 mg/dL
postmeal 100–180 mg/dL
Target glycosylated hemoglobin (HgbA$_{1c}$) level: 6–7.5%
Self-monitoring (method, frequency, education, evaluation): refer to diabetes education program.

Education Completed Physician explained the definition and etiology of type II diabetes and provided the client with a brochure on "What Is Diabetes?" that summarized this information. He also emphasized the importance of moderate weight loss, healthy eating, and increased physical activity for the management of type II diabetes. He provided Sarah with a copy of *The First Step in Diabetes Meal Planning* as an initial step to make some changes in her current food habits.

Nutrition Assessment

Clinical Data Physical information: Height: 64 inches
Weight: 210 pounds
Body frame: medium
Reasonable body weight: 190–200 pounds
Estimated daily energy needs: approximately 2,000 calories

*Nutrition History** Usual food intake: Breakfast: seldom eats before 11 AM
Lunch (11 AM–1 PM): refried tepary beans, squash, tomato, flour tortilla
PM snack: two 20-oz soft drinks, homemade cookies
Dinner (7–8 PM, usually at home): red chili stew with beef and potatoes, fry bread, canned peaches or pineapple, iced tea
HS snack (9–10 PM, at home): taco chips or cookies, 20-oz soft drink
Nutrition evaluation: Energy intake: 2,250 calories
Frequency and timing of meals: no breakfast, inclusion of PM and HS snacks
Other nutritional concerns: high-calorie, simple-carbohydrate, high-fat, low-nutrient-density snacks
Weight history: at maximum weight of 210 pounds; stable for the past 5 years
Appetite/eating/digestion problems: N/A

*Information summarized from the Lifestyle Change Questionnaire, a resource from *Facilitating Lifestyle Change*.

Eating outside the home: seldom eats out
Alcohol intake: N/A
Use of vitamins/minerals/supplements: N/A

None; interested in increasing physical activity.   *Exercise History*

Sarah is married and lives with her three children (ages 6, 10, 18), one grandchild (age 1 year), husband, and 65-year-old father. Sarah is responsible for food preparation and shopping.   *Psychosocial and Economic Issues*

None; interested in learning.   *Blood Glucose Monitoring*

Sarah is a high school graduate. She has some knowledge about diabetes, but has some misconceptions about it from experience with her mother's diabetes.   *Knowledge, Skills, Attitudes, and Motivation*

- ➤ Review the healthy eating guidelines in *The First Step in Diabetes Meal Planning* brochure; ask Sarah to put a check mark by each statement that describes her current eating behavior.
- ➤ Review the serving sizes using the inside of *The First Step in Diabetes Meal Planning*; emphasize eating a higher number of servings from food groups at the base of the pyramid.

Initial Nutrition Intervention (with RN)

Food/Meal Planning

- ➤ Demonstrate the technique of self-monitoring of blood glucose using a glucose meter; ask Sarah to monitor her blood glucose level 3–4 times a week at random times throughout the day.
- ➤ Review target blood glucose levels.

Blood Glucose Monitoring

- ➤ Encourage Sarah to start a walking program of daily walks up to 15 minutes in duration.

Exercise

Nutrition/behavior goals are developed collaboratively by the client and diabetes educator. A number of goals have been noted, but in actual practice only one or two may be established at each visit. The number of visits and circumstances will dictate what goals can be accomplished.

Short-Term Goals

Sarah will:
- ➤ reduce her calorie intake by using foods from the lower portion of the Diabetes Food Guide Pyramid introduced in *The First Step in Diabetes Meal Planning*.
- ➤ observe and reduce food portions.
- ➤ walk daily for a minimum of 10–15 minutes.
- ➤ test her blood glucose levels 3–4 times a week at random times throughout the day.
- ➤ identify two eating behavior changes that she would be willing to work on until she is seen by the dietitian in 2 weeks: 1) drink less regular or try diet soft drinks; 2) begin to eat breakfast.

Diabetes Medical Nutrition Therapy

Follow-up
➤ Provide Sarah with record-keeping forms for food, exercise, SMBG (ie, Lifestyle Change: Food and Physical Activity Records from *Facilitating Lifestyle Change*) and ask her to complete for 2–3 days in preparation for the follow-up visit with the dietitian.

First Follow-up Visit
(with RD)
Follow-up Data

Lab data: N/A
Medications: none
Blood glucose monitoring: see record-keeping forms
Weight: 208 pounds
Exercise: see record-keeping forms
Food records: see record-keeping forms

Nutrition Progress
Sarah has begun to drink diet soft drinks or water for snacks, is eating a tortilla with beans for breakfast (at about 8:30 AM) and eating less food for lunch, and has walked a total of 5 days (10 minutes each session) over the past 2 weeks.

Food/Meal Planning
➤ Provide Sarah with a copy of "Portions: How Much Is Enough?" from *Single-Topic Diabetes Nutrition Resources*; review content and establish behavioral objectives for portion control.

Blood Glucose Monitoring
➤ Review blood glucose monitoring technique.
➤ Review blood glucose, food intake, and physical activity records; discuss patterns that may be apparent with food intake and/or exercise activity and their effect on Sarah's blood glucose levels.

Exercise
➤ Recommend an increase in walking to every other day for 15 minutes.

Short-Term Goals
➤ Sarah will monitor and record her blood glucose, food intake, and physical activity to identify patterns in her glucose results.
➤ Sarah decided that the additional behavior changes she would like to work on until her next appointment were 1) exercise more frequently and for a longer period of time and 2) eat healthier snacks between meals.

Follow-up
➤ Provide Sarah with copies of Lifestyle Change: Summary Records (from *Facilitating Lifestyle Change*) and ask her to summarize her daily self-management activities (blood glucose monitoring, eating plan information, physical activity) for review at next follow-up.
➤ Make follow-up appointment in 1 month to review records, assess progress with behavior changes, and provide additional structure with meal planning (ie, individualized eating plan using *The First Step in Diabetes Meal Planning*), if Sarah is receptive.

Lifestyle Change
Food and Physical Activity Record

Name: Sarah – 1st visit

Time	Food Eaten — Day: Tuesday	Nutr. Info.	Time	Food Eaten — Day: Wednesday	Nutr. Info.	Time	Food Eaten — Day: Thursday	Nutr. Info.
8:30 am	Refried beans, 1 flour tortilla, water		8:30 am	Refried beans, 1 flour tortilla, water		8:30 am	Refried beans, 1 flour tortilla, water	
1:00 pm	1 bean tortilla, squash, iced tea c̄ sweetener		1:00 pm	1 bean tortilla, stewed tomatoes, iced tea c̄ sweetener		1:00 pm	1 bean tortilla, squash and tomatoes, iced tea c̄ sweetener	
3:00 pm	Diet soda, 1 homemade cookie		3:00 pm	Diet soda, 2 homemade cookies		3-4:00 pm	2 diet sodas	
7:00 pm	Red chili stew with beef and potatoes, Fried bread, Canned fruit cocktail		7:00 pm	Red chili stew with beef and potatoes, Fried bread, Unsweetened pineapple		7:00 pm	2 Chicken enchiladas with cheese, Lettuce and tomato, Canned peaches	
10:00 pm	Water, 2 handfuls taco chips		9:30 pm	Water, 2 handfuls taco chips		10:00 pm	Water, 2 handfuls taco chips	

Nutrient Totals

Physical Activity	Type	Walking	Walking		Walking
	Amt.	10 minutes	12 minutes		15 minutes
Other Information		Blood glucose (before breakfast) 130 mg			Blood glucose (before dinner) 112 mg

Instructions: Test blood glucose randomly.

Comments:

Start Date:

205

Case Study 2

Demographic Information	Mattie is a 75-year-old widow.
Referral Data	Client is referred by internist to a home health agency for a home visit to provide nutrition/diabetes education.
Diabetes Treatment Regimen	Oral glucose-lowering medication; recently started Diabeta 10 mg twice a day.
Laboratory Values	Fasting blood glucose: 167 mg/dL Glycosylated hemoglobin (HgbA$_{1c}$): 9.3% Cholesterol: 288 mg/dL HDL cholesterol: 32 mg/dL LDL cholesterol: 162 mg/dL Triglycerides: 270 mg/dL Blood pressure: 130/90 Microalbumin: N/A
Medical History	Hyperlipidemia; had a stroke 9 months ago with some residual hemiparesis.
Diabetes History	Has had type II diabetes for 7 years; older sister died of diabetes complications.
Medications That Affect Therapy	None.
Exercise Guidelines	Client is limited in ability to perform physical activity because of recent stroke; is challenged in completing activities of daily living.
Medical Treatment Goals for Client	Target blood glucose levels: fasting: 80–140 mg/dL postmeal: 100–180 mg/dL Target glycosylated hemoglobin (HgbA$_{1c}$) level: 6–7.5% Self-monitoring (method, frequency, education, evaluation): client obtained blood glucose meter at the local pharmacy and was taught how to use it by the pharmacist; usually tests twice each day, before breakfast and before dinner. Diabetes educator to review glucose monitoring technique and records, and make recommendation regarding suggested times for glucose testing.
Education Completed	Mattie has had no specific diabetes education other than being taught how to use a glucose meter by the local pharmacist; referring physician considers Mattie's control to be acceptable.

Nutrition Assessment
 Clinical Data
	Physical information: Height: 65 inches
	                              Weight: 205 pounds
	                              Body frame: medium
	 Reasonable body weight: 185–195 pounds
	 Estimated daily energy needs: approximately 2,000 calories

Nutrition History*

Usual food intake:
- Breakfast (7:30–8:30 AM): coffee with 3 heaping teaspoons of sugar, Danish
- Lunch (11:30 AM–12:30 PM): 1 package oriental noodles, 2 hot dogs with 2 slices of bread, 12 oz whole milk
- PM snack: ½ bag potato chips, 1 can regular soda
- Dinner (5:30–6:30 PM): beef pot pie, gelatin dessert, 2 slices bread with butter, tea with 2 teaspoons sugar
- HS snack: large bowl of ice cream

Nutrition evaluation:
- Energy intake: approximately 3,900 calories
- Frequency and timing of meals: eats 3 meals, evenly spaced with the inclusion of high-fat, high-calorie PM and HS snacks
- Other nutritional concerns: high-calorie, high-fat food choices with limited intake of fresh fruits and vegetables

Weight history: weight stable for the past 5 years; gained approximately 30 pounds after husband's death 7 years ago
Appetite/eating/digestion problems: N/A
Eating outside the home: seldom eats out
Alcohol intake: N/A
Use of vitamins/minerals/supplements: N/A

Exercise History

None; very limited in her ability to increase level of physical activity.

Psychosocial and Economic Issues

Mattie is widowed and lives alone. She is limited in her ability to shop for and prepare meals. A neighbor takes her food shopping once a week and she has a son in a neighboring town who visits her on weekends. She is on a limited income, receiving only social security and Medicare benefits.

Blood Glucose Monitoring

See referral data (under method and frequency of self-monitoring).

Knowledge, Skills, Attitudes, and Motivation

Mattie is a high school graduate. She has received very little formal education about diabetes; what she has learned has been from her sister's experiences. She is fearful of diabetes because of her sister's death from diabetes complications. She is also frustrated with her inability to self-manage her diabetes because of physical limitations and is under stress because of financial problems.

Initial Nutrition Intervention

Food/Meal Planning

- ➤ Work with Mattie to complete the Lifestyle Questionnaire (specifically the Lifestyle Change, Nutrition History, Food Record, Weight History, and Stress History sections) from *Facilitating Lifestyle Change*. Have Mattie identify areas of specific interest and those in which she needs more information and/or assistance.
- ➤ Introduce "Food, Diabetes, and the Older Person" from *Single-Topic Diabetes Resources*. Have Mattie verbalize her feelings and concerns about having diabetes.

---

*Information summarized from the Lifestyle Change Questionnaire, a resource from *Facilitating Lifestyle Change*.

Diabetes Medical Nutrition Therapy

➤ Introduce the *Guide to Good Eating* educational resource to assist Mattie with the development of a food plan, a section discussed in the "Food, Diabetes, and the Older Person" resource.

Blood Glucose Monitoring

➤ Discuss the suggested target blood glucose ranges with Mattie; assess whether she is keeping blood glucose records and if she understands how to interpret her blood glucose records.

Exercise

➤ Determine Mattie's ability, interest, and long-term limitations in regard to increasing physical activity.

Short-Term Goals

Nutrition/behavior goals are developed collaboratively by the client and diabetes educator. A number of goals have been noted, but in actual practice only one or two may be established at each visit. The number of visits and circumstances will dictate what goals can be accomplished.

Mattie will:
➤ identify three eating habit changes she is interested in working on until next follow-up visit: 1) increase servings of fruits and vegetables; 2) try sugar substitutes and sugar-free products such as soda and gelatin; 3) substitute lower-calorie, lower-fat choices for afternoon and evening snacks.
➤ determine target range for blood glucose.

Follow-up

➤ Home health nurse will provide follow-up in 1 month to assess and review her feelings about diabetes, glucose monitoring technique, alternative schedule of glucose testing, progress with eating habit changes, and need for additional structure and/or additional behavioral goals.
➤ Recommend referral to physical therapist to further assess abilities and limitations with physical movement and make recommendations for appropriate exercise activity and schedule.
➤ Discuss American Diabetes Association Standards of Care with referring physician.

Lifestyle Questionnaire

Name Mattie   **Date**

Do You Want to Change Your Lifestyle?

The time you take to provide this information will help your health care team work better for you. Thank you for taking an important step to manage your health.

- Have you made any changes in your lifestyle that you feel good about? ( ) Yes (X) No
  If yes, what changes have you made? _____

- If you and your nutritionist discover changes you could make in your lifestyle to improve your health (e.g., eating, exercise, or self-monitoring plan), would you be open to the changes?

  uncertain   ( ) Yes   ( ) No

    If yes, who will support and encourage you as you make these changes? family – my son sees me on weekends

    If no, what would keep you from making these changes? limited income and physical limitations

- What information would you like from the nutritionist?

  (X) Meal planning   (X) Weight management
  ( ) Eating out   ( ) Exercise
  (X) Food label reading/supermarket shopping   ( ) Record keeping
  ( ) Eating less fat   ( ) Other _____

- What changes would you like to make?

  (X) Improve my eating habits   ( ) Get more information
  ( ) Improve my activity level   (X) Feel better about my health
  (X) Improve my blood glucose control   (X) Learn how to manage my weight
  ( ) Lower my blood pressure   (X) Improve my energy level
  (X) Improve my cholesterol, triglyceride levels (X) Control food cravings
  ( ) Learn how to prevent high or low blood glucose levels
  ( ) Other _____

American Diabetes Association   The American Dietetic Association

Diabetes Medical Nutrition Therapy

Lifestyle Questionnaire

Name Mattie **Date**

Nutrition History

- Have you ever wanted to make changes in what you eat? (X) Yes ( ) No
  If yes, what advice have you been given? *lose weight and avoid sugar*

- Are you following any type of meal plan, such as exchange lists, calorie counting, carbohydrate counting, low cholesterol, low fat, or low sodium? ( ) Yes (X) No
  If yes, please describe. *given exchange lists in the past – didn't understand or follow*
  If yes, how much of the time are you able to follow your meal plan?
  (X) Rarely ( ) Sometimes ( ) Often ( ) Usually

- How many people live in your household? (0) Ages ( )

- Who usually does the cooking? *myself* The shopping? *myself*

- How many times each week do you eat away from home? (0)
  a. Which meals are usually eaten away from home?
  b. In which type of restaurant do you usually eat or carry out? (mark **F** for Frequently, **O** for Occasionally, **N** for Never)
     ( ) Fast food (hamburger, chicken, seafood, pizza, subs, tacos)
     ( ) Buffets/All-you-can-eat
     ( ) Sit-down restaurant (Types:)
     ( ) Sweets/Dessert Shops

- Do you drink alcohol? (NO) Beer ( ) Wine ( ) Liquor
  How often?   How much?

- Do you take vitamins, minerals, herbs, or any other food or nutritional supplement? ( ) Yes (X) No
  If yes, please list.

- Do you regularly skip meals? ( ) Yes (X) No
  If yes, list which meals you skip most often and why.

- Do you have "trigger" foods that often cause you to overeat? (X) Yes ( ) No
  If yes, please list. *snack foods – potato chips, ice cream*

- Have you ever been on an extreme diet (such as fasting) or a fad diet? ( ) Yes (X) No
  If yes, please describe.

- Do you eat for other reasons than hunger? (X) Yes ( ) No
  If yes, please describe. *when I am lonely or bored*

American Diabetes Association

THE AMERICAN DIETETIC ASSOCIATION

210

Case Studies of Clinical Application

Lifestyle Questionnaire

Name: Mattie **Date:**

Food Record

- This food record can help you and your nutritionist better understand how food affects your health.

- Please write down everything you eat and drink from the time you wake up to the time you go to bed. Include meals, snacks, and drinks. If you eat or drink anything when you wake up, that should be added to the list.

Time	Type of Food / Beverage	Amount
7:30 – 8:30	Danish or cinnamon roll Coffee with sugar (1 tbsp)	1 2–3 cups
11:30 – 12:30	Hot dogs with catsup and mustard Bread Oriental noodles Whole milk	2 2 slices 1 package 1½ cups
2:30 – 4:00	Potato chips Soda	approx. ½ bag 1
5:30 – 6:30	TV dinner: beef pot pie, etc. Gelatin dessert with fruit and marshmallows Bread with butter Iced tea with 2 teaspoons sugar	 2 slices
8:30 – 9:00	Chocolate chip mint ice cream	large bowl

Diabetes Medical Nutrition Therapy

Lifestyle Questionnaire

Name: Mattie   Date:

Weight History

- Height: 5'5"   Present weight: 205   Usual weight: 200-210

- Has your weight changed any over the past year?   ◯ Yes   (X) No

    If yes, please describe how. ....

    How do you feel about your weight now? need to lose weight

- What has been your weight range as an adult? 175-200

- What would you consider to be a healthy weight for you? 175-185

    Would you feel comfortable at that weight?   (X) Yes   ◯ No

- Have you ever tried to change your weight before?   (X) Yes   ◯ No

    If yes, what have you tried? exchange lists

    Have you been successful? no

- Are you interested in working to change your weight?

    (X) Yes, right now
    ◯ Yes, but I can't right now
    ◯ No, but I will think it over
    ◯ No, not now
    ◯ No, I'm not interested

American Diabetes Association

THE AMERICAN DIETETIC ASSOCIATION

Lifestyle Questionnaire

Name Mattie   **Date**

Physical Activity History

- What type of activities do you do regularly and how much time each week do you spend doing them? Examples include walking, dancing, golf, tennis, biking, aerobics, and swimming.

Activity	Times per Week	Minutes per Activity
NO		

- Do you like to do these activities alone or with others? ....

- Do you perform other physical activities of daily living, such as housework, gardening, or climbing stairs? If yes, list type and amount. ....

- Are you interested in becoming more physically active?

  ( ) Yes, right now
  ( ) Yes, but I can't right now
  (X) No, but I will think it over
  ( ) No, not now
  ( ) No, I'm not interested

  If yes, what type of physical activity could you see yourself doing regularly?
  ......?......

  If no, why? because of my recent stroke, unable to do any physical activity

213

Diabetes Medical Nutrition Therapy

Lifestyle Questionnaire

Name Mattie   **Date**

Stress History

- Have you had a significant change in life events (such as marriage, divorce, death of a family member, new home, or change in employment) over the past year? (X) Yes ( ) No
  If yes, please describe.

- How does stress affect you physically or emotionally (e.g., headaches, neckaches, sleeping difficulties, eating too much or too little, fear, depression)? _eating too much, depression_

- How do you deal with stress (e.g., meditation, exercise, avoidance)? _avoidance_

Record Keeping

	Yes	No	How Often
Do you keep food records?	( )	(X)	
Do you keep blood glucose records?	(X)	( )	
Do you keep exercise records?	( )	(X)	
Do you keep any other kind of records? (for example, blood pressure) Type	( )	(X)	

- Who benefits from your record keeping?
  (X) Self
  ( ) Family
  ( ) Doctor
  ( ) Other

American Diabetes Association

THE AMERICAN DIETETIC ASSOCIATION

Case Study 3

John is 48 years old, divorced, and lives alone.	**Demographic Information**
Client has been referred by his primary care physician to the outpatient dietitian at a local hospital for nutrition counseling for newly diagnosed type II diabetes.	**Referral Data**
5 mg glyburide plus medical nutrition therapy and exercise.	**Diabetes Treatment Regimen**
Random blood glucose (2½ hrs postmeal): 267 mg/dL Glycosylated hemoglobin (HgbA$_{1c}$): 9% Cholesterol: 325 mg/dL HDL cholesterol: 25 mg/dL LDL cholesterol: 215 mg/dL Triglycerides: 370 mg/dL Blood pressure: 135/83 Microalbumin: N/A	**Laboratory Values**
No previous health problems noted.	**Medical History**
No family history of diabetes.	*Diabetes History*
None.	**Medications That Affect Therapy**
Client has no exercise limitations and has been encouraged to begin a daily routine of exercise.	**Exercise Guidelines**
Target blood glucose levels: fasting: 80–140 mg/dL postmeal: 100–180 mg/dL Target glycosylated hemoglobin (HgbA$_{1c}$): 6–7.5% Self-monitoring (method, frequency, education, evaluation): Using meter to check blood glucose levels 2 times a day (fasting and postdinner). Had been instructed on use of meter by physician's office nurse practitioner.	**Medical Treatment Goals for Client**
Physician reviewed basic information about diabetes with client. Client was referred to the nurse practitioner for self-monitoring of blood glucose education.	**Education Completed**

Physical information: Height: 72 inches
                       Weight: 220 pounds
                       Body frame: medium
Reasonable body weight: 180–190 pounds
Estimated daily energy needs: 2,000–2,500 calories
	Nutrition Assessment
	
	Clinical Data

Diabetes Medical Nutrition Therapy

Nutrition History* Usual food intake: Breakfast: 3-egg omelet, 2 slices buttered toast (white), 6 oz orange juice, coffee with cream.
AM snack: 1 package snack chips, 1 can fruit juice
Lunch: 1–2 slices of pizza (thick crust with everything on it), diet soft drink, or 3 hot dogs on buns, diet pop. Usually skips lunch on Fridays.
PM snack: same as AM snack
Dinner: Frozen dinner or 2 pieces frozen fried chicken or 6–8 oz hamburger, 2–3 slices of bread with butter, 1–2 light beers
HS snack: 1½–2 cups dry cereal with 2% milk

Nutrition evaluation: Energy intake: 3,355 calories
Frequency and timing of meals: skips lunch once a week, eats three snacks a day
Other nutritional concerns: eats many high-fat foods; limited fruit and vegetable intake

Weight history: at maximum weight of 220 pounds; has gained 15 pounds since his divorce
Appetite/eating/digestion problems: N/A
Eating outside the home: eats his breakfast and lunch away from home daily
Alcohol intake: 1–2 light beers per day; usually drinks more on weekends.
Use of vitamin/mineral supplements: N/A

Exercise History Has not engaged in any form of regular physical activity during the last 5 years.

Psychosocial and Economic Issues John has been divorced for 6 months and lives alone in an apartment. He is employed in a factory on an assembly line (7 AM–3:30 PM). Has no children. Has adequate finances.

Blood Glucose Monitoring Using a meter 2 times a day. Client reported ranges of blood glucose levels:
Fasting: 160–200 mg/dL
Postdinner: 200–250 mg/dL

Knowledge, Skills, Attitudes, and Motivation John is a high school graduate and has taken some night classes. He has very limited knowledge of diabetes. Does not know how to cook, but is willing to learn. He hates the idea of "dieting," as his ex-wife had been on "every diet in the book" and it drove him crazy.

Initial Nutrition Intervention

Food/Meal Planning
➤ Review relationship of food, medication, and exercise to blood glucose.
➤ Explain the purpose of individualized menus and emphasize the fact the menus provide a short-term solution to modifying food intake.
➤ Assist John in developing two menus, with three meals and three snacks. Show John how menus can be used alternatively from one day to the next.
➤ Using food models, measuring equipment, and real food whenever possible, demonstrate how to determine accurate food portion sizes.

*Information summarized from the Lifestyle Change Questionnaire, a resource from *Facilitating Lifestyle Change.*

➤ Provide John with "Eating Out: From Burgers to Burritos" from *Single-Topic Diabetes Resources*.
➤ Discuss the need for further education through the diabetes education program. Client agrees to attend.

➤ No records available.

Blood Glucose Monitoring

➤ Discuss the need for daily physical activity and the impact on blood glucose and lipid levels, as well as weight. John is asked the type and frequency of activity he is willing to engage in.

Exercise

Nutrition/behavior goals are developed collaboratively by the client and diabetes educator. A number of goals have been noted, but in actual practice only one or two may be established at each visit. The number of visits, his circumstances, and what John is willing to do will dictate what goals can be accomplished.

Short-Term Goals

John will:
➤ use individualized menus developed with the assistance of dietitian.
➤ monitor the portions of foods eaten at each meal and snack.
➤ begin his individualized exercise program.
➤ attend the diabetes education program classes at the hospital.

The dietitian enrolls John in the diabetes education program classes, which start in 2 weeks. A letter introducing John to the diabetes education program dietitian is sent, providing background information and client's goals. John will keep blood glucose and exercise records to be reviewed with the RD/CDE at the diabetes education program classes.

Follow-up

Case Study 4

Marion is a 56-year-old homemaker with three children.

Demographic Information

Client is referred by her internist to the diabetes education program for evaluation and possible initiation of insulin therapy.

Referral Data

20 mg glipizide bid. Consider the initiation of insulin therapy if control does not improve in the next 2 months.

Diabetes Treatment Regimen

Fasting blood glucose: 342 mg/dL
Cholesterol: 183 mg/dL
LDL cholesterol: N/A
Blood pressure: 125/85

Glycosylated hemoglobin (HgbA$_{1c}$): 14%
HDL cholesterol: N/A
Triglycerides: 334 mg/dL
Microalbumin: 9 µg/mL

Laboratory Values

Diabetes Medical Nutrition Therapy

Medical History History of hypothyroidism and hypertriglyceridemia.

Diabetes History Type II diabetes for 6 years. For last 3 years, her diabetes was controlled with oral glucose-lowering medications and intermittent dieting. Has seen a dietitian in the past and was given an exchange list meal plan, but became frustrated with the limited food choices and lack of flexibility. Had been utilizing the visual method of blood glucose monitoring until just recently.

Medications That Affect Therapy
20 mg glipizide
.05 mg synthroid
20 mg lovastatin

Exercise Guidelines Client is encouraged to walk daily or to participate in physical activity program offered by the local hospital.

Medical Treatment Goals for Client
Target blood glucose levels: fasting: 80–140 mg/dL
                               postmeal: 100–180 mg/dL
Target glycosylated hemoglobin (HgbA$_{1c}$): 6–7.5%
Self-monitoring (method, frequency, education, evaluation): Started using a meter in the last week. Checking blood glucose levels 3 times a day (fasting, before dinner, before bed). Was instructed on the use of meter by nurse educator in the diabetes education program.

Education Completed Physician discussed the pros and cons of initiating insulin therapy. Reviewed the need for regular exercise and consistent eating habits. Physician discussed the need for Marion to attend the diabetes education program to learn how to self-manage her diabetes.

Nutrition Assessment

Clinical Data
Physical information: Height: 63 inches
                        Weight: 194 pounds
                        Body frame: large
Reasonable body weight: 174 pounds
Estimated daily energy needs: 1,700 calories

Nutrition History*
Usual food intake: Breakfast (7:30–9:00 AM): 1–2 eggs or 2–3 Tbsp peanut butter, 2 slices of toast with margarine, 6 oz juice, black coffee
Lunch (12–1:30 PM): ½ cup cottage cheese and fresh fruit or ½ cup tuna salad (with low-fat mayonnaise) and salad with raw vegetables, 12 oz juice
PM snack (3–4 PM): 2 homemade cookies with 4–6 oz 2% milk or ½–1 cup frozen yogurt

*Information summarized from the Lifestyle Change Questionnaire, a resource from *Facilitating Lifestyle Change*.

	Dinner (5–6 PM): 4–6 oz poultry or fish, 1 cup rice or pasta, 1 cup vegetable, salad with low-calorie dressing, 1 slice bread with margarine, 1½ cup 2% milk
	HS snack (9–10 PM): 3–4 cup oil-popped popcorn or 1 cup dry cereal with ¾ cup 2% milk
Nutrition evaluation:	Energy intake: 2,275 calories
	Frequency, timing of meals: meal times are close together.
	Nutritional concerns: food portions are large and meals/snacks are too close together, which may be affecting blood glucose levels.

Weight history: has gained 15 pounds since her husband's early retirement 1 year ago. Has gained and lost weight over the last 6 years. Highest weight was 215 pounds, and lowest weight was 163 pounds.

Appetite/eating/digestion problems: N/A

Eating outside the home: eats out with husband and daughter 3 times a week; once is usually at the local pizza parlor.

Alcohol intake: usually has a cocktail or glass of wine with dinner in a restaurant.

Use of vitamins/mineral supplements: N/A

No current pattern of exercise; has an exercise bike, but rarely uses it. Has done swimming and walking in the past.

Exercise History

Marion has never worked outside the home. She loves to cook and bake, and does volunteer work at her church. Her husband is retired, and income and health insurance are adequate. Her teenage daughter lives at home.

Psychosocial and Economic Issues

Uses a meter 3 times a day since seeing the nurse educator at the diabetes education program. Review of blood glucose records reveals:
Fasting: 223–320 mg/dL
Pre-dinner: 300–375 mg/dL
Pre-HS snack: 289–392 mg/dL

Blood Glucose Monitoring

Marion has a high school education and has attended junior college. She is concerned about the possibility of taking insulin and is afraid of complications from her diabetes. She is eager to improve her lifestyle in order to manage her diabetes. Marion is especially open to learning how to manage her food intake and to identify emotional eating triggers. Her family appears to be supportive of her efforts, and her husband attends all appointments.

Knowledge, Skills, Attitudes, and Motivation

➤ Discuss the impact of food, medication/insulin, and exercise on blood glucose and blood lipids.
➤ Review the calorie-counting approach to meal planning; establish calorie level, and develop plan of spacing calories more equally between meals and snacks; provide reference book of calorie information.
➤ Discuss timing of meals and snacks and impact on blood glucose levels.
➤ Review record keeping. Provide with Lifestyle Change Summary Record from *Facilitating Lifestyle Change*.

Initial Nutrition Intervention

Food/Meal Planning

Diabetes Medical Nutrition Therapy

Blood Glucose Monitoring
➤ Review Marion's technique of blood glucose monitoring and review her log book.

Exercise
➤ Discuss various physical activities that could be worked into her daily routine, and establish an exercise plan.

Short-Term Goals

Nutrition/behavior goals are developed collaboratively by the client and diabetes educator. A number of goals have been noted, but in actual practice only one or two may be established at each visit. The number of visits and circumstances will dictate what goals can be accomplished.

Marion will:
➤ spread calories more equally between meals and snacks.
➤ eliminate her afternoon snack.
➤ reduce the number of high-fat food choices.
➤ walk 3 times a week for 20 minutes after her evening meal.
➤ continue to keep food and blood glucose records.

Follow-up
➤ Schedule for follow-up appointment in 2 weeks with dietitian and nurse.

First Follow-up Visit

Follow-up Data

Lab data: N/A
Medications: continues on current medications
Blood glucose monitoring: see Lifestyle Change Summary Record
Exercise: client has walked 3 times per week for 30 minutes after dinner. No problems noted. Blood glucose at bedtime and fasting have improved.

Nutrition Progress

Marion has kept detailed records and has reduced her calorie intake to 1,600 calories a day. She is eating at more set mealtimes (breakfast at 7:30; lunch at 12:30; dinner at 5:00, and a bedtime snack at 9:30). She is eating less fat. Has many questions about baking and eating away from home.

Food/Meal Planning

➤ Review food and exercise record. Reinforce positive changes in eating behavior, and point out how her modified eating habits and regular activity are having an effect on her blood glucose levels. Provide with additional Lifestyle Change Summary Records.
➤ Review the handout "Eating Out: From Burgers to Burritos" from *Single-Topic Diabetes Resources*. Using local restaurant menus, practice ordering a meal in a restaurant.
➤ Provide client with the handout "Cooking, Baking and Diabetes" from *Single-Topic Diabetes Resources* for review at home.

Blood Glucose Monitoring
➤ Review record book. Client will be seeing the nurse for follow-up.

Exercise
➤ Discuss increasing the frequency of her walks and the positive benefits it will have on blood glucose.

Short-Term Goals

Marion will:
- continue to keep food, exercise and blood glucose records using the Lifestyle Change Summary Record form.
- walk for 30 minutes daily after dinner.
- eat lower-fat entrees when eating out.
- attempt to modify some of her recipes to reduce their fat content.

Follow-up

- Marion will return for a final individual session with the dietitian in 4 weeks and then will attend the type II diabetes education classes with her husband.
- Marion is scheduled to see her physician in 6 weeks.

Lifestyle Change
Summary Record

Name: Marion

Day	Nutrient Information		Physical Activity		Blood Glucose Records			Comments
		Calories	Type	Amount	Fasting	Pre-dinner	Pre-HS	
1st		1745	walked	30 min	250	275	271	
2nd		1685	—	—	220	263	250	
3rd		1635	walked	30 min	227	254	259	
4th		1605	—	—	210	241	245	
5th		1615	walked	30 min	200	223	231	
6th		1600	—	—	202	215	224	
7th		1695	—	—	209	221	220	
8th		1620	walked	30 min	199	209	210	
9th		1615	—	—	193	200	206	
10th		1625	walked	30 min	187	198	203	
11th		1600	—	—	194	202	200	
12th		1605	walked	30 min	191	200	198	
13th					195			Appt. with RD
14th								
15th								
16th								
17th								
18th								
19th								
20th								
21st								
22nd								
23rd								
24th								
25th								
26th								
27th								
28th								

Instructions:

Case Study 5

Joey is an 11-year-old, in the 5th grade.	**Demographic Information**
Client is admitted to hospital with newly diagnosed type I diabetes. The pediatric endocrinologist writes order for dietitian to assess and develop nutrition prescription.	**Referral Data**
Insulin therapy initiated, along with medical nutrition therapy, exercise, and blood glucose monitoring. AM insulin: 10 units NPH, 3 units Regular PM insulin: 14 units NPH, 5 units Regular	***Diabetes Treatment Regimen***
Blood glucose on admission: 574 mg/dL Glycosylated hemoglobin (HgbA$_{1c}$): 16.5% Urine ketones: 3+ Cholesterol: 148 mg/dL HDL cholesterol: N/A LDL cholesterol: N/A Triglycerides: 139 mg/dL Blood pressure: 110/70 Microalbumin: 3 µg/mL	***Laboratory Values***
No previous health problems noted.	***Medical History***
Elevated blood glucose (450 mg/dL 2 hours postmeal) was obtained during a routine sports physical. Has experienced a 5-lb weight loss following the flu. Has had symptoms of excess thirst, hunger, and has been urinating five times a day. No family history of diabetes.	*Diabetes History*
None.	***Medications That Affect Therapy***
No restrictions.	***Exercise Guidelines***
Target blood glucose levels: fasting: 80–140 mg/dL postmeal: 100–180 mg/dL Target glycosylated hemoglobin: 6–7.5% Self-monitoring (method, frequency, education, evaluation): was taught the use of a meter and to check blood glucose levels 4 times a day (fasting, before lunch, before dinner, and at bedtime). Was instructed and evaluated by the diabetes nurse educator.	***Medical Treatment Goals for Client***
The following was provided by the nursing staff: blood glucose monitoring; insulin injection technique; diabetes overview; and hypoglycemia treatment.	***Education Completed***

Diabetes Medical Nutrition Therapy

Nutrition Assessment

Clinical Data

Physical information: Height: 60 inches (90th percentile for height)
                        Weight: 89 pounds (75th percentile for weight)
Estimated daily energy needs: minimum 2,500 calories

Nutrition History

Usual food intake:
- Breakfast (usually 6:30 AM): 3 cups sweetened cereal with 1½ cups 2% milk
- AM snack (usually 9:30 AM): 1 carton chocolate milk
- Lunch (usually 11:45 AM): (school lunch) fish sandwich with tartar sauce, green beans, canned fruit, cookie or cake, and 1 carton 2% milk
- PM snack (usually 3:30 PM): meat sandwich (2 slices bread, 2 slices lunch meat, 1–2 slices cheese, low-fat mayonnaise) and 1 can of soda, or crackers (20–25) with peanut butter (2–4 Tbsp) and 1 can of soda
- Dinner (usually 6:00–7:30 PM): 2 cups casserole, 2 dinner rolls or slices of bread with butter, 2 cups 2% milk
- HS snack (usually 9:30 PM): 2 scoops of ice cream or 6–7 cookies or 1 container of pudding

Nutrition evaluation:
- Energy intake: 3,000–3,200 calories
- Frequency and timing of meals: adequate
- Other nutritional concerns: many high-fat foods utilized; need to make sure client receives adequate calories for growth and development.

Weight history: had lost 5 pounds prior to diagnosis. Client underweight.
Appetite/eating/digestion problems: N/A
Eating outside the home: eats away from home 1–2 times a week, usually in fast-food restaurant.
Alcohol intake: N/A
Use of vitamins/mineral supplements: N/A

Exercise History

Participates in a variety of school sports (flag football, basketball, and baseball).

Psychosocial and Economic Issues

Parents divorced for 2 years, lives with mother, no siblings. Adequate finances and complete health insurance. Attends public school.

Blood Glucose Monitoring

Just taught to use meter.

Knowledge, Skills, Attitudes, and Motivation

Currently in the 5th grade and earns good grades. Client and family have no prior knowledge of diabetes. Client and family anxious to learn about diabetes and self-management skills.

Initial Nutrition Intervention

Food/Meal Planning

- Review the nutrient content of foods and impact on blood glucose.
- Review nutrition goals for diabetes.
- Develop and review meal plan using *Healthy Food Choices*.
- Develop several days of sample menus.
- Review school lunch menus and demonstrate how they fit into the meal plan.

Blood Glucose Monitoring

- Review the importance of monitoring for making adjustments to the meal plan.

Exercise

- Review the handout "Exercise and Diabetes: On the Move" from *Single-Topic Diabetes Resources*.

Short-Term Goals

Nutrition/behavior goals are developed collaboratively by the client and diabetes educator. A number of goals have been noted, but in actual practice only one or two may be established at each visit. The number of visits and circumstances will dictate what goals can be accomplished.

- Joey will be consistent with the timing of his meals.
- Joey and mother will follow meal plan and identify problems and questions related to following it.
- Joey and mother will keep food, exercise, and blood glucose records using the Lifestyle Change Food and Physical Activity Record forms for review during outpatient diabetes education appointment with dietitian.

Follow-up

- Joey and family to be seen in the outpatient diabetes education program by the nurse and dietitian in 10 days. The necessary referral documents will be forwarded to the program before his first appointment.

First Follow-up Visit

Follow-up Data

Lab data: N/A
Medications: insulin regimen adjusted during physician visit.
Blood glucose monitoring: N/A
Exercise: has participated in physical education class four times since discharge without incident. The school nurse checked blood glucose levels before and after exercise.
Food records: detailed records kept. A number of questions were noted on the records regarding how certain foods fit into the meal plan.

Nutrition Progress

Client and family are planning meals in advance. They have a number of questions about how certain foods fit into the meal plan. Also, there are many questions about eating away from home. Client is obtaining adequate calories and does not feel hungry. No adjustment in calories or meal plan needed.

Food/Meal Planning
- ➤ Provide additional information on how certain foods fit into the meal plan. Reinforce the positive eating behaviors.
- ➤ Discuss tips for dining out using "Eating Out: From Burgers to Burritos" from *Single-Topic Diabetes Resources*.

Blood Glucose Monitoring
- ➤ Review blood glucose records along with food and exercise records and discuss some ways to manage several situations.

Exercise
- ➤ Reinforce information about the impact of exercise on blood glucose levels and ways to prevent and treat hypoglycemia.

Short-Term Goals

Joey will:
- ➤ continue to keep intermittent food records (2 days a week), along with blood glucose and exercise records.
- ➤ make decisions about school lunch and discuss with his mother.
- ➤ make appropriate choices in a fast-food restaurant with assistance from his mother.

Follow-up
- ➤ Schedule return visit in 1 month. Mother expresses interest in learning more about the use of exchanges.

Second Follow-up Visit

Follow-up Data

Lab data: glycosylated hemoglobin (HgbA$_{1c}$): N/A
Medication: switched to new insulin regimen:
    AM: 8 units Regular   Noon: 4 units Regular
    PM: 6 units Regular   HS: 3 units Regular, 10 units Ultralente
Blood glucose monitoring: N/A
Exercise: no incidents of hypoglycemia or hyperglycemia with participation in flag football
Food records: reviewed detailed food records

Nutrition Progress

Client desires more detail about exchange list values of foods. Food records reveal consistent timing of meals/snacks and calorie intake. There is sufficient calorie intake. No complaints of hunger. Joey is using fewer high-fat foods and is requesting information about reading food labels.

Food/Meal Planning
- ➤ Counsel Joey and his mother on the use of the *Exchange Lists for Meal Planning*. Make modifications to the meal plan. Identify additional resource materials.
- ➤ Discuss label reading and review how the information may be used to identify exchange values for foods.

Short-Term Goals
- ➤ Joey and his mother will use the revised meal plan using the *Exchange Lists for Meal Planning*.

- ➤ Joey and his mother will use the information on food labels to determine the exchange value for foods not found in the exchange list booklet provided.
- ➤ Joey will continue with record keeping.

- ➤ Dietitian will contact Joey's mother in 1 week to check for questions. *Follow-up*
- ➤ Return visit in 2 months.

Lab: glycosylated hemoglobin: 8%   **Third Follow-up**
Medication: insulin regimen adjusted   **Visit**
             AM: 9 units Regular
             Noon: 7 units Regular   *Follow-up Data*
             PM: 6 units Regular
             HS: 10 units Ultralente
Blood glucose monitoring: blood glucose records are reviewed
Exercise: several episodes of hypoglycemia during basketball practice and games
Food records: N/A

Using *Exchange Lists for Meal Planning* without problem. Continues to be consistent with the timing of meals and the amount of food consumed. Calorie intake appears to be sufficient. Concern expressed about hypoglycemia and basketball practice and games.   **Nutrition Progress**

- ➤ Review ways for client to adjust calorie intake for basketball practice and games. Adjustment of insulin for practices and games will need to be discussed with physician.   ***Food/Meal Planning***
- ➤ Review signs/symptoms of hypoglycemia and treatment guidelines. Stress the importance of blood glucose monitoring during exercise.

Joey will: ***Short-Term Goals***
- ➤ increase the carbohydrate content of meals/snacks for days he has basketball practice or a game.
- ➤ plan snacks for after school and at bedtime.

- ➤ Dietitian will contact Joey's mother to see how adjustment to carbohydrate intake for games and practices has reduced the incidence of hypoglycemia.   ***Follow-up***
- ➤ Return in 6 months. Consider use of carbohydrate counting.

Glycosylated hemoglobin: 7.5%   **Fourth Follow-up**
Medication: no change to current regimen   **Visit**
Blood glucose records: blood glucose records are reviewed
Exercise: playing baseball with no incidence of hypoglycemia
Food records: N/A   ***Follow-up Data***

Diabetes Medical Nutrition Therapy

Nutrition Progress Joey and his mother are asking questions about adjusting carbohydrate intake at meals/snacks. Continues to be consistent with eating pattern. Three-pound weight gain noted. Good food choices.

Food/Meal Planning
- Introduce *Carbohydrate Counting: Getting Started.* Review booklet.
- Set up carbohydrate grams for each meal and snack.
- Plan sample menu demonstrating use of carbohydrate counting.
- Discuss the importance of food portions with carbohydrate counting. Instruct Joey to begin weighing and measuring all food portions and keep food and blood glucose records again.

Short-Term Goals
- Joey will weigh and measure all foods eaten at home.
- Joey will keep food and blood glucose records.
- Joey and his mother will identify blood glucose patterns and consider strategies to adjust food, insulin, or exercise.

Follow-up
- Joey will return for visit in 2 weeks and will attend a food lab to work on measuring and weighing foods.
- Joey will progress to *Carbohydrate Counting: Moving On* in the next month, after further education.

Case Study 6

Demographic Information Sheri is a 20-year-old who is married and pregnant with her first child.

Referral Data Client referred by family physician to hospital dietitian for newly diagnosed gestational diabetes.

Diabetes Treatment Regimen Medical nutrition therapy and blood glucose monitoring.

Laboratory Values
3-hr oral glucose tolerance test (OGTT):
    Fasting: 220 mg/dL
    1-hr: 198 mg/dL
    2-hr: 182 mg/dL
    3-hr: 148 mg/dL
Glycosylated hemoglobin ($HgbA_{1c}$): 7%
HDL cholesterol: N/A
Triglycerides: N/A
Microalbumin: N/A
Cholesterol: N/A
LDL cholesterol: N/A
Blood pressure: 125/75

Medical History Currently at 25 weeks gestation, uncomplicated pregnancy to date. No other medical problems.

Family history of diabetes.	*Diabetes History*
N/A	***Medications That Affect Therapy***
Encouraged to walk 3 times a week for 30 minutes.	***Exercise Guidelines***
Target blood glucose levels: fasting: < 105 mg/dL 2 hr postmeal: < 120 mg/dL Target glycosylated hemoglobin (HgbA$_{1c}$): 6–7.5% Self-monitoring (method, frequency, education, evaluation): Will use meter (on loan from hospital) and will check 4 times a day for 1 week. To be instructed by nurse after nutrition consultation.	***Medical Treatment Goals for Client***
Physician briefly explained definition of gestational diabetes and impact on mother and infant. Stressed importance of medical nutrition therapy and self-monitoring to treat gestational diabetes.	***Education Completed***

Physical information: Height: 63 inches
                               Weight: 170 pounds
                               Prepregnancy weight: 155 pounds
                               Body frame: medium
	Nutrition Assessment
	
	Clinical Data

Estimated daily energy needs: 1,900 calories	*Nutrition History**

Usual food intake: Breakfast: None
                            AM snack (10:00 AM): large muffin with margarine and
                                12 oz juice
                            Lunch (12:00 PM): quarter-pound hamburger with
                                cheese, small french fries, regular soda, or 1 cup
                                casserole, ½ cup vegetable, small dinner roll with
                                margarine, tea with 3 packets sugar
                            PM snack (3:00 PM): candy bar, crackers or regular soda
                            Dinner (6:30 PM): pork chop, fried chicken, or fish,
                              1 cup mashed potatoes with gravy, 1 cup coleslaw,
                              large dinner roll with butter, tea with 3 packets
                              sugar. Dessert (pie or cake) 2–3 times a week.
                            HS snack (8:30 PM): 1 scoop ice cream or sherbet
Nutrition evaluation: Energy intake: 3,000 calories
                            Frequency and timing of meals: skips breakfast daily;
                              2–3 hours between meals and snacks
                            Other nutritional concerns: uses many high-fat foods;
                              poor intake of milk, fruits, and vegetables
Weight history: weight stable for 2 years at 150–155 pounds. Has gained 15 pounds during pregnancy, which is higher than prenatal weight-gain grid goal of 10 pounds for overweight women at 25 weeks gestation.

---

*Information summarized from the Lifestyle Change Questionnaire, a resource from *Facilitating Lifestyle Change.*

Appetite/eating/digestion problems: none
Eating outside the home: eats out for lunch daily; dinner meal eaten out 3–4 times a week.
Alcohol intake: none
Use of vitamins/minerals/supplements: prenatal vitamin supplement

Exercise History   No routine exercise prior to pregnancy.

Psychosocial and Economic Issues   Has been married for 2 years. Works part-time as a billing clerk for a local pharmacy. Worries about expenses of having a child. Limited insurance coverage. Does not know how to cook; usually eats out or has carry-out food. Overwhelmed by diagnosis; concerned with being taught the exchange system.

Blood Glucose Monitoring   Has not been taught use of meter.

Knowledge, Skills, Attitudes and Motivation   Sheri is a high school graduate. She is convinced she cannot follow any type of diet, and is worried about the health of her baby.

Initial Nutrition Intervention

Food/Meal Planning
- ➤ Review the impact of food on blood glucose.
- ➤ Review the nutrient content of foods.
- ➤ Review "Diabetes Just During Pregnancy" from *Single-Topic Diabetes Resources*, emphasizing eating 3 meals and 2 snacks (PM and HS).
- ➤ Provide copy of "Portions: How Much Is Enough?" from *Single-Topic Diabetes Resources*.

Blood Glucose Monitoring
- ➤ Stress the importance of daily self-monitoring.

Exercise
- ➤ Discuss the impact of exercise on blood glucose levels. Encourage to walk daily for 30 minutes.

Short-Term Goals   Nutrition/behavior goals are developed collaboratively by the client and diabetes educator. A number of goals have been noted, but in actual practice only one or two may be established at each visit. The number of visits and circumstances will dictate what goals can be accomplished.

Sheri will:
- ➤ eat breakfast daily.
- ➤ eliminate AM snack.
- ➤ be consistent with the timing of meals.
- ➤ use the section What and How Much to Eat of the "Diabetes Just During Pregnancy" resource for meal planning.
- ➤ keep food records.
- ➤ walk 5 days a week for 30 minutes.

➤ Sheri will return in 1 week.	*Follow-up*
	First Follow-up Visit
Lab data: N/A Medications: none Blood glucose monitoring: blood glucose records reviewed Food records: food records reviewed Exercise: walking 3–4 times a week	*Follow-up Data*
Sheri has started to eat a light breakfast, has skipped AM snack, and has reduced her calorie intake by 400–600 calories a day. She is drinking more milk, eating more fruits and vegetables, and eating fewer high-fat foods. Has difficulty making good food choices when eating out. Blood glucose levels within target ranges. Weight stable since last visit. Has been attempting to walk more frequently.	*Nutrition Progress*
➤ Reinforce positive changes in eating and exercise habits. ➤ Discuss the handout "Eating Out: From Burgers to Burritos" from *Single-Topic Diabetes Resources*. Develop three menus for evening meals based on the usual restaurants Sheri frequents.	*Food/Meal Planning*
➤ Review record book; Sheri is seeing nurse for follow-up today.	*Blood Glucose Monitoring*
➤ Encourage Sheri to continue her walking program.	*Exercise*
Sheri will: ➤ use sample dinner menus to lower calorie and fat intake at PM meals. ➤ continue to modify food portions and utilize foods that have higher nutrient content. ➤ walk 4 times a week for 30 minutes.	*Short-Term Goals*
➤ Due to limited finances and insurance coverage, Sheri is not willing to return for further follow-up with dietitian. Will see her physician in 1 week. Dietitian will call her in 2 weeks.	*Follow-up*

Case Study 7

Jackie is a 23-year-old single woman.	**Demographic Information**
Client was seen by her endocrinologist approximately 2 weeks ago for evaluation of her diabetes. The client is interested in improving her diabetes control and will be working with the endocrinologist to adjust her insulin schedule for more intensive management. She is being referred to a local private practice dietitian/diabetes educator to assist the client with fine-tuning her diabetes control with the addition of carbohydrate counting.	**Referral Data**

Diabetes Medical Nutrition Therapy

Diabetes Treatment Regimen	AM: 18 units NPH; 7 units Regular PM: 10 units NPH, 9 units Regular

Laboratory Values	Blood glucose ranges:
	    Fasting: 65-210 mg/dL
	    Before lunch (weekdays): 40-100 mg/dL
	    Before lunch (weekends): 90-160 mg/dL
	    Before dinner: 50-180 mg/dL
	    Before bed: 150-200 mg/dL
	Glycosylated hemoglobin (HgbA$_{1c}$): 9.7% Cholesterol: 160 mg/dL
	HDL cholesterol: 57 mg/dL LDL cholesterol: 118 mg/dL
	Triglycerides: 85 mg/dL Blood pressure: 115/68
	Microalbumin: normal

Medical History	Unremarkable.
Diabetes History	14-year history of type I diabetes.
Other Medications That Affect Therapy	None.
Exercise Guidelines	Client is currently physically active, using a step machine or stationary bike 2 nights/week after work and on Saturday morning. She is very interested in continuing this schedule of physical activity.
Medical Treatment Goals for Client	Target blood glucose levels: premeal: 80–140 mg/dL bedtime: 100–180 mg/dL Target glycosylated hemoglobin level: 6–7.5% Self-monitoring (method, frequency, education, evaluation): has been using a glucose meter and testing glucose levels 1–2 times a day; instructed to increase frequency of monitoring and test blood glucose levels four times/day (before meals, snacks, and bedtime).
Education Completed	She received general updated information about diabetes at her physician's office. The diabetes nurse educator focused education on assessing Jackie's current diabetes self-management skills (testing, recording, and interpreting result of blood glucose levels; experience and ability in adjusting insulin levels based on glucose results; and coordinating food intake and physical activity with insulin schedules. She provided Jackie with diabetes self-care records for charting and evaluating medication and glucose results.
First Visit (with RD 2 weeks later) **Clinical Data**	Lab data: N/A Medications: NPH insulin was increased by 2 units in the PM because of persistently high fasting blood glucose levels; Regular insulin was also increased by 2 units in the PM because of high bedtime blood glucose levels.

Blood glucose monitoring: log book results show the following:
 Fasting: 115–220 mg/dL
 Before lunch (weekdays): 98–129 mg/dL
 Before dinner: 40–80 mg/dL
 Before bed: 64–199 mg/dL
 Blood glucose levels continue to be high before bedtime
Exercise: Jackie reported that she had exercised twice this past week after work and felt hypoglycemic each time. Glucose levels on these days prior to evening meals were 40 and 50 mg.
Food records: See Diabetes Self-Care Daily Record (first visit).

Nutrition Assessment
Clinical Data

Physical information: Height: 66 inches
         Weight: 125 pounds
         Body frame: medium
Reasonable body weight: 125 pounds
Estimated daily energy needs: approximately 1,800–2,000 calories

Nutrition History*

Usual food intake: Breakfast (7:30–8:00 AM): 2 slices toast, orange juice, hot tea
       Lunch (12:00–1:00 PM): yogurt, crackers/chips, fresh fruit or deli sandwich with chips, diet soda
       Dinner (6:00–7:00 PM): stir-fry, egg roll, rice, tea
       HS snack: 3–4 cookies
Nutrition evaluation: Energy intake: approximately 1,800–2,000 calories
       Frequency and timing of meals: limited time to eat lunch; lunch sometimes delayed until midafternoon
       Other nutritional concerns: low glucose levels before meal times indicate need for food-insulin adjustment—ie, less insulin, additional and/or higher-calorie snacks PM and HS may also need additional information regarding eating-out choices
Weight history: weight stable over past 10 years
Appetite/eating/digestion problems: N/A
Eating outside the home: stops for carryout food 1–2 times a week (Chinese or pizza)
Alcohol intake: 1–2 drinks at "happy hour" on Friday afternoons after work
Use of vitamins/minerals/supplements: N/A

Exercise History

Step machine or stationary bike 2 nights a week after work; biking or hiking on Saturday morning.

Psychosocial and Economic Issues

Client is single, works as accountant for large firm. Enjoys outdoor activities, such as hiking, during her free time. Often meets friends for "happy hour" on Fridays after work.

Blood Glucose Monitoring

See *Medical Treatment Goals for Client.*

---
*Information summarized from the Lifestyle Change Questionnaire, a resource from *Facilitating Lifestyle Change.*

Diabetes Medical Nutrition Therapy

Knowledge, Skills, Attitudes and Motivation

Jackie is a college graduate. She is very interested in improving her diabetes control and is anxious to learn more about intensive insulin management, carbohydrate counting, and the skills necessary for better diabetes self-management; she desires to continue her usual lifestyle and schedule of activities.

Food/Meal Planning

- Introduced the concept of carbohydrate counting using the educational resource *Carbohydrate Counting: Getting Started* (Level 1). A meal plan of approximately 240 g/day was developed with Jackie. The method of carbohydrate choices was discussed and a carbohydrate distribution plan as listed below, based on her caloric needs and typical eating pattern, was provided to get Jackie started with carbohydrate counting. Recommended that Jackie use measuring cups and spoons to measure foods.
  - Breakfast: 4 CHO choices
  - Lunch: 4–5 CHO choices
  - Dinner: 5–6 CHO choices
  - HS snack: 1–2 CHO choices
- Provided Jackie with Diabetes Self-Care Daily Record forms, which include more specific nutrient information for her to record carbohydrate choices, as well as medication and blood glucose results.

Exercise

- Emphasized the importance of exercise and continuing her usual patterns of exercise. Discussed the importance of glucose monitoring with exercise to prevent hypoglycemia and the inclusion of a small snack in the afternoon before her after-work exercise sessions. Also provided sample pack of glucose replacement tablets to have as an accessible treatment of hypoglycemia.
- Discussed precautions to use when including alcohol; recommended that Jackie not exercise on the Fridays she goes to "happy hour."

Short-Term Goals

- Jackie will keep combined glucose, food, and exercise records intermittently over the next 2 weeks using the Diabetes Self-Care Record forms provided in the Level 1 carbohdyrate counting booklet in order to record food intake intake, calculate carbohydrate choices, evaluate effects of foods and exercise on glucose level, and begin to detect patterns in daily glucose levels. She was provided with multiple copies of this form for record keeping.
- Jackie will incorporate PM snack on days she exercises, and as needed.
- Jackie will test blood glucose levels prior to exercise and when she feels hypoglycemic; recommended that Jackie decrease her NPH insulin in AM by 2 units on the days she exercises in the afternoons.

Follow-up

- Schedule follow-up appointment in 2 weeks with Jackie to review self-care records, evaluate any problems with hypoglycemia, and continue progress with carbohydrate counting.
- Follow up with endocrinologist to discuss use of carbohydrate counting, issues with hypoglycemia, and plans for altering insulin regimen—decreasing AM intermediate-acting insulin and switching PM intermediate-acting insulin to bedtime.

Lab data: N/A
Medication:
 (new insulin regimen)
  AM: 16 units NPH; 7 units Regular
  PM: 9 units Regular
  HS: 12 units NPH
Blood glucose monitoring: see Diabetes Self-Care Record (second visit)
Exercise: added PM snack on exercise days; no problem with hypoglycemia in the afternoon
Food records: see Diabetes Self-Care Record (2nd visit)

Second Visit

Follow-up Data

Nutrition Progress

Client has attempted to eat at consistent times this past week, especially at lunch. She has eaten all her evening meals at home, avoiding take-out foods. She has been using the *Carbohydrate Counting: Getting Started* (Level 1) booklet to become familiar with carbohydrate content of foods, is following the meal plan using the carbohydrate choices method at meals, and is keeping self-care records. She is interested in additional information about estimating portion sizes of foods, interpreting food labels, and learning carbohydrate content of snack foods and alcohol.

Food/Meal Planning

- Reinforced healthy eating habits and positive changes that have occurred.
- Provided client with blank food record form and asked to complete 24-hour food recall. Assessed ability to calculate carbohydrate intake of her food record using food lists provided in the Level 1 booklet. Jackie has good working knowledge of how to use carbohydrate choices method to estimate carbohydrate intake at meals. She is unsure about how to estimate portion sizes of some foods, especially portions of meat and amounts of specific foods in mixed dishes such has pizza and casseroles. Jackie was provided with food scale and encouraged to practice weighing foods at meals to gain experience with accurately estimating portion sizes, and also to continue measuring foods.
- Jackie was also given book with comprehensive listing of calorie and carbohydrate values of foods, including convenience foods, fast-food restaurants, and alcoholic beverages. She was also encouraged to bring food labels of commonly purchased foods at next visit to discuss how to interpret food labels.
- Jackie was introduced to the next level of carbohydrate counting, which introduces pattern management, and provided with *Carbohydrate Counting: Moving On* (Level 2). Recommended that she keep combined food, glucose, and exercise records and begin to count grams of carbohydrate instead of using carbohydrate as follows for meals and snacks:
    Breakfast: 60 g carbohydrate
    Lunch: 70–75 g carbohydrate
    Dinner: 85–90 g carbohydrate
    HS snack: 15 g carbohydrate if blood glucose < 150 mg/dL
- Discussed snack choices and emphasize the importance of including PM snack, especially when exercising, to prevent hypoglycemia.

Diabetes Medical Nutrition Therapy

Blood Glucose Monitoring
- Discuss target glucose range as 70–150 mg premeal.
- Review glucose records and patterns with Jackie.
- Discuss possible actions or strategies for low and high blood glucose levels, such as adjusting food, activity, and/or medication.

Short-Term Goals

Jackie will:
- continue to keep combined glucose, food, and exercise records intermittently over the next month using the Diabetes Self-Care Record form provided in the Level 2 carbohdyrate counting booklet in order to evaluate effects of foods and exercise on glucose level and to begin to detect patterns in daily glucose levels. She was provided with multiple copies of this form for record keeping.
- use the resource *Carbohydrate Counting: Moving On* to assist in understanding patterns and problem-solving with her own diabetes self-care.
- record carbohydrate intake in grams using the recommendations listed above.

Follow-up
- Schedule follow-up appointment in 1 month with Jackie to review self-care records, establish CHO/insulin ratio, evaluate any problems with hypoglycemia, and discuss additional issues, such as eating out and food labeling.
- Jackie will emphasize consistency of carbohydrate at meals and snacks and measure foods at meals to develop better accuracy at estimating portion sizes.
- Jackie will work with endocrinologist and/or diabetes nurse educator on insulin supplementation and decision-making for adjusting Regular insulin based on glucose results. Jackie's individualized insulin supplement formula is BG: 100/40 = supplement (refer to Chapter 7, page 55 for insulin supplement formula)
- Follow up with endocrinologist to discuss additional changes that have been made to intensive insulin regimen.

Third Visit

Follow-up Data

Lab data: random blood glucose (2 hours postprandical): 132 mg/dL
Medication: AM: 8 units NPH; 7 units Regular
(switched to new Noon: 6 units Regular
insulin regimen) PM: 9 units Regular
  Bedtime: 12 units NPH
Blood glucose monitoring: see Diabetes Self-Care Record (3rd visit)
Exercise: exercising 2–3 days/week, usually in late afternoons on weekdays and in morning on weekend day; no problem with hypoglycemia when including snack before exercise
Food records: see Diabetes Self-Care Record (3rd visit)

Diabetes Self-Management Progress

Jackie has kept daily records of CHO intake, insulin dosage, and glucose levels prior to meals, snacks, and exercise sessions. She is now making adjustments with Regular insulin before meals based on her blood glucose levels. She is interested in making some adjustment with food intake and meals and is expressing concern about making good choices and knowing how to count carbohydrates when eating out.

Food/Meal Planning

- Introduce the concept of developing a carbohydrate:insulin ratio using CHO worksheet from Level 3 carbohydrate counting booklet *Carbohydrate Counting: Using Carbohydrate/Insulin Ratios.* Determine carbohydrate/insulin ratio using the CHO gram method and based on Jackie's CHO intake at meals and insulin dose before meals (see attached worksheet for calculations of Jackie's individualized CHO/insulin ratio). Use examples of meals and snacks to practice using ratio to adjust for carbohydrate.
- Provide Jackie with a copy of the resource *The Restaurant Companion* for obtaining carbohydrate values of foods in several national chain and popular fast-food, American style, and upscale restaurants; suggest that she also purchase a resource listing nutritive values of foods, specifically calories and carbohodyrates (eg, Corrine Netzer's *Complete Book of Food Counts*).
- Review the food labels Jackie provided by discussing the Nutrition Facts panel. Have Jackie determine total grams of carbohydrate based on serving size.
- Discuss effects of protein, fat, and fiber on blood glucose results. Caution discretion with using larger amounts of carbohydrate at meals and snacks to avoid weight gain.

Short-Term Goals

- Jackie will keep daily Diabetes Self-Care Records over the next week, recording CHO intake at each meal, insulin dosage, physical activity, and blood glucose results prior to each meal, snack, and exercise session.
- Jackie will begin adjusting Regular insulin based on carbohydrate intake and using the CHO/insulin ratio established at this visit.

Follow-up

- Follow up by phone and faxing self-care records in 2 weeks; review records and evaluate progress with using CHO/insulin ratio and adjusting insulin and CHO intake based on glucose results.
- Contact endocrinologist to update on Jackie's progress, establish CHO/insulin ratio and her interest in self-adjustment of food and insulin. Client is scheduled to see MD 1 week prior to next follow-up consultation and will have a glycosylated hemoglobin test completed at that time.

Fourth Visit
(by phone and fax)

Follow-up Data

Lab data: glycosylated hemoglobin: 7.8%
Medication: current regimen: AM: 8 units NPH; 4 units Regular
　　　　　　　　　　　　　　　Noon: 5 units Regular
　　　　　　　　　　　　　　　PM: 9 units Regular
　　　　　　　　　　　　　　　Bedtime: 12 units NPH
Blood glucose monitoring: see Blood Glucose Record (4th visit)
CHO records: see Blood Glucose Record (4th visit)

Diabetes Self-Management Progress

Jackie is doing well with self-adjustment of insulin based on carbohydrate intake and glucose results. Most of her blood glucose values are within her target range.

Education

➤ Confirm CHO/insulin ratio and determine whether it is working; fine-tune ratio to promote blood glucose results within blood glucose target of 70–150 mg/dL.
➤ Reemphasize portion control and continuing development in ability to estimate carbohydrate amounts.

Follow-up

➤ Jackie will send intermittent records on a monthly basis to review and follow up by phone if she has questions or problems arise.
➤ Monitor weight and glycosylated hemoglobin through contact with endocrinologist.

Diabetes Self-Care Record

Jackie – 1st visit

Date	Time	Insulin Dose	Blood Glucose Test	Ketones	Activity, Feelings, Comments	Foods Eaten/Amounts
Monday	8:00 am	18u NPH; 7u Reg	220 mg			
	12:00 pm	—	124			
	6:00 pm	10u NPH; 9u Reg	78			
	9:00 pm	—	181			
Tuesday	8:00 am	18u NPH; 7u Reg	170			
	12:00 pm	—	142			
	6:30 pm	10u NPH; 9u Reg	78			
	9:00 pm	—	192			
Wednesday	8:00 am	—	160			
	12:00 pm	—	98			
	5:30 pm	10u NPH; 9u Reg	40		Tested glucose after exercise – felt hypoglycemic	Ate dinner early; took insulin after eating
	9:00 pm	—	164			
Thursday	8:00 am	18u NPH; 7u Reg	150			
	12:00 pm	—	137			
	6:15 pm	10u NPH; 9u Reg	50		Felt hypoglycemic again after exercise	Ate dinner as soon as arrived home; took insulin after meal
	9:00 pm	—	157			
Friday	8:00 am	18u NPH; 7u Reg	115			
	12:00 pm	—	129			
	6:00 pm	10u NPH; 9u Reg	69		Happy hour with friends after work – 2 beers before dinner	Ate bedtime snack late
	10:00 pm	—	64			
Saturday	9:00 am	18u NPH; 7u Reg	170			
	12:30 pm	—	112			
	5:00 pm	10u NPH; 9u Reg	61		Biking for ½ hour in afternoon	Ate larger dinner than usual
	9:30 pm	—	199			

Diabetes Medical Nutrition Therapy

Jackie — 2nd visit

Diabetes Self-Care Daily Record

Day of week: **Saturday**   Date: _____

Time	Medication type	Medication amount	BG Results am	BG Results pm	Food Intake amount	Food Intake type of food/drink	Carbohydrate choices	Carbohydrate grams	Physical Activity type	Physical Activity amount
8:30 am	NPH / Reg	16u / 7u	49 mg		1 / ½	Cranberry English muffin / grapefruit / hot tea	2 / 1		hiking	1½ hrs
10:30 am			42		½ pkg	M&Ms	?			
12:00 pm				60	1 / 20 / 1 small / 2 / 1	Peanut butter & fruit spread on oatmeal bread / Low-fat cheese crackers (minis) / Banana / Low-fat sandwich cookies / Diet soda	2 / 1 / 1 / 1			
6:00 pm	Reg	9u		127	1½ cups / 2 slices / / 1 glass	Pasta Primavera / French bread-plain / Lettuce salad with fat-free dressing / Red wine	3 / 2 / ?			
9:00 pm	NPH	10		78	½ cup	Frozen yogurt	1			

Daily Totals:

Comments: Felt hypoglycemic during hike — ate some M&Ms

Jackie – 2nd visit

Diabetes Self-Care Record

Day of week __Monday__   Date _____

Time	Medication type	Medication amount	BG Results am	BG Results pm	Food Intake amount	Food Intake type of food/drink	Carbohydrate Information choices	Carbohydrate Information grams	Physical Activity type	Physical Activity amount
7:30am	NPH Reg	8u 7u	72mg		2 slices 2 tsp 2 tsp 4 oz.	whole-wheat toast diet margarine fruit spread orange juice		34 — 8 15 /57	step machine	30 min
12:15pm	Reg	6u (+1u Supplement)		160	½ ½ pkg 1 1	turkey sub low-fat potato chips apple diet soda		37 18 15 — /70		
5:00pm				62						
6:30pm	Reg	9u		110		stir-fry (vegetable) egg roll rice tea		15 40 30 — /85		
9:00pm	NPH	10u		137	2 ½ cup	Fortune cookies milk		8 6 /14		

Daily Totals: 226g CHO

Comments:

Visit 3

Practice Worksheet

How to Figure Your Carbohydrate-to-Insulin Ratio Using the Carbohydrate Gram Method

1. Record the grams (g) carbohydrate that you consistently eat at each meal based on your BG and food records.

   Breakfast __60__ g   Lunch __70__ g   Supper __90__ g

2. Record the Regular (R) insulin meal doses that consistently meet target BGs. (u = units of insulin)

   Breakfast __7__ u   Lunch __6__ u   Supper __9__ u

3. Determine the carbohydrate g per u insulin for each meal by dividing the total g carbohydrate for each meal by the number of u R.

   Breakfast = B   Lunch = L   Supper = S

   $\dfrac{\_\_\_\text{ g carbohydrate}}{\_\_\_\text{ u R insulin}} = \_\_\_$ g/u

   B $\dfrac{60 \text{ g}}{7 \text{ u}} = \dfrac{9}{}$ g/u

   L $\dfrac{70 \text{ g}}{6 \text{ u}} = \dfrac{12}{}$ g/u

   S $\dfrac{90 \text{ g}}{9 \text{ u}} = \dfrac{10}{}$ g/u

4. If your answers to step 3 vary from each other by no more than 1 g carbohydrate, add the 3 answers together and divide by 3 to get the average grams carbohydrate per unit of insulin.

   B ____
   L ____
   + S ____
   ____ total divided by 3 = ____ g/unit

5. If your answers to step 3 vary from each other by more than 1 g carbohydrate and you and your health-care team agree that your basal insulin doses are well adjusted, then use your answers to step 3 as your carbohydrate-to-insulin ratios for each meal.

   My carbohydrate-to-insulin ratios are
   B __9__ g/u   L __12__ g/u   S __10__ g/u

6. To make insulin adjustments for more or less carbohydrate eaten, add up the total carbohydrate and divide by the appropriate carbohydrate-to-insulin ratio.

   Total carbohydrate __60__ g ÷ __10__ g/u (ratio) = __6__ u R

   Example:
   Smaller supper = 60 gm carbohydrate

Level 4 Jackie - 4th visit

Blood Glucose Records

Name: _____ Phone Number: _____ Physician: _____

BG = Blood Glucose **Carb** = Grams Carbohydrate **Ins** = Insulin BG target = 70-150

| | 8 am |||| 12 pm |||| 6 pm |||| 9 pm ||| Comments |
Date/Time	BG	Carb	Ins	BG	Carb	Ins	BG	Carb	Ins	BG	Carb	Ins	Comments
Mon	120	60	8N / 5R	80	70	6R	140	90	9R (+1)	130	15	12N	Breakfast CHO: insulin ratio is now 12:1
Tues	115	60	8N / 5R	96	70	6R	110	90	9R	120	15	12N	L & D confirmed
Wed	96	60	8N / 5R	118	70	6R	136	90	9R	140	15	12N	ratio L=12:1, D=10:1
Thurs	160	45	6N* / 4R(+1)	130	60	5R (+1)	120	75	7R (+1)	116	15	12N	Step machine - 30 min. 3pm
Fri	175	60	8N / 5R(+2)	120	70	6R	80	90	9R	156	∅	14N	
Sat	130	90	6N* / 7R	130	45	4R (+1)	60	100	10R (-1)	130	15	14N	Hiking - 2 hrs. 2-4pm
Sun	110	60	8N / 5R	76	90	7R	170	90	9R (+2)	104	15	14N	

*Reduced N for planned exercise.

Conclusion 23

Diabetes Medical Nutrition Therapy

A major message of this publication is the importance of nutrition in the management of diabetes mellitus. Maximizing the role of diabetes medical nutrition therapy requires considerably more than having a dietitian or physician develop a nutrition prescription. It is important for the client with diabetes to acquire the information necessary and become able to achieve self-management of his or her own nutrition care plan.

A second message highlights the importance of individualizing the nutrition care plan. The nutrition care plan must meet the client's individual physiologic needs and must be adapted to the client's lifestyle, rather than requiring a change of lifestyle to accommodate the regimen.

A third major message supports the registered dietitian as the nutrition expert and the health care provider responsible for developing the nutrition care plan. The registered dietitian is also the provider who can teach the client with diabetes the necessary information and skills for self-management of the plan. This includes recommendations about medications, exercise, and the self-monitoring of blood glucose.

Finally, dietitians should be proactive, along with other members of the diabetes care team, in identifying outcomes and continually documenting the effectiveness of their intervention, as reflected in:

- improved SMBG results, glycated hemoglobin levels, blood lipids, blood pressure, renal function, and weight management;
- reduced need for medications;
- less hypoglycemia;
- less hospitalization; and
- lower cost of overall health care.

Diabetes Nutrition Education Resources

The long-term aspects of a life with diabetes need to be taken into account when selecting and tailoring meal-planning resources for clients. The use of a variety of meal-planning resources by the diabetes educator/dietitian is crucial for providing appropriate diabetes medical nutrition therapy. The diabetes educator/dietitian needs to individualize diabetes self-management training based on a comprehensive nutrition assessment of each client, which includes diabetes regimen, health status, learning ability, motivation, and lifestyle. Each meal-planning resource represented in this book, as well as others not mentioned, has advantages and disadvantages for use with various clients. Therefore, the diabetes educator is encouraged to use several different meal-planning resources in his or her practice setting to meet the unique needs of each client.

Clients may often need to have adjustments made in their original diabetes self-management training plan. For example, changes occur in personal relationships, careers, and work schedules, and adjustments in insulin and medications need to be made. All of these changes affect the diabetes self-management training plan. In addition, a change is sometimes needed just to achieve a new level of interest and motivation. Therefore, the meal-planning resource may need to be changed by the diabetes educator/dietitian based on reassessment and mutually agreed-upon goals. It is important to remember that there is no set time frame for eating changes, nor is there any standard formula for determining which meal-planning resource should be tried next to promote a particular change. Changing the meal-planning resource is based on assessment and goal-setting information, with the client's input as a key component of the decision-making process.

A combination of different meal-planning resources and teaching strategies may need to be used over a period of time to enable the client to make permanent changes in his or her eating and lifestyle behaviors. Ideally, a client will be able to see the diabetes educator/dietitian over a period of time in order to accomplish the diabetes self-management training plan, but this may not always be realistic. Regardless of the situation, the educator should use his or her creativity and various meal-planning resources to assist a client in achieving the goals of diabetes management.

Table 23.1 summarizes the meal-planning approaches that have been discussed, indicating the degree of emphasis on glucose control, weight loss, healthy eating, literacy required, structure, and complexity. *Table 23.2* shows which meal-planning approaches are best suited to each type of diabetes.

There is no one "right" or "wrong" method for meal planning. Any method, technique, or teaching tool that supports the nutrition self-management goals of achieving or maintaining appropriate serum glucose and lipid levels, reasonable body weight, and good nutrition that is realistic and workable for the client should be considered an acceptable approach to diabetes medical nutrition therapy. Many approaches can be individualized for use with different clients.

Using the four-pronged approach of diabetes medical nutrition therapy with a client represents the ideal. However, discounting this approach by saying "my clients are all elderly and are incapable of setting goals and making lifestyle changes" or "my work setting doesn't allow me to provide follow-up" may be accepting mediocrity. Providing information without incorporating this step-by-step approach, regardless of the quality of the educational material, is a setup for noncompliance.

When providing nutrition self-management training, the educator should be flexible and creative. Boredom can set in with any regimen and can lead to noncompliance. It is the responsibility of the diabetes educator to promote continuity of learning by introducing new ideas and concepts and altering the learning environment.

As educators, we also need to remember that we cannot force our values and knowledge on clients and assume that they will make changes in their eating behaviors because we think they should. Rather, we need to try to diminish the distance between "where they are" and "what we know." We can help them to discover new choices and make them aware of new possibilities. Taking the time to listen to clients, hear what they are telling us, and provide

Table 23.1
Summary of Meal-Planning Approaches

	Degree of emphasis on metabolic control	Degree of emphasis on weight loss	Degree of literacy required	Degree of structure	Degree of complexity
*Facilitating Lifestyle Change Manual**	moderate	high	moderate to high	moderate	moderate
Guideline Approaches					
Guide to Good Eating	low	low to moderate	low	low	low
Dietary Guidelines for Americans	low	low to moderate	low	low	low
Food Guide Pyramid	low	low to moderate	low	low	low
Healthy Food Choices (Guideline Section)	low	moderate	low	low	low
The First Step in Diabetes Meal Planning	low	low to moderate	low	low	low
Single-Topic Diabetes Resources	individualized depending on the resource				
Meal-Planning Approaches					
Individualized Menus	moderate to high	moderate to high	low	moderate	low
Month of Meals 1–5	moderate	moderate	low	moderate	low
Exchange Lists for Meal Planning	moderate to high	moderate	moderate to high	moderate to high	moderate to high
Calorie Counting	low	high	moderate	moderate to high	moderate
Fat Counting	low	high	moderate	moderate to high	moderate
Carbohydrate Counting: Getting Started	moderate to high	low	high	high	high
Carbohydrate Counting: Moving On	high	low	high	high	high
Carbohydrate Counting: CHO/Insulin Ratios	high	low	high	high	high

This table represents the authors' judgment and experience with meal-planning approaches. Readers are encouraged to modify the table based on each client's lifestyle and metabolic goals.
*This manual can be used for all four steps of the diabetes medical nutrition therapy model, but it is particularly useful for assessment, goal setting, and evaluation.

Adapted with permission from *Diabetes Educator,* 1987;13:146, as referenced in Powers MA, ed, *Handbook of Nutritional Management* (Rockville, Md: Aspen Publishers, Inc; 1987).

Table 23.2

Selection of Meal-Planning Approaches According to Type of Diabetes

		Type I	Type II Non-obese	Type II Obese
	Facilitating Lifestyle Change	X	X	X
Guideline Approaches				
Basic Nutrition	*Guide to Good Eating*	X	X	X
	Dietary Guidelines for Americans	X	X	X
	Food Guide Pyramid	X	X	X
Diabetes Nutrition Guidelines	*Healthy Food Choices* (Guideline Section)	X	X	X
	The First Step in Diabetes Meal Planning	X	X	X
	Single-Topic Diabetes Resources	X	X	X
Meal-Planning Approaches				
Menus	Individualized Menus		X	X
	Month of Meals 1–5		X	X
Exchanges	Exchange Lists for Meal Planning	X	X	X
Counting	Calorie Counting			X
	Fat Counting			X
	Carbohydrate Counting	X	X	

This table represents the authors' judgment and experience with meal-planning approaches. Readers are encouraged to modify the table based on each client's individualized lifestyle and metabolic goals.

---

them with new possibilities will promote more permanent behavior changes than just giving them a standardized or structured tool for meal planning.

For additional information about diabetes care and education and ways to obtain client and professional education resources, contact the following organizations:

➤ American Diabetes Association
National Center
1660 Duke Street
Alexandria, VA 22314
1-800-232-3472

➤ The Diabetes Care and Education Practice Group of
The American Dietetic Association
216 West Jackson Boulevard
Chicago, IL 60606-6995
1-800-877-1600

➤ American Association of Diabetes Educators
500 North Michigan Avenue
Chicago, IL 60611
1-800-338-3633

Nutrition is integral to total diabetes care and management, but it is also its most challenging aspect. It is essential for glycemic control and overall good health. The educator must incorporate the four-pronged approach of diabetes medical nutrition therapy for successful self-management training. We challenge you to consider your approach to nutrition self-management training, as well as the existing systems within which you provide diabetes care, to maximize your effort to improve the quality of life and longevity of clients with diabetes.

Appendixes

Appendix 1 Laboratory Values for Diabetes Mellitus

Table 1

Lipid and Glucose Measurements

Test	Normal	Acceptable	Improvement Attempted	Unacceptable
Type I Diabetes				
Hemoglobin A_1C (%)	< 6	6–7	8–9	11–13
Mean blood glucose (mg/dL)	80–120	120–160	160–240	> 300
Premeal self-monitored blood glucose (SMBG)	80–120	120–160	160–200	
Bedtime SMBG	—	100–140	—	—
Type II Diabetes				
Hemoglobin A_1C (%)	< 6	6–7.5	7.5–9	> 9
Fasting plasma glucose (mg/dL)	< 115	80–140	140–200	> 200
2-hr postprandial blood glucose (mg/dL)	< 140	100–180	180–235	> 235
Fasting plasma cholesterol (mg/dL)	< 200	< 200	200–240	> 240
Fasting LDL cholesterol (mg/dL)	< 130	< 130	130–160	> 160
Fasting plasma triglyceride (mg/dL)	< 200	< 200	200–250	> 250

Reprinted with permission from HE Lebovitz, Goals for treatment, in: *Therapy for Diabetes Mellitus & Related Disorders,* 2nd ed (Alexandria, Va: American Diabetes Association, Inc; 1994).

Appendix 2 Clinical Data

Table 1
Body Weight (in pounds) According to Height (in inches) and Body Mass Index

Body mass index is weight in kilograms divided by height in meters squared. Each entry gives the body weight in pounds for a person of a given height and body mass index. Pounds have been rounded off. To use the table, find the appropriate height in the left-hand column. Move across the row to a given weight. The number at the top of the column is the body mass index for that weight and height.

Body Mass Index

Height	19	20	21	22	23	24	25	26	27	28	29	30	31	32	33	34
								Body Weight								
58	91	95	100	105	110	114	119	124	129	133	138	143	148	152	157	162
59	94	99	104	109	114	119	124	129	134	139	144	149	154	159	164	169
60	97	102	107	112	117	122	127	132	138	143	148	153	158	163	168	173
61	101	106	111	117	122	127	132	138	143	148	154	159	164	169	175	180
62	103	109	114	120	125	130	136	141	147	152	158	163	168	174	179	185
63	107	113	119	124	130	135	141	147	152	158	164	169	175	181	186	192
64	111	117	123	129	135	141	146	152	158	164	170	176	182	187	193	199
65	114	120	126	132	138	144	150	156	162	168	174	180	186	192	198	204
66	118	124	131	137	143	149	156	162	168	174	180	187	193	198	205	212
67	121	127	134	140	147	153	159	166	172	178	185	191	198	204	210	217
68	125	132	139	145	152	158	165	172	178	185	191	198	205	211	218	224
69	128	135	142	149	155	162	169	176	182	189	196	203	209	216	223	230
70	133	140	147	154	161	168	175	182	189	196	203	210	217	224	231	237
71	136	143	150	157	164	171	179	186	193	200	207	214	221	229	236	243
72	140	148	155	162	170	177	185	192	199	207	214	221	229	236	244	251
73	143	151	158	166	174	181	189	196	204	211	219	226	234	241	249	257
74	148	156	164	171	179	187	195	203	210	218	226	234	242	249	257	265
75	151	159	167	175	183	191	199	207	215	223	231	239	247	255	263	271
76	156	164	172	181	189	197	205	214	222	230	238	246	255	263	271	279

Body Mass Index

Height	35	36	37	38	39	40	41	42	43	44	45	46	47	48	49	50
								Body Weight								
58	167	172	176	181	186	191	195	200	205	210	214	219	224	229	233	238
59	174	179	184	188	193	198	203	208	213	218	223	228	233	238	243	248
60	178	183	188	194	199	204	209	214	219	224	229	234	239	244	250	255
61	185	191	196	201	207	212	217	222	228	233	238	244	249	254	260	265
62	190	196	201	206	212	217	223	228	234	239	245	250	255	261	266	272
63	198	203	209	214	220	226	231	237	243	248	254	260	265	271	277	282
64	205	211	217	223	228	234	240	246	252	258	264	269	275	281	287	293
65	210	216	222	228	234	240	246	252	258	264	270	276	282	288	294	300
66	218	224	230	236	243	249	255	261	268	274	280	286	292	299	305	311
67	223	229	236	242	248	255	261	268	274	280	287	293	299	306	312	319
68	231	238	244	251	257	264	271	277	284	290	297	304	310	317	323	330
69	236	243	250	257	263	270	277	284	290	297	304	311	317	324	331	338
70	244	251	258	265	272	279	286	293	300	307	314	321	328	335	342	349
71	250	257	264	271	279	286	293	300	307	314	321	329	336	343	350	357
72	258	266	273	281	288	295	303	313	317	325	332	340	347	354	362	369
73	264	272	279	287	294	302	309	317	324	332	340	347	355	362	370	377
74	273	281	288	296	304	312	319	327	335	343	351	358	366	374	382	390
75	279	287	294	302	310	318	326	334	342	350	358	366	374	382	390	398
76	287	296	304	312	320	328	337	345	353	361	370	378	386	394	402	411

Source: Adapted and expanded from National Institute of Diabetes and Digestive and Kidney Diseases, *Understanding Adult Obesity* (Rockville, Md: National Institutes of Health; 1993). NIH Publ No 94-3680.

Table 2
Healthy Weight Ranges for Men and Women

Height*	Weight (lb)†
4'10"	91–119
4'11"	94–124
5'0"	97–128
5'1"	101–132
5'2"	104–137
5'3"	107–141
5'4"	111–146
5'5"	114–150
5'6"	118–155
5'7"	121–160
5'8"	125–164
5'9"	129–169
5'10"	132–174
5'11"	136–179
6'0"	140–184
6'1"	144–189
6'2"	148–195
6'3"	152–200
6'4"	156–205
6'5"	160–211
6'6"	164–216

*Without shoes
†Without clothes

Source: *Report of the Dietary Guidelines Advisory Committee on the Dietary Guidelines for Americans* (Washington, DC: US Department of Agriculture, Agriculture Research Service; 1995), 23–24.

Table 3
Reasonable Body Weight

Desirable body weight (DBW) is the ideal body weight for a person based on height and frame size and can be calculated with the following formula[1]:

- *Adult women* 100 lb for first 5 ft of height and 5 lb for each inch over 5 ft (ie, DBW for a 5 ft 4 in woman is 120 lb) at medium body frame; subtract 10% for small frame and add 10% for large frame.
- *Adult men* 106 lb for first 5 ft of height and 6 lb for each inch over 5 ft (ie, DBW for a 5 ft 10 in man is 166 lb) at medium body frame; subtract 10% for small frame and add 10% for large frame.

Establishing a *reasonable body weight* may be a more appropriate goal than the client's desirable body weight. Reasonable body weight is defined as an achievable and maintainable weight goal. This reasonable goal may not be in the range of published desirable weights. For example, a reasonable weight goal for a 5 ft 2 in obese woman with diabetes weighing 180 lb may be 160 lb, although her desirable body weight may actually be closer to 110 lb. Losing even 10 lb to 20 lb may dramatically improve glucose tolerance and may be a maintainable weight loss. Weight loss goals should be individualized for every client.

Another resource used for determining weight is the *Recommended Dietary Allowances*.[2] Suggested weights for adults from that publication appear in Table 1.

1. Powers MA, ed. *Nutrition Guide for Professionals: Diabetes Education and Meal Planning*. Alexandria, Va: American Diabetes Association, Inc; 1988:29.
2. National Research Council, National Academy of Sciences. *Recommended Dietary Allowances*. 10th ed. Washington, DC: National Academy Press; 1989.

Table 4
Estimating Daily Energy Needs for Adults and Children

There are many formulas available for calculating calorie needs. More important than what method is used for the calculation is that consideration be given to the individual needs of the client. The following questions should be considered:

- What calorie level is realistic for the client?
- How much weight does the client need or, more importantly, want to lose?
- Is a calorie level and meal plan necessary to accomplish the nutrition goals established with the client?

Estimating Caloric Intake for Adults

Basal Calories: 10–12 kcal/lb desirable body weight
20–25 kcal/kg desirable body weight

Add Calories for Activity:
If sedentary	30% more calories
If moderately active	50% more calories
If strenuously active	100% more calories

Adjustments:*
Add 300 kcal/d during pregnancy
Add 500 kcal/d during lactation
Add 500 kcal/d to gain one lb/wk
Subtract 500 kcal/d to lose one lb/wk

*Adjustments are approximate: weight changes should be monitored and compared to caloric intake.

Reprinted with permission from M Joyce, Issues in prescribing calories, in: MA Powers, *Handbook of Diabetes Medical Nutrition Therapy* (Gaithersburg, Md: Aspen Publishers, Inc; 1996), p 368.

National Research Council RDAs 1989: Recommended Energy Intake for Infants and Children

	Age in Years	Calories /kg	Calories /day
Infants	0–0.5	108	650
	0.5–1.0	98	850
Children	1–3	102	1,300
	4–6	90	1,800
	7–10	70	2,000
Males	11–14	55	2,500
	15–18	45	3,000
	19–24	40	2,900
Females	11–14	47	2,200
	15–18	40	2,200
	19–24	38	2,200

Note: From birth to age 10 years, no distinction between sexes is made regarding energy requirements. Separate allowances are recommended for boys and girls older than 10 years because of differences in the age of onset of puberty and patterns of physical activity. Considerable variability is seen in the timing and magnitude of the adolescent growth spurt and in activity patterns. Consequently, the range of the recommendation for children older than 20 years is wider, and energy allowances should be adjusted individually to take into account body weight, physical activity, and rate of growth.

Reprinted with permission from *Recommended Dietary Allowances*, 10th ed. Copyright 1989 by the National Academy of Sciences. Courtesy of the National Academy Press, Washington, DC.

Appendix 3   Nutrition History

Table 1
Food Record Form

This food record can help you and your nutritionist better understand how food affects your health. Please write down everything you eat and drink from the time you wake up to the time you go to bed. Include meals, snacks, and drinks.

Time	Type of Food/Beverage	Amount

Table 2

Diabetes Self-Care Daily Record

Day of week _____ Date _____

Time	Medication		Blood Glucose Results		Food Intake		Nutrient Information	Physical Activity	
	type	amount	am	pm	amount	type of food/drink		type	amount

Comments: Daily Totals:

Diabetes Medical Nutrition Therapy

Table 3
Simplified Form for Assessment of Food Intake

Questions to Assess Nutritional Adequacy

Review the usual food intake or food records with the client and ask the following questions to identify nutrition problems and potential solutions:

- ➤ Are there enough or too many food choices from each category in the Food Guide Pyramid?
- ➤ Are many of the food choices high in fat? (margarine/butter, salad dressing, mayonnaise, gravy, sauce, olives, nuts, snack chips, cheeses, luncheon meats, sausage, desserts, ice cream, whole milk)
- ➤ Are many of the food choices high in fiber? (whole-grain breads, cereals, crackers, pastas, long-grain/brown rice, dried beans and peas, fresh/frozen fruits and vegetables)
- ➤ Is there more than 7 oz meat, poultry, fish, or meat alternatives? (Remember, the Food Guide Pyramid recommends 4–6 oz of protein per day. This will help maintain a lower fat intake.)
- ➤ Are there many carbohydrate food choices that are high-calorie and/or low-nutrient-density? (sugar, jam, candy, regular soft drinks, dessert)

Sample Nutrition History

Breakfast	Lunch	Dinner	HS Snack
1 c orange juice	Sandwich:	**5 oz fried chicken**	**1 c CHOCOLATE**
1 biscuit	2 slices white bread	(1 breast + 1 thigh)	**ICE CREAM**
1 fried egg	**½ c tuna, packed in oil**	½ c mashed potatoes	
2 fried sausage links	**3 tsp mayonnaise**	with **gravy**	
1 tsp margarine	**1½ oz potato chips**	1 c *green beans*	
1 tsp JELLY	HOSTESS TWINKIE	seasoned with **bacon**	
Coffee with	COKE	1 dinner roll	
half and half		**1 tsp margarine**	
		½ c salad	
		(pineapple,	
		MARSHMALLOW)	

Assessment of the Sample Nutrition History*

1. The nutrition history reveals a low intake of milk and milk products and grains.
2. The nutrition history reveals an intake of 12 food items that are sources of fat (**boldface** food items).
3. The nutrition history reveals only one food source of fiber (*italic* food item).
4. The nutrition history reveals an intake of 8 oz of meat or meat substitutes.
5. The nutrition history reveals an intake of 5 food items that are sources of carbohydrate that are high-calorie and/or low-nutrient-density (CAPITALIZED food items).

*This is a crude assessment based only on a food record or nutrition history. This assessment does not take into account the person's caloric needs.

Appendix 4   Diabetes Knowledge Checklist

The following checklist was developed to reflect the 1994 American Diabetes Association Nutrition Recommendations. This can be used as a tool for the dietitian/diabetes educator to assess current understanding of the nutrition-related aspects of diabetes management. This worksheet can be filled out by the professional as part of a detailed assessment of what the client knows and needs to know. The date can be added by the topic under "Needs Info" when the client is counseled.

Nutrition Topic	Knows	N/A	Needs Info
A simple definition of carbohydrate			
Foods containing carbohydrate do not have to be restricted			
Food sources of starch (bread, pasta, cereals)			
Food sources of sugar (candy, carbonated beverages, jelly, syrup)			
How to incorporate sugars into the meal plan			
The effects of large amounts of fiber on blood lipid levels			
Food sources of soluble and insoluble fiber			
Food sources of protein (meat, poultry, seafood, eggs, dairy, dried beans and peas)			
Types of fat (saturated, poly, and mono)			
Main food sources of the three types of fat			
The effects of each type of fat on blood lipids			
Caloric contribution of fat as compared to carbohydrate and protein			
Goals of balanced nutrition			
The relationship of weight loss, exercise, nutrition, and medication to blood glucose management			
The benefits of exercise			
The desired range for fasting blood glucose			
The desired range for glycated hemoglobin			
Goal or target range for blood glucose levels			
Weight goal, if appropriate			
Lipid goal (total cholesterol, HDL, LDL, triglycerides)			

Diabetes Medical Nutrition Therapy

Appendix 5 Goal Setting

CLINICAL/METABOLIC GOALS

	Target Range	*Individualized Goal*
Weight		
Glucose		
Lipids		
Other		

LIFESTYLE CHANGE GOALS

	Individualized Goals
Eating	
Physical Activity	
Monitoring	
Other	

EDUCATION GOALS

Type of Nutrition Intervention	
Education Resource(s)	
Follow-up • Frequency • Teaching Format • Specific Needs	

Appendix 6 Sample Completed *Single-Topic Diabetes Resources* Handouts

FOOD, DIABETES, AND THE OLDER PERSON

👉 What about you?

- Do you test your blood glucose levels? (yes)/no *2 times a week*
  What is your target range? __100__ to __150__ mg/dl
- Do you take diabetes medicine? (yes)/no
  What medicine do you take? __Diabeta__
  What times do you take it? __7:30 am 4:30 pm__
  How much do you take? __10 mg twice a day__
- How many times a week do you exercise or do physically active things? __Ø__
- How many times a day do you eat? __5__
  Do you skip meals and snacks? (yes)/no *Sometimes*
- Do you have problems with any foods?
  __Dislikes cooking / eating alone__

❓ Why learn how to take care of your diabetes?

- Learning to take care of your diabetes helps you feel well and stay healthy.
- Making healthy food choices and staying active helps you keep your blood glucose in your target range.
- Keeping your diabetes under control can help prevent damage to your eyes, heart, nerves, and kidneys.

💡 What will you learn?

- How to control your blood glucose level. *Bring your levels closer to your target.*
- What you need to know about diabetes medicine, exercise, and food.
- What to do if you have problems with seeing, shopping, preparing food, appetite, or chewing.
- How your food choices can affect your blood pressure, bones, weight, and health.

Your blood glucose

- Your blood glucose changes all day long. You want your blood glucose to stay in the range you and your health care team set as a goal.
- High blood glucose damages your eyes, heart, nerves, kidneys, and blood vessels.
- Low blood glucose can cause shakiness, trouble concentrating, headache, dizziness, clumsiness, extreme hunger, or irritability. Very low blood glucose can make you pass out.
- Test your blood glucose at different times each day and write down the results. If your blood glucose is often too high or too low, ask your health care team if you need to change your food, medicine, or activity routine.

Test at lunch 2 times a week. Test at bedtime 2 times a week. Test at breakfast and dinner everyday.

Your food plan

- Your registered dietitian (RD) can help you work out a food plan that works for you. Let your RD know what and when you like to eat. He or she can show you how to make small changes to help control your diabetes.
- Include food from all the food groups to make sure you get all the nutrients you need:

the number I have ↓

Food Group	Servings Per Day ↓	
1 slice bread, 1 6" tortilla, 1/2 cup cooked pasta or rice	6 or more	12
1 cup raw or 1/2 cup cooked vegetables	3-5	0
1 small fresh fruit or 1/2 cup canned or juice	3-4	0
1 cup nonfat or low-fat milk or yogurt	2-3	1-2
2-3 oz lean meat, poultry, or fish or low-fat cheese, 1 egg	2-3	2

- Eat at least 3 times a day.
- Eat the same types and amounts of food at about the same time each day to help control your blood glucose.
- Find out how to include foods with sugar on occasion in your food plan.

Your diabetes medicine

- Always take your diabetes medicine, unless your doctor has told you not to.
- Take your medicine at about the same time each day.
- Eat regularly when you take diabetes medicine to keep your blood glucose in your target range. *Don't forget to eat snacks.*

Diabetes Medical Nutrition Therapy

Your exercise plan

- Plan to do something active each day. _Walk, garden_
- Choose activities you enjoy. You may prefer a formal exercise class, a sport such as tennis or golf, social activities like dancing, or informal activities such as _gardening_ or walking the dog.
- Before you start a new exercise plan, discuss it with your physician.

How to get help

- Talk to your health care team if you cannot see well or have problems shopping or preparing food. They may give you large-print publications or refer you for help in your community. _Ask about Meals on Wheels for lunch._
- If you have trouble chewing, visit your dentist. Your RD can suggest foods that are easy to eat.
- If you just don't feel like eating much, ask your RD for ideas to make food more appealing. Eat with friends or family or have _lunch at your local senior citizen center._

Special health concerns

- If you have problems with constipation, eat plenty of fiber from whole-wheat bread and tortillas, whole-grain cereals and pasta, brown rice, beans, vegetables, and fruit. Drink at least 8 cups of liquid (water, sugar-free, or calorie-free drinks and other beverages) a day. _Use diet soda._
- If you have high blood pressure, eat less salt and sodium. Use herbs and spices to season foods; use fresh, frozen, or low-sodium canned vegetables; and choose reduced-sodium soups and convenience foods.
- Eat plenty of high-calcium foods to keep your bones strong. Drink skim or low-fat _milk_ and eat nonfat or low-fat yogurt, low-fat cheese, _broccoli_, kale, and turnip and mustard greens. _Add milk or yogurt to breakfast._
- Control your weight and help keep your blood cholesterol down by staying active and choosing low-fat foods. _Use turkey instead of hot dogs._
- Learn how to have a sweet food as part of your food plan once in a while, rather than as an extra. _Small bowl of ice cream._
- Talk to your diabetes health care team at least twice a year and more often if you have problems.
- Visit your eye doctor once a year and your dentist twice a year. Check your feet every day.

Courtesy of _Julie Smith, RD, CDE_
Paradise Lane Home Health Care

This handout gives general guidelines for everyone with diabetes. Your educator can help you learn more and decide what will work for you.

Set your sights

1. My target range for blood glucose is _100_ to _150_ mg/dl.
2. I will test my blood glucose level at these times: _7:30am_   _4:30pm_   _9:00pm (2 times a week)_
* 3. I will do some type of physical activity at least 3 days a week, such as _walk around the block._
4. One change I will make to my food plan is _Use low-fat milk. Use low-calorie sweetener in coffee._
5. _Decrease serving size of ice cream and use sugar-free ice cream. Eat at least 4 servings of fruits and vegetables._

*Discuss with physician.

Keep track

Date _July 10_
Medicine: name _Diabeta_
   number of pills _____ time(s) _7:30am_ _4:30pm_
Meal and snack times _7:30am_ _11:30am_ _4:30pm_ _2:00pm_ _8:00pm_
Activity: type _walk around the block_ time _15 min._
Blood glucose level: time _7:30am_ _4:30pm_ _9:00pm_
   mg/dl _170_   _210_   _180_

Here's the challenge; What's your solution?

1. You have just started to take diabetes medicine in the morning. You do not usually eat breakfast and have been feeling dizzy before lunch. What food plan changes will you make?
Eat breakfast: shredded wheat and low-fat milk.
2. You like to have a small scoop of ice cream or a cookie before you go to bed. Your blood glucose level has been high first thing in the morning. What could you do?
In my case: Use smaller serving of ice cream and use sugar-free ice cream.
3.

American Diabetes Association.

THE AMERICAN DIETETIC ASSOCIATION

Developed by Sue McLaughlin, RD, CDE

Appendixes

DIABETES MEDICINES (pills and insulin)

👉 What about you?

- What diabetes medicine do you take?
  Name(s) _NPH and regular insulin_
  Time(s) _6:30am, 6:00pm, 9:00pm_
  Amount(s) _am: 18 NPH, 7 regular pm: 9 regular_
  HS: 10 NPH
- Do you take your medicine every day? (yes)/no
  If no, why? _____
- How often do you talk to your health care team about your diabetes medicine? _new diagnosis_
- Do you write down when you take your medicine in a record book? yes/(no)
- What concerns or questions do you have about your diabetes medicine? _Why do I take 3 injections instead of 2 like my cousin? Why do I have a reaction before dinner?_

❓ Why learn about diabetes medicine?

- If you understand how your diabetes medicine works, you can more easily balance ~~pills or~~ insulin, food, and exercise to control your diabetes.
- You need to know how and when to take your diabetes medicine.
- Diabetes medicines lower blood glucose. You need to know what to do if your blood glucose goes too low.

💡 What will you learn?

- ~~What you need to know about diabetes pills.~~
- ~~Why you may need to switch from diabetes pills to insulin.~~
- What you need to know about insulin.
- What you need to know about balancing food, exercise, and diabetes medicine.
- _How to plan for exercise._
- _How to manage low blood glucose._

What to know about diabetes pills

- Diabetes pills are not insulin. They help your pancreas make insulin and/or help your body use insulin or glucose. You still need to follow a food and exercise plan when you take diabetes pills.
- You might take 1 or 2 types of diabetes pills.
- Take diabetes pills at the same time each day, unless your doctor tells you not to. If you forget to take your pills, do not double up on the next dose. Call your doctor.
- Take diabetes pills 30 minutes before a meal. Do not wait longer than an hour to eat after you take your medicine.
- Learn the possible side effects of diabetes pills, such as low blood glucose, and know how to treat.
- You may be able to stop taking diabetes pills if you lose weight and follow your meal plan.

Switching from pills to insulin

- After you have had type II diabetes for a few years, your pancreas may not make enough insulin.
- If you can't keep your blood glucose in your target range balancing pills, food, and exercise, you may need insulin injections instead of or in addition to pills.
- Don't be alarmed. Many people with type II diabetes eventually need to take insulin by injection.

What to know about insulin

- Insulin is normally made by your pancreas. When you eat, your blood glucose goes up. Your pancreas puts out the right amount of insulin to let the glucose go from your blood into your body's cells. In the cells, the glucose is stored or used for energy.
- People with type I diabetes and some people with type II diabetes do not make any insulin and need insulin by injection every day.
- Insulin does not control your blood glucose; it just lowers it.
- Your food plan, insulin injections, and exercise program work together to control your diabetes.
- Several types of insulin exist. They work at different speeds. The chart on page 2 describes their action curves.
- Your doctor can use different amounts of different insulins to get the right amount of insulin working when your blood glucose goes up.
- The number of injections you need each day and the amount of each type of insulin you use depends on how much you eat, when you eat, your exercise routine, and your blood glucose goals.
- Insulin should be injected 30 minutes before a meal. Even short-acting insulin needs 30 minutes to have an effect.
- Save an empty plastic bottle to throw out your syringes and blood glucose monitoring needles and strips.
- _Take a mid-afternoon snack, such as fruit and crackers, every day._

263

Diabetes Medical Nutrition Therapy

Types of insulin

- Know the onset, peak, and duration of the types of insulin you use.
  - **Onset:** time before the insulin starts to work.
  - **Peak:** time when the insulin works best.
  - **Duration:** total time the insulin keeps working.

Type of insulin	Onset (hrs)	Peak (hrs)	Duration (hrs)
Short-acting - regular	1/2	2-5	5-8
Intermediate-acting - NPH and lente	1-3	6-12	16-24
Long-acting ultralente	4-6	8-20	24-28
Premixed 70/30	1/2	7-12	16-24

Diabetes medicine and exercise

- Do not inject insulin close to a muscle that you will exercise within the next hour. Exercise may make the insulin act more quickly. Inject insulin in your arms or abdomen if you will be exercising your legs.
- You may need an extra snack when you exercise if you use diabetes pills or insulin.
- If you try to lose weight, ask your health care team if you can take fewer pills instead of eating more.
- Check your blood glucose before and after you exercise.
- Call your health care provider if you have problems with high or low blood glucose.

Low blood glucose reactions

- Your blood glucose can go too low (hypoglycemia) if
  - you miss or delay a meal or snack or eat less food than the amount in your meal plan,
  - you take too many pills or inject too much insulin,
  - you exercise more than usual without eating extra food.
- Check your blood glucose if you feel sweaty, shaky, nervous, faint, or dizzy.
- Keep a food or drink with you, such as 2 to 3 glucose or dextrose tablets or 1/2 cup fruit juice, to treat low blood glucose.
- If you go out to eat, take your pills or inject your insulin after you get to the restaurant in case the meal is delayed.
- Call your health care provider if you have 2 or more low blood glucose test results per week.

This handout gives general guidelines for everyone with diabetes. Your educator can help you learn more and decide what will work for you.

Set your sights

1. I will take my diabetes pills/inject insulin at these times each day 6:30am 6:00pm 9:00pm
2. I will eat meals and snacks at these times each day 7:00am 12:30pm 3:00pm (snack) 6:30pm 9:00pm (snack)
3. I will keep a record of when I take my medicine and how much I take. (and my blood glucose level)
4. When lunch is delayed, add a morning snack of fresh fruit and a breakfast bar and decrease afternoon snack by 1/2.

Keep track

(10/2/95)

Time	Name of pills or insulin	Amount
6:30am	NPH/regular	18/7
6:00pm	regular	9
9:00pm	NPH	10

Here's the challenge; What's your solution?

1. You forgot to take your pills or insulin this morning. It is now lunchtime. What should you do? Test your blood glucose. Take your regular breakfast insulin dose now.
2. You have been told to take diabetes medicine in the morning. You usually eat breakfast when you get to work. When will you take your medicine and eat your meal? Move breakfast and insulin to before you leave the house.
3. On Fridays, you usually stop for happy hour after work. When should you take your insulin? Test your blood glucose and take your insulin at the restaurant/bar. Eat dinner 1/2 hour later. Order non-alcoholic beverage until appetizer or dinner arrives.

Courtesy of Cindy Smith, RN, CDE
Diabetes Care Center

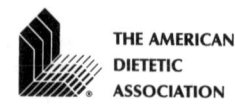

American Diabetes Association

THE AMERICAN DIETETIC ASSOCIATION

Developed by Deborah K. Sanden, RD, CDE

Appendix 7   Database for the *Exchange Lists for Meal Planning*

The nutrient information in this appendix was used to determine the food categories in The American Dietetic Association and American Diabetes Association's 1995 *Exchange Lists for Meal Planning*. Note that the database contains more foods than the *Exchange Lists* because some averaging was done to determine final portion sizes for the booklet. The database represents food nutrient information up to April 1995.

➤ The following are explanations of the nutrient sources:
  • Five-digit numbers identify the food nutrient source as the USDA nutrient database.[1]
  • Four-digit numbers identify the food nutrient source as coming mainly from USDA Handbook 456.[2]
  • B&C indicates that the food nutrient information comes from *Bowes and Church,* 16th edition.[3]
  • Some nutrient information comes directly from food labels, and thus the term *Label* or *Avg* is used.
  • Some nutrition information comes directly from the maker or a food association and is labeled with the company name or *Assoc.*
➤ Total dietary fiber values are from the USDA or *Plant Fiber in Foods*.[1,4]
➤ All values are based on edible portion (eg, grams per serving or per portion) rather than as purchased except for ingredients such as flour and cornmeal.
➤ All meats are trimmed of fat and cooked, unless noted.
➤ All values for canned fruits (in juice pack) include some liquid as well as the fruit.
➤ Numbers in parentheses indicate approximations.
➤ Dashes (missing values) indicate unavailable information.
➤ Abbreviations used in the database are:
  pro: protein   *cho:* carbohydrate
  SFA: saturated fatty acids   *MUFA:* monounsaturated fatty acids
  PUFA: polyunsaturated fatty acids *chol:* cholesterol
  ck: cooked   *fz:* frozen, cooked (except for
  raw: raw or fresh   frozen foods and yogurts)
  cn: canned, drained, except for canned fruits and those listed as s + l
  s + l: canned, both solids and liquids included in analysis

This database was compiled by Madelyn L. Wheeler MS, RD, Diabetes Research and Training Center (DRTC), Indiana University School of Medicine. DRTC support is through the National Institute of Diabetes and Digestive and Kidney Diseases (PHS P60-AM-20542). Invaluable assistance, support, and information were provided by Phyllis Barrier, MS, RD; Nancy Cronmiller, MMSc, RD; Linda Delahanty, MS, RD; Marion Franz, MS, RD; and Harold Holler, RD.

References

1. USDA Nutrient Data Base for Standard Reference, Full Version, Release 10, July 1993.
2. Adams CF. *Nutritive Values of American Foods in Common Units.* Agriculture Handbook No. 456. Washington, DC: US Government Printing Office; 1975.
3. Pennington JAT. *Bowes and Church's Food Values of Portions Commonly Used.* 16th ed. Philadelphia, Pa: JB Lippincott; 1994.
4. Anderson JW. *Plant Fiber in Foods.* 2nd ed. Lexington, Ky: HCF Nutrition Research Foundation; 1990.

STARCH: BREAD

Nutrient	Food Source	Quantity	Grams per Serving	Cal	Cho (g)	Pro (g)	Fat (g)	SFA (g)	MUFA (g)	PUFA (g)	Chol (mg)	Na (mg)	K (mg)	Total Dietary Fiber (g)
18001	Bagel	0.50 bagel	35	98	19.0	3.7	0.6	0.1	0.1	0.3	0	190	36	0.7
18057	Bread, reduced-calorie white	2.00 slices	46	96	20.4	4.0	1.2	0.3	0.5	0.3	0	208	36	4.2
18069	Bread, white (inc French & Italian)	1.00 slice	25	67	12.4	2.0	0.9	0.2	0.4	0.2	0	134	30	0.6
18075	Bread, whole-wheat	1.00 slice	28	70	13.1	2.7	1.2	0.3	0.5	0.3	0	149	71	2.0
18044	Bread, pumpernickel	1.00 slice	32	80	15.2	2.8	1.0	0.1	0.3	0.4	0	215	67	1.9
18060	Bread, rye	1.00 slice	32	83	15.5	2.7	1.1	0.2	0.4	0.3	0	211	53	2.0
18080	Bread sticks (4" × ½")	2.00 sticks	20	82	13.7	2.4	1.9	0.3	0.8	0.7	0	131	25	0.6
18258	English muffin	0.50 muffin	28	67	13.0	2.2	0.5	0.1	0.1	0.3	0	132	37	0.8
18350	Hot dog bun	0.50 bun	22	61	10.8	1.8	1.1	0.3	0.5	0.2	0	120	30	0.6
18350	Hamburger bun	0.50 bun	22	61	10.8	1.8	1.1	0.3	0.5	0.2	0	120	30	0.6
18041	Pita bread (6" across)	0.50 pita	30	83	16.7	2.7	0.4	0.1	0.0	0.2	0	161	36	0.5
18342	Roll, plain small	1.00 roll	28	85	14.3	2.4	2.1	0.5	1.0	0.4	0	148	38	0.8
18047	Rasin bread, unfrosted	1.00 slice	26	71	13.6	2.1	1.1	0.3	0.6	0.2	0	101	59	1.1
18363	Tortilla, corn, 6" across	1.00 tortilla	25	56	11.6	1.4	0.6	0.1	0.2	0.3	0	40	38	1.3
18364	Tortilla, flour, 7-8" across	1.00 tortilla	35	114	19.5	3.0	2.5	0.4	1.0	1.0	0	167	46	1.1
Label	Waffle, red-fat, 4½" square	1.00 waffle	37	80	16.5	2.5	0.5	0.0	0.0	0.2	0	270	62	0.5

Appendixes

STARCH: CEREALS and GRAINS

Nutrient	Food Source	Quantity	Grams per Serving	Cal	Cho (g)	Pro (g)	Fat (g)	SFA (g)	MUFA (g)	PUFA (g)	Chol (mg)	Na (mg)	K (mg)	Total Dietary Fiber (g)
08029	40% Bran flakes cereal	0.50 cup	24	78	19.0	2.7	0.4	0.0	0.0	0.0	0	220	128	4.7
08001	All Bran cereal	0.50 cup	30	75	22.0	4.0	1.0	0.3	0.3	0.3	0	280	340	10.0
08005	Bran Buds cereal	0.50 cup	42	112	32.9	6.0	1.1	—	—	—	0	265	721	16.2
Label	Fiber One cereal	0.50 cup	30	60	24.0	3.0	1.0	—	—	—	0	140	220	13.0
08060	Raisin bran cereal	0.50 cup	23	85	21.5	2.0	0.5	0.0	0.0	0.0	0	215	170	3.5
20013	Bulgur	0.50 cup	91	76	16.9	2.8	0.2	0.0	0.0	0.1	0	5	62	4.1
08101	Cream of rice cereal, ck	0.50 cup	122	63	14.0	1.1	0.1	0.0	0.0	0.0	0	1	24	0.1
08103	Cream of wheat cereal, ck	0.50 cup	126	67	13.9	1.9	0.3	0.0	0.0	0.0	0	1	21	0.9
08121	Oatmeal cereal, ck	0.50 cup	117	73	12.6	3.0	1.2	0.2	0.4	0.4	0	1	65	2.0
08145	Whole-wheat natural cereal, ck	0.50 cup	121	75	16.6	2.4	0.5	0.0	0.0	0.0	0	0	86	1.9
	Cereals, unsweetened, ready-to-eat													
08013	Cheerios	0.75 cup	23	90	15.9	3.5	1.5	0.3	0.5	0.6	0	210	82	1.6
08020	Cornflakes	0.75 cup	23	89	19.8	1.9	0.1	0.0	0.0	0.0	0	235	21	0.6
08039	Grape Nuts	0.75 cup	29	104	23.7	3.1	0.3	0.0	0.0	0.0	0	164	101	2.9
08048	Kix	0.75 cup	17	66	14.0	1.5	0.4	0.1	0.1	0.2	0	174	27	0.3
08058	Product 19	0.75 cup	23	88	19.1	2.3	0.2	0.0	0.0	0.0	0	264	36	0.9
08065	Rice Krispies	0.75 cup	18	71	15.7	1.2	0.1	0.0	0.0	0.0	0	216	19	0.3
08089	Wheaties	0.75 cup	23	80	18.3	2.2	0.4	0.1	0.1	0.2	0	219	86	2.1
20022	Cornmeal, dry, degermed, enriched	3.00 Tbsp	26	97	20.5	2.3	0.5	0.1	0.1	0.2	0	1	43	1.9
20029	Couscous, ck	0.33 cup	59	67	13.8	2.2	0.1	0.0	0.0	0.0	0	3	34	0.9
20081	Flour, white	3.00 Tbsp	24	87	18.3	2.5	0.2	0.0	0.0	0.1	0	0	26	0.6
Label	Granola cereal, low-fat	0.25 cup	27	105	21.3	2.5	1.5	(0.2)	(0.3)	(0.9)	0	61	67	1.5
08038	Grape Nuts cereal	0.25 cup	29	105	24.0	3.5	0.1	0.0	0.0	0.0	0	177	97	2.5
08091	Grits, ck	0.50 cup	121	73	15.7	1.7	0.2	0.0	0.1	0.1	0	0	27	0.2
20010	Kasha (buckwheat groats), ck	0.50 cup	99	91	19.7	3.4	0.6	0.1	0.2	0.2	0	4	88	(2.2)
20032	Millet, ck	0.25 cup	60	72	14.2	2.1	0.6	0.1	0.1	0.3	0	1	37	(0.8)
Label	Muesli	0.25 cup	20	75	15.5	1.5	1.1	0.0	0.5	0.4	0	71	75	1.5
08121	Oats (rolled/oatmeal), ck	0.50 cup	117	73	12.6	3.0	1.2	0.2	0.4	0.4	0	1	65	2.0
20100	Macaroni, ck firm	0.50 cup	70	99	19.8	3.3	0.5	0.1	0.1	0.2	0	1	22	0.9
20110	Noodles, enriched egg, ck	0.50 cup	80	106	19.9	3.8	1.2	0.3	0.3	0.3	26	6	22	0.9
20121	Spaghetti, ck firm	0.50 cup	70	99	19.8	3.3	0.5	0.1	0.1	0.2	0	1	22	1.2
08066	Puffed Rice cereal	1.50 cup	24	90	21.5	1.5	0.1	0.0	0.0	0.0	0	1	22	0.4
08146	Puffed Wheat cereal	1.50 cup	21	76	15.0	3.1	0.3	0.0	0.0	0.0	0	1	75	0.9
Label	Rice milk	0.50 cup	113	85	19.0	0.5	1.5	(0.3)	(0.3)	(0.3)	0	40	(40)	—
20045	Rice, white, long-grain, ck, hot	0.33 cup	53	69	14.9	1.4	0.1	0.0	0.1	0.0	0	1	19	0.2
20037	Rice, brown, ck	0.33 cup	65	72	14.9	1.7	0.6	0.1	0.2	0.2	0	3	28	1.2
08148	Shredded Wheat cereal	0.50 cup	25	90	20.0	2.8	0.6	0.1	0.1	0.3	0	3	90	2.5
08069	Sugar-frosted flakes	0.50 cup	18	67	15.8	0.9	0.0	0.0	0.0	0.0	0	142	13	0.3
Label	Sugar-frosted cereal	0.50 cup	26	90	22.5	2.0	0.5	0.1	0.1	0.1	0	100	(24)	(0.5)
08084	Wheat germ, toasted	3.00 Tbsp	21	80	10.4	6.1	2.2	0.4	0.3	1.4	0	1	199	2.7

Diabetes Medical Nutrition Therapy

Nutrient	Food Source	Quantity	Grams per Serving	Cal	Cho (g)	Pro (g)	Fat (g)	SFA (g)	MUFA (g)	PUFA (g)	Chol (mg)	Na (mg)	K (mg)	Total Dietary Fiber (g)
STARCH: STARCHY VEGETABLES
16006	Beans, baked	0.33 cup	84	79	17.3	4.1	0.4	0.1	0.0	0.1	0	335	249	4.2
11179	Corn, fz, ck	0.50 cup	82	66	16.8	2.5	0.1	0.0	0.0	0.0	0	4	114	2.0
11176	Corn, whole-kernel, vac pack	0.50 cup	105	83	20.4	2.5	0.5	0.1	0.2	0.3	0	286	195	6.0
11168	Corn on cob, ck, med	1.00 cob (5 oz)	77	83	19.3	2.6	1.0	0.2	0.3	0.5	0	13	192	2.2
Label	Corn on cob, fz, 3"	1.00 cob	61	70	14.0	2.0	0.5	—	—	—	0	5	—	1.0
Label	Mixed vegetables with corn	1.00 cup	135	80	18.0	4.0	0.0	0.0	0.0	0.0	0	80	230	(4.0)
Label	Mixed vegetables with pasta	1.00 cup	112	80	15.0	3.0	0.0	0.0	0.0	0.0	0	85	(189)	5.0
11308	Peas, green, cn	0.50 cup	85	59	10.7	3.8	0.3	0.1	0.0	0.1	0	186	147	3.5
11313	Peas, green, fz	0.50 cup	80	62	11.4	4.1	0.2	0.0	0.0	0.1	0	70	134	4.4
11305	Peas, green, fresh ck	0.50 cup	80	67	12.5	4.3	0.2	0.0	0.0	0.1	0	2	217	4.4
09278	Plantain, ck slices	0.50 cup	77	89	24.0	0.6	0.1	0.0	0.0	0.0	0	4	358	1.8
11674	Potato, baked with skin	3.00 oz	85	93	21.5	2.0	0.1	0.0	0.0	0.0	0	7	355	2.0
11367	Potato, white, peeled, boiled	3.00 oz	85	73	17.0	1.5	0.1	0.0	0.0	0.0	0	4	279	1.5
11379	Potato, mashed, flakes (milk & fat)	0.50 cup	105	119	15.8	2.0	5.9	3.6	1.7	0.3	15	349	245	2.4
11484	Squash, winter	1.00 cup	244	83	21.5	1.6	0.1	0.0	0.0	0.1	0	8	641	7.1
11512	Potato, sweet, cn, vac pack	0.50 cup	102	92	21.5	1.7	0.2	0.0	0.0	0.2	0	53	317	3.0
11602	Yam, plain, ck	0.50 cup	68	79	18.7	1.1	0.2	0.0	0.0	0.0	0	6	454	2.4
STARCH: BEANS/PEAS/LENTILS
16057	Beans, garbanzo (chickpeas), ck	0.50 cup	82	134	22.5	7.3	2.1	0.2	0.5	0.9	0	6	239	4.3
16043	Beans, pinto, ck	0.50 cup	85	117	21.8	7.0	0.4	0.1	0.1	0.2	0	1	398	7.3
16029	Beans, kidney, cn, s+l	0.50 cup	129	105	19.1	6.7	0.4	0.0	0.0	0.3	0	447	332	4.2
16028	Beans, kidney, ck	0.50 cup	88	112	20.1	7.6	0.4	0.1	0.0	0.2	0	2	355	5.6
16050	Beans, white, ck	0.50 cup	91	126	22.9	8.8	0.3	0.2	0.0	0.2	0	6	511	5.8
16038	Beans, navy, ck	0.50 cup	91	129	24.0	7.9	0.5	0.1	0.0	0.2	0	1	335	6.5
16086	Peas, split, ck	0.50 cup	98	117	20.8	8.2	0.4	0.0	0.2	0.2	0	2	356	8.2
16063	Peas, black-eyed, ck	0.50 cup	86	100	17.9	6.7	0.4	0.2	0.0	0.2	0	3	239	5.6
11033	Beans, lima, cn, s+l	0.67 cup	166	125	23.0	7.5	0.5	0.1	0.0	0.3	0	414	448	5.4
11038	Beans, lima, fz	0.67 cup	114	114	21.4	7.0	0.4	0.1	0.0	0.1	0	60	465	8.2
16070	Lentils, ck	0.50 cup	100	117	20.2	9.1	0.4	0.0	0.0	0.2	0	2	370	7.9
16112	Miso	3.00 Tbsp	52	106	14.5	6.1	3.1	0.5	0.7	1.8	0	1887	85	2.8

268

Appendixes

Nutrient	Food Source	Quantity	Grams per Serving	Cal	Cho (g)	Pro (g)	Fat (g)	SFA (g)	MUFA (g)	PUFA (g)	Chol (mg)	Na (mg)	K (mg)	Total Dietary Fiber (g)
	STARCH: CRACKERS/SNACKS													
18150	Animal crackers	8.00 crackers	20	89	14.8	1.4	2.8	0.7	1.5	0.4	0	79	20	0.5
18173	Graham crackers	3.00 crackers	21	89	16.1	1.4	2.1	0.5	1.0	0.3	0	127	28	0.6
18217	Matzoh	0.75 oz	21	83	17.6	2.1	0.3	0.1	0.0	0.1	0	0	23	0.6
18220	Melba toast	4.00 slices	20	78	15.3	2.4	0.6	0.1	0.2	0.2	0	166	41	1.3
18228	Oyster crackers	24.0 crackers	18	78	12.9	1.7	2.1	0.4	1.2	0.3	0	234	23	0.5
19034	Popcorn, popped, no fat added	3.00 cups	24	92	18.7	2.9	1.0	0.1	0.3	0.5	0	1	72	3.6
Label	Popcorn, microwave light	3.00 cups	24	65	11.2	1.8	2.1	0.3	—	—	0	143	—	1.8
19047	Pretzels, sticks/rings	0.75 oz	21	80	16.6	1.9	0.7	0.2	0.3	0.3	0	360	31	0.7
19051	Rice cake, regular	2.00 cakes	18	70	14.7	1.5	0.5	0.1	0.2	0.2	0	59	52	0.8
18228	Saltine type crackers	6.00 crackers	18	78	12.9	1.7	2.1	0.4	1.2	0.3	0	234	23	0.5
Label	Snack chips, tortilla, fat-free	17.0 chips	21	82	18.0	2.2	0.8	0.0	—	—	0	120	(41)	3.0
Label	Snack chips, potato, fat-free	23.0 chips	21	82	17.2	2.2	0.0	0.0	0.0	0.0	0	135	(268)	1.5
	Whole-wheat crackers, no fat added													
18216	Crispbread	2.00 slices	20	73	16.4	1.6	0.3	0.0	0.0	0.1	0	53	64	3.2
Label	Crispbread, Wasa (Golden Rye)	2.00 slices	22	70	14.0	2.0	0.0	0.0	0.0	0.0	0	100	—	4.0
18226	Rye Krisp	3.00 slices	25	86	20.5	2.5	0.2	0.0	0.1	0.1	0	202	126	2.0
Label	Triscuits, reduced-fat	5.00 wafers	20	81	15.0	1.9	1.9	0.3	0.6	0.0	0	112	(37)	2.5
	STARCH: STARCHY FOODS PREPARED WITH FAT													
18009	Biscuit, baked	1.00 biscuit	35	127	17.0	2.2	5.8	0.9	2.4	2.2	0	368	78	0.6
20113	Chow mein noodles	0.50 cup	22	116	12.7	1.8	6.8	1.0	1.7	3.8	0	97	26	0.9
18024	Cornbread, baked	2.00 oz	57	152	24.8	3.8	4.0	0.9	1.0	1.8	23	375	84	1.4
18229	Crackers, round butter type	6.00 crackers	18	90	11.0	1.3	4.6	0.9	1.9	1.5	0	152	24	0.4
18242	Croutons	1.00 cup	30	122	22.0	3.6	2.0	0.5	1.0	0.3	0	209	37	0.9
Label	French fries, fz, oven-heated, no salt	≈20.0 fries	84	120	20.0	2.0	4.0	1.0	(1.5)	(0.3)	0	25	260	2.0
19020	Granola	0.25 cup	28	126	19.0	2.1	4.9	2.0	1.1	1.5	0	79	92	1.3
18273	Muffin, baked	1.00 muffin	45	133	18.6	3.1	5.1	1.0	1.2	2.6	18	210	54	1.2
18292	Pancakes, prepared from mix	2.00 pancakes	76	166	22.0	5.9	5.9	1.5	1.6	2.2	54	384	151	1.0
Label	Popcorn, microwave	3.00 cups	(24)	103	14.6	2.6	4.3	0.4	—	—	0	206	(72)	2.5
18230	Sandwich crackers, cheese	3.00 crackers	21	99	12.9	2.1	4.5	1.2	2.4	0.6	0	294	90	(0.3)
18231	Sandwich crackers, peanut butter	3.00 crackers	21	102	12.3	2.4	5.1	1.2	2.7	0.9	0	198	48	(0.3)
18082	Stuffing, bread, prepared	0.33 cup	66	117	14.4	2.1	5.7	1.2	2.5	1.7	0	359	49	2.0
18360	Taco shells	2.00 shells	26	122	16.2	1.9	5.9	0.9	2.5	2.2	0	95	47	2.1
18367	Waffle, prepared from mix	1.00 waffle	50	145	16.5	4.0	7.1	1.4	1.8	3.4	35	256	80	0.7
	Whole wheat crackers, fat added													
18232	Triscuits	6.00 crackers	27	128	17.5	2.3	5.6	1.0	3.2	0.8	0	215	49	1.5

269

FRUITS: FRESH, CN, DRIED

Nutrient	Food Source	Quantity	Grams per Serving	Cal	Cho (g)	Pro (g)	Fat (g)	SFA (g)	MUFA (g)	PUFA (g)	Chol (mg)	Na (mg)	K (mg)	Total Dietary Fiber (g)
09003	Apple, unpeeled, small	1.00 apple	106	63	16.2	0.2	0.4	0.1	0.0	0.1	0	0	122	2.9
09019	Applesauce, unsweetened	0.50 cup	122	52	13.8	0.2	0.1	0.0	0.0	0.0	0	2	91	1.5
09011	Apples, dried	4.00 rings	26	63	17.1	0.2	0.1	0.0	0.0	0.0	0	23	117	2.3
09021	Apricots, fresh	4.00 apricots	141	68	15.7	2.0	0.5	0.0	0.2	0.1	0	1	417	3.4
09032	Apricots, dried	8.00 halves	28	66	17.3	1.0	0.1	0.0	0.1	0.0	0	2	386	2.5
09024	Apricots, cn, juice pack	0.50 cup	124	60	15.3	0.8	0.0	0.0	0.0	0.0	0	5	205	1.6
09025	Apricots, cn, extra light syrup	0.50 cup	124	60	15.4	0.7	0.1	0.0	0.0	0.0	0	2	173	1.6
09040	Banana, fresh	1.00 small	70	64	16.4	0.7	0.3	0.1	0.0	0.1	0	1	277	1.7
09042	Blackberries, fresh	0.75 cup	108	56	13.8	0.8	0.4	0.0	0.0	0.0	0	0	212	5.4
09048	Blackberries, fz, unsweetened	0.75 cup	113	73	17.7	1.3	0.5	0.1	0.1	0.1	0	2	158	5.6
09050	Blueberries, fresh	0.75 cup	109	61	15.4	0.7	0.4	—	—	—	0	7	97	2.9
09054	Blueberries, fz, unsweetened	0.75 cup	116	58	14.1	0.5	0.7	—	—	—	0	1	62	3.1
09181	Cantaloupe, fresh	1.00 cup	160	56	13.4	1.4	0.4	0.0	0.0	0.0	0	14	494	1.3
	Cantaloupe, fresh	0.33 melon	159	56	13.3	1.4	0.4	—	—	—	0	14	491	1.3
09070	Cherries, sweet, fresh	12.0 cherries	82	59	13.6	1.0	0.8	0.2	0.2	0.2	0	0	184	1.9
09072	Cherries, sweet, cn, juice pack	0.50 cup	125	68	17.3	1.1	0.0	0.0	0.0	0.0	0	4	164	0.9
09087	Dates	3.00 dates	25	68	18.3	0.5	0.1	0.0	0.0	0.0	0	0	162	1.9
09089	Figs, fresh	1.50 figs, large	96	71	18.4	0.7	0.3	0.1	0.1	0.1	0	1	222	3.3
09094	Figs, dried	1.50 figs, dried	28	71	18.3	0.9	0.3	0.1	0.1	0.2	0	3	199	2.6
09097	Fruit cocktail, cn, juice pack	0.50 cup	124	57	14.7	0.6	0.0	0.0	0.0	0.0	0	5	118	1.4
09089	Fruit cocktail, cn, extra light syrup	0.50 cup	124	55	14.3	0.5	0.1	0.0	0.0	0.0	0	5	128	1.4
09111	Grapefruit, fresh	0.50 grapefruit	160	51	12.9	1.0	0.2	0.0	0.0	0.0	0	0	222	1.7
09120	Grapefruit, sections, cn	0.75 cup	186	69	17.1	1.3	0.2	0.0	0.0	0.0	0	13	314	0.7
09132	Grapes, fresh seedless	17.0 grapes	85	60	15.1	0.6	0.5	0.2	0.0	0.1	0	2	157	0.9
09184	Honeydew melon, fresh	1.00 cup	170	59	15.6	0.8	0.2	0.0	0.0	0.0	0	17	461	1.0
	Honeydew melon, fresh	1.00 slice	150	53	13.8	0.7	0.2	0.0	0.0	0.0	0	15	407	0.9
09148	Kiwi, fresh	1.00 kiwi	91	56	13.5	0.9	0.4	0.0	0.0	0.0	0	5	302	3.1
09219	Mandarin oranges, cn, juice pack	0.75 cup	186	69	17.8	1.2	0.1	0.0	0.0	0.1	0	9	247	1.3
09176	Mango, fresh	0.50 cup	104	68	17.7	0.5	0.3	0.1	0.1	0.1	0	2	162	1.9
	Mango, fresh	0.50 cup	83	54	14.0	0.4	0.2	0.1	0.1	0.0	0	2	129	1.5
09191	Nectarine, fresh	1.00 nectarine	136	67	16.0	1.3	0.6	0.0	0.0	0.0	0	0	288	2.2
09200	Orange, fresh	1.00 orange	131	62	15.4	1.2	0.2	0.0	0.0	0.0	0	0	237	3.1
09226	Papaya, fresh	1.00 cup cubes	140	55	13.7	0.9	0.2	0.1	0.1	0.0	0	4	360	2.5
	Papaya, fresh, medium	0.50 papaya	152	59	14.9	0.9	0.2	0.1	0.1	0.0	0	4	390	2.7
09236	Peach, fresh, medium	1.00 peach	132	57	14.7	0.9	0.1	0.0	0.1	0.1	0	0	260	2.6
09238	Peaches, cn, juice pack	0.50 cup	124	55	14.4	0.8	0.0	0.0	0.0	0.0	0	5	159	1.2
09239	Peaches, cn, extra light syrup	0.50 cup	124	52	13.7	0.5	0.1	0.0	0.1	0.1	0	6	92	1.2
09252	Pear, fresh, large	0.50 pear	100	59	15.1	0.4	0.4	0.0	0.1	0.1	0	0	125	2.4
09254	Pears, cn, juice pack	0.50 cup	124	62	16.0	0.4	0.1	0.0	0.0	0.0	0	5	119	2.5
09255	Pears, cn, extra light syrup	0.50 cup	124	58	15.1	0.4	0.1	0.0	0.0	0.0	0	3	55	2.5

Appendixes

Nutrient	Food Source	Quantity	Grams per Serving	Cal	Cho (g)	Pro (g)	Fat (g)	SFA (g)	MUFA (g)	PUFA (g)	Chol (mg)	Na (mg)	K (mg)	Total Dietary Fiber (g)
	FRUITS: FRESH, CN, DRIED, continued													
09266	Pineapple, fresh	0.75 cup	116	57	14.4	0.5	0.5	0.0	0.1	0.2	0	1	131	1.4
09268	Pineapple, cn, juice pack	0.50 cup	124	74	19.5	0.1	0.0	0.0	0.0	0.0	0	1	150	0.9
09279	Plums, fresh, small	2.00 plums	132	73	17.2	1.0	0.8	0.1	0.5	0.2	0	0	227	2.0
09280	Plums, cn, juice pack	0.50 cup	126	73	19.1	0.6	0.0	0.0	0.0	0.0	0	2	194	1.3
09291	Prunes, dried, uncooked	3.00 prunes	25	60	15.7	0.7	0.1	0.0	0.1	0.0	0	1	186	1.8
09298	Raisins, dark, seedless	2.00 Tbsp	18	54	14.2	0.6	0.1	0.0	0.0	0.0	0	2	135	0.7
09302	Raspberries, black, fresh	1.00 cup	123	60	14.2	1.1	0.7	0.0	0.1	0.4	0	0	187	8.4
09316	Strawberries, fresh	1.25 cups	186	56	13.1	1.1	0.7	0.0	0.1	0.4	0	2	309	4.3
09318	Strawberries, fz, unsweetened	1.25 cups	186	65	17.0	0.8	0.2	0.0	0.0	0.1	0	4	275	3.9
09218	Tangerine, fresh, small	2.00 fruits	168	74	18.8	1.1	0.3	0.0	0.1	0.1	0	2	264	3.9
09218	Watermelon, fresh, cubes	1.25 cup	200	64	14.4	1.2	0.9	—	—	—	0	4	232	(1.0)
09326	Watermelon, fresh	1.00 slice	202	65	14.5	1.3	0.9	—	—	—	0	4	234	(2.0)
	FRUITS: JUICES													
09016	Apple juice or cider, cn/bottled	0.50 cup	124	58	14.5	0.1	0.1	0.0	0.0	0.0	0	4	148	0.1
09080	Cranberry juice cocktail, bottled	0.33 cup	84	48	12.1	0.0	0.1	0.0	0.0	0.0	0	2	15	0.0
14243	Cranberry juice cocktail, red-cal	1.00 cup	237	45	11.1	0.0	0.0	0.0	0.0	0.0	0	7	52	0.0
Label	Fruit juice blends, 100% juice	0.33 cup	85	50	12.3	0.5	0.1	0.0	0.0	0.0	0	10	111	0.5
09135	Grape juice, bottled	0.33 cup	84	51	12.6	0.5	0.1	0.0	0.0	0.0	0	3	111	0.1
09123	Grapefruit juice, cn	0.50 cup	124	47	11.1	0.6	0.1	0.0	0.0	0.0	0	1	190	0.1
09207	Orange juice, cn	0.50 cup	124	52	12.2	0.7	0.2	0.0	0.0	0.0	0	3	217	0.2
09206	Orange juice, fresh	0.50 cup	124	56	12.9	0.9	0.2	0.0	0.0	0.1	0	1	248	0.2
09215	Orange juice, fz, reconstituted	0.50 cup	124	56	13.4	0.8	0.1	0.0	0.0	0.0	0	1	236	0.2
09273	Pineapple juice, cn	0.50 cup	125	70	17.2	0.4	0.1	0.0	0.0	0.0	0	1	167	0.1
09294	Prune juice	0.33 cup	85	60	14.8	0.5	0.0	0.0	0.0	0.0	0	3	235	0.9
	MILK: SKIM and VERY LOW FAT													
01085	Milk, skim	1.00 cup	245	86	11.9	8.4	0.4	0.3	0.1	0.0	4	126	406	0.0
Label	Milk, 1/2% milkfat	1.00 cup	245	90	11.0	8.0	1.0	0.6	0.3	0.0	7	125	406	0.0
01082	Milk, 1%	1.00 cup	244	102	11.7	8.0	2.6	1.6	0.8	0.1	10	123	381	0.0
01088	Buttermilk, low-fat/nonfat	1.00 cup	245	99	11.7	8.1	2.2	1.3	0.6	0.1	9	257	371	0.0
01097	Evaporated skim milk	0.50 cup	128	100	14.5	9.7	0.3	0.2	0.1	0.0	5	147	424	0.0
01092	Milk, dry, nonfat	0.33 cup	23	82	12.0	8.1	0.2	0.1	0.0	0.0	4	126	392	0.0
Label	Yogurt, nonfat plain	0.75 cup	186	90	13.0	10.0	0.0	0.0	0.0	0.0	4	128	450	0.0
Label	Yogurt, nonfat/low-fat fruit-flavored with nonnutritive sweetener	1.00 cup	248	100	17.0	9.0	0.0	0.0	0.0	0.0	(4)	140	430	0.0

271

Diabetes Medical Nutrition Therapy

Nutrient	Food Source	Quantity	Grams per Serving	Cal	Cho (g)	Pro (g)	Fat (g)	SFA (g)	MUFA (g)	PUFA (g)	Chol (mg)	Na (mg)	K (mg)	Total Dietary Fiber (g)
	MILK: LOW-FAT													
01079	Milk, 2%	1.00 cup	244	121	11.7	8.1	4.7	2.9	1.4	0.2	18	122	377	0.0
Label	Yogurt, plain low-fat	0.75 cup	186	112	12.8	9.8	3.0	1.9	(0.8)	0.1	15	128	442	0.0
Label	Sweet acidophilus milk	1.00 cup	244	110	12.0	8.0	3.5	2.5	(.9)	(0.1)	15	120	(377)	0.0
	MILK: WHOLE													
01077	Whole milk	1.00 cup	244	150	11.4	8.0	8.1	5.1	2.3	0.3	33	120	370	0.0
01096	Evaporated milk	0.50 cup	126	169	12.6	8.6	9.5	5.8	2.9	0.3	37	133	382	0.0
01106	Goat's milk, whole	1.00 cup	244	168	10.9	8.7	10.1	6.5	2.7	0.4	28	122	499	0.0
Label	Kefir	1.00 cup	(233)	(151)	(7.8)	(8.9)	(8.7)	(5.2)	(2.4)	(0.3)	(18)	(49)	(201)	0.0
	OTHER CARBOHYDRATE													
18089	Angel food cake	0.08 cake	53	142	31.5	4.0	0.1	0.0	0.0	0.0	0	96	116	0.6
18151	Brownie, small	1.00 brownie	28	115	18.1	1.4	4.6	1.2	2.4	0.7	5	88	42	0.7
Avg	Cake, unfrosted	1.00 2" square	32	97	16.6	1.5	3.1	0.6	1.3	1.0	18	168	53	(0.5)
Avg	Cake, frosted	1.00 2" square	50	175	29.2	1.6	6.4	1.6	3.0	1.4	18	194	75	(0.9)
Label	Cookies, fat-free	2.00 cookies	23	68	16.0	2.0	0.1	0.0	0.0	0.0	0.0	51	(27)	1.8
Avg	Cookie, 3" diameter	1.00 cookie	30	142	19.0	1.8	7.0	1.9	3.4	0.8	10	103	30	0.9
Avg	Cookies, small (1¾" diameter)	2.00 cookies	24	114	15.2	1.4	5.6	1.5	2.7	0.6	8	82	24	0.7
18166	Cookie, sandwich w/cream filling	2.00 cookies	20	94	14.0	1.0	4.2	0.8	2.4	0.6	—	120	36	(0.6)
B&C	Cupcake, frosted, small	1.00 cupcake	48	172	28.4	2.2	6.0	(1.6)	(3.0)	(1.4)	1	161	56	(0.9)
09081	Cranberry sauce, jellied	0.25 cup	57	86	22.2	0.1	0.1	0.0	0.0	0.0	0	17	15	0.6
18248	Donut, plain cake	1.00 donut	47	198	23.4	2.3	10.8	1.8	4.5	3.8	18	257	60	0.8
18255	Donut, glazed (3¾" diameter)	2.00 oz	60	242	26.6	3.8	13.7	3.5	7.7	1.7	4	205	65	1.3
19263	Fruit juice bar, fz, 100% juice	1.00 bar (3 oz)	92	75	18.6	1.1	0.1	0.0	0.0	0.0	0	3	48	0.0
19014	Fruit snacks (pureed fruit conc)	1.00 roll (¾ oz)	21	78	18.0	0.2	1.0	0.1	0.3	0.1	0	38	54	(0.5)
Label	Fruit spreads, 100% fruit	1.00 Tbsp	19	43	11.0	0.0	0.0	0.0	0.0	0.0	0	5	(15)	(0.2)
19173	Gelatin, reg (Jello)	0.50 cup	135	80	18.9	1.6	0.0	0.0	0.0	0.0	0	57	1	(0.0)
18172	Gingersnaps	3.00 cookies	21	87	16.1	1.2	2.1	0.4	1.2	0.3	0	137	73	0.5
19015	Granola bar	1.00 bar	28	133	18.2	2.9	5.6	0.7	1.2	3.4	0	83	95	1.5
Label	Granola bar, fat-free	1.00 bar	42	140	35.0	2.0	0.0	0.0	0.0	0.0	0	5	—	3.0
16137	Hummus	0.33 cup	82	140	16.5	4.0	6.9	1.0	2.9	2.6	0	200	142	(4.2)
19095	Ice cream, 10% fat	0.50 cup	66	133	15.6	2.3	7.3	4.5	2.1	0.3	29	53	131	0.0
Label	Ice cream, light	0.50 cup	60	100	14.0	3.0	4.0	2.5	(0.5)	—	25	35	(141)	1.0
Label	Ice cream, fat-free, no sugar added	0.50 cup	71	95	20.0	3.5	0.0	0.0	0.0	0.0	0	53	(150)	(0.5)
19297	Jam or preserves, regular	1.00 Tbsp	20	48	12.9	0.1	0.0	0.0	0.0	0.0	0	8	15	—
19300	Jelly, regular	1.00 Tbsp	19	52	13.5	0.1	0.0	0.0	0.0	0.0	0	7	12	0.2
01102	Milk, chocolate, whole	1.00 cup	250	208	25.8	7.9	8.5	5.3	2.5	0.3	30	149	417	0.0
Avg	Pie, fruit, 2 crusts	0.16 pie	117	290	43.3	2.2	12.9	2.4	7.0	2.4	0	300	86	(2.0)

Nutrient	Food Source	Quantity	Grams per Serving	Cal	Cho (g)	Pro (g)	Fat (g)	SFA (g)	MUFA (g)	PUFA (g)	Chol (mg)	Na (mg)	K (mg)	Total Dietary Fiber (g)
OTHER CARBOHYDRATE (continued)														
Avg	Pie, pumpkin or custard	0.12 pie	80	168	19.3	3.8	8.4	1.1	2.7	0.8	21	209	105	(1.6)
19411	Potato chips	1.00 oz (12–18)	28	152	15.0	2.0	9.8	3.1	2.8	3.4	0	168	361	1.3
Avg	Pudding, regular	0.50 cup	140	144	26.5	4.3	2.6	1.6	0.7	0.1	9	201	209	—
Label	Pudding, sugar-free (low-fat milk)	0.50 cup	142	90	13.0	4.0	2.0	1.5	0.7	0.1	9	420	188	(0.5)
Label	Salad dressings, fat-free	0.25 cup	64	80	18.0	0.0	0.0	0.0	0.0	0.0	0	580	52	(0.4)
19097	Sherbet	0.50 cup	96	132	29.2	1.1	1.9	1.1	0.5	0.1	5	44	92	0.0
Label	Sorbet	0.50 cup	92	130	31.0	0.4	0.0	0.0	0.0	0.0	0	0.0	3.0	(0.0)
11455	Spaghetti sauce, cn	0.50 cup	125	136	19.9	2.3	6.0	0.8	3.0	1.6	0	620	480	(4.3)
Label	Pasta sauce, cn	0.50 cup	128	110	17.0	2.0	4.0	0.5	(2.0)	(1.0)	0	480	(492)	4.0
18356	Sweet roll or Danish, 2½ oz	1.00 roll	71	293	36.1	4.4	11.0	3.0	6.5	1.5	47	272	79	0.9
19128	Syrup, pancake, light	2.00 Tbsp	30	49	13.3	0.0	0.0	0.0	0.0	0.0	0	60	1	0.0
19353	Syrup, maple, regular	1.00 Tbsp	20	52	13.4	0.0	0.0	0.0	0.0	0.0	0	2.0	41	0.0
19129	Syrup, pancake, regular	1.00 Tbsp	20	57	15.1	0.0	0.0	0.0	0.0	0.0	0	17	0	0.0
19056	Tortilla chips	1.00 oz (6–12)	28	142	17.8	2.0	7.4	1.4	4.4	1.0	0	150	56	1.8
Label	Yogurt, fz, low-fat	0.33 cup	47	70	13.4	2.0	1.0	0.7	(0.3)	0.0	5	26	89	0.7
Label	Yogurt, fz, fat-free	0.33 cup	44	60	11.9	2.6	0.0	0.0	0.0	0.0	0	58	141	—
Label	Yogurt, fz, fat-free, no sugar add	0.50 cup	72	90	18.0	4.0	0.0	0.0	0.0	0.0	0	65	(152)	—
Label	Yogurt, low-fat with fruit	1.00 cup	248	253	47.2	10.0	2.8	1.7	0.7	0.1	10	145	482	(1.0)
18212	Vanilla wafers	5.00 wafers	20	88	14.7	1.0	3.0	0.7	1.2	0.8	12	62	19	0.3
19335	Sugar	1.00 Tbsp	12	46	12.5	0.0	0.0	0.0	0.0	0.0	0	0	0	0.0
19296	Honey	1.00 Tbsp	21	64	17.3	0.1	0.0	0.0	0.0	0.0	0	1	11	0.0

VEGETABLES

Nutrient	Food Source	Quantity	Grams per Serving	Cal	Cho (g)	Pro (g)	Fat (g)	SFA (g)	MUFA (g)	PUFA (g)	Chol (mg)	Na (mg)	K (mg)	Total Dietary Fiber (g)
11008	Artichoke, ck	0.50 artichoke	60	30	6.7	2.1	0.1	0.0	0.0	0.0	0	57	212	3.2
11009	Artichoke hearts	0.50 cup	80	36	7.3	2.5	0.4	0.1	0.0	0.2	0	42	211	0.5
11019	Asparagus, fz	0.50 cup	83	23	4.0	2.4	0.3	0.1	0.0	0.2	0	3	181	2.8
11015	Asparagus, spears, cn, drained	0.50 cup	121	23	3.0	2.6	0.8	0.2	0.0	0.3	0	472	208	1.9
11056	Beans (green, wax), cn, drained	0.50 cup	68	14	3.1	0.8	0.1	0.0	0.0	0.0	0	171	74	1.3
11061	Beans, green, fz	0.50 cup	68	18	4.2	0.9	0.1	0.0	0.0	0.1	0	9	76	2.2
11043	Bean sprouts, raw	1.00 cup	104	31	6.2	3.2	0.2	0.1	0.0	0.0	0	6	155	1.9
11084	Beets, cn, drained, sliced	0.50 cup	85	26	6.1	0.8	0.1	0.0	0.0	0.0	0	233	126	1.5
11095	Broccoli, spears, fz	0.50 cup	92	26	4.9	2.9	0.1	0.0	0.0	0.1	0	22	166	2.8
11090	Broccoli, raw, chopped	1.00 cup	88	25	4.6	2.6	0.3	0.1	0.0	0.2	0	24	286	2.6
11101	Brussels sprouts, fz	0.50 cup	78	33	6.5	2.8	0.3	0.1	0.0	0.2	0	18	253	3.3
11110	Cabbage, fresh, ck	0.50 cup	75	16	3.3	0.8	0.3	0.0	0.0	0.2	0	6	73	2.1
11119	Cabbage, Chinese, raw	1.00 cup	76	12	2.5	0.9	0.2	0.0	0.0	0.1	0	7	181	0.8
11109	Cabbage, raw, green	1.00 cup	70	18	3.8	1.0	0.2	0.0	0.0	0.1	0	13	172	1.6
11128	Carrots, cn, drained	0.50 cup	73	17	4.0	0.5	0.1	0.0	0.0	0.1	0	176	131	1.1
11125	Carrots, fresh, ck	0.50 cup	78	35	8.2	0.9	0.1	0.0	0.0	0.1	0	52	177	2.6
11124	Carrots, raw	1.00 cup	110	47	11.1	1.1	0.2	0.0	0.0	0.1	0	38	355	3.3
11138	Cauliflower, fz	0.50 cup	90	17	3.4	1.4	0.2	0.0	0.0	0.1	0	16	125	2.0
11135	Cauliflower, raw	1.00 cup	100	25	5.2	2.0	0.2	0.0	0.0	0.1	0	30	303	2.5
11144	Celery, fresh, ck	0.50 cup	75	14	3.0	0.6	0.1	0.0	0.0	0.1	0	68	213	1.3
11143	Celery, raw	1.00 cup	120	19	4.4	0.9	0.2	0.0	0.1	0.1	0	104	344	2.0
11205	Cucumber, raw	1.00 cup	104	14	2.9	0.7	0.1	0.0	0.0	0.1	0	2	150	0.8
11210	Eggplant, fresh, ck	0.50 cup	48	13	3.2	0.4	0.1	0.0	0.0	0.0	0	1	119	1.2
11291	Green onion, raw	1.00 cup	100	32	7.3	1.8	0.2	0.0	0.0	0.1	0	16	276	2.6

Greens

Nutrient	Food Source	Quantity	Grams per Serving	Cal	Cho (g)	Pro (g)	Fat (g)	SFA (g)	MUFA (g)	PUFA (g)	Chol (mg)	Na (mg)	K (mg)	Total Dietary Fiber (g)
11162	Collard greens, fresh, ck	0.50 cup	64	17	3.9	0.9	0.1	0.0	0.0	0.0	0	10	84	1.3
11234	Kale, fresh, ck	0.50 cup	65	21	3.7	1.2	0.3	0.0	0.0	0.1	0	15	148	1.3
11271	Mustard greens, fresh, ck	0.50 cup	70	10	1.5	1.6	0.2	0.0	0.0	0.0	0	11	141	1.4
11569	Turnip greens, fresh, ck	0.50 cup	72	14	3.1	0.8	0.2	0.0	0.0	0.1	0	21	146	2.2
11242	Kohlrabi, ck	0.50 cup	82	24	5.5	1.5	0.1	0.0	0.0	0.0	0	17	279	0.9
11247	Leeks, ck	0.50 cup	52	16	4.0	0.4	0.1	0.0	0.0	0.0	0	6	46	—
Label	Mixed veg (no corn, peas, pasta)	0.50 cup	54	20	3.3	1.0	0.0	0.0	0.0	0.0	0	15	(60)	1.3
11264	Mushrooms, cn, drained	0.50 cup	78	19	3.9	1.5	0.2	0.0	0.0	0.1	0	331	101	1.9
11261	Mushrooms, fresh, ck	0.50 cup	78	21	4.0	1.7	0.4	0.1	0.0	0.1	0	2	278	1.7
11260	Mushrooms, raw	1.00 cup	70	18	3.3	1.5	0.3	0.0	0.0	0.1	0	3	259	0.8
11281	Okra, fz	0.50 cup	92	34	7.5	1.9	0.3	0.1	0.1	0.1	0	3	215	2.6
11283	Onions, fresh, chopped, ck	0.50 cup	105	46	10.7	1.4	0.2	0.0	0.0	0.1	0	3	174	1.5
11282	Onions, raw	1.00 cup	160	61	13.8	1.9	0.3	0.0	0.0	0.1	0	5	251	2.9
11301	Pea pods, fresh, ck	0.50 cup	80	34	5.6	2.6	0.2	0.0	0.0	0.1	0	3	192	2.2
11300	Pea pods, raw	1.00 cup	145	61	11.0	4.1	0.3	0.1	0.0	0.1	0	6	290	(3.8)

Appendixes

Nutrient	Food Source	Quantity	Grams per Serving	Cal	Cho (g)	Pro (g)	Fat (g)	SFA (g)	MUFA (g)	PUFA (g)	Chol (mg)	Na (mg)	K (mg)	Total Dietary Fiber (g)
	VEGETABLES, *continued*													
11334	Peppers, green, fresh, ck	0.50 cup	68	19	4.6	0.6	0.1	0.0	0.0	0.1	0	1	113	0.8
11333	Pepper, green, raw	1.00 cup	100	27	6.4	0.9	0.2	0.0	0.0	0.1	0	2	177	1.8
11670	Pepper, hot green chile, raw	1.00 cup	150	60	14.2	3.0	0.3	0.0	0.0	0.2	0	10	510	2.3
11429	Radishes	1.00 cup	116	20	4.2	0.7	0.6	0.0	0.0	0.1	0	28	269	1.9
	Salad greens													
11213	Endive/escarole, raw	1.00 cup	50	9	1.7	0.6	0.1	0.0	0.0	0.0	0	11	157	1.5
11252	Lettuce, iceberg, raw	1.00 cup	56	7	1.2	0.6	0.1	0.0	0.0	0.1	0	5	89	0.8
11251	Romaine, raw	1.00 cup	56	9	1.3	0.9	0.1	0.0	0.0	0.1	0	5	162	1.3
11457	Spinach, raw	1.00 cup	56	12	2.0	1.6	0.2	0.0	0.0	0.1	0	44	313	1.5
11439	Sauerkraut, cn	0.50 cup	118	22	5.1	1.1	0.2	0.0	0.0	0.1	0	780	201	3.0
11461	Spinach, cn, drained	0.50 cup	107	25	3.6	3.0	0.5	0.1	0.0	0.2	0	29	370	2.6
11464	Spinach, fz	0.50 cup	95	27	5.1	3.0	0.2	0.0	0.0	0.1	0	82	283	2.8
11642	Squash, summer, fresh, ck	0.50 cup	90	18	3.9	0.8	0.3	0.1	0.0	0.1	0	1	173	1.3
11641	Squash, summer, raw	1.00 cup	130	26	5.7	1.5	0.3	0.1	0.0	0.1	0	3	253	2.5
11529	Tomatoes, raw	1.00 cup	180	38	8.4	1.5	0.6	0.1	0.1	0.2	0	16	400	2.0
11529	Tomato, raw, small	1.00 small	123	26	5.7	1.0	0.4	0.1	0.1	0.2	0	11	273	(1.4)
11531	Tomatoes, cn, s + l	0.50 cup	120	24	5.2	1.1	0.3	0.0	0.0	0.1	0	196	265	1.2
11540	Tomato juice	0.50 cup	122	21	5.2	0.9	0.1	0.0	0.0	0.0	0	440	268	0.5
11549	Tomato sauce	0.50 cup	122	37	8.8	1.6	0.2	0.0	0.0	0.1	0	738	453	1.7
11578	Vegetable juice	0.50 cup	121	23	5.5	0.8	0.1	0.0	0.0	0.1	0	442	233	1.0
11565	Turnips, fresh, ck, cubed	0.50 cup	78	14	3.8	0.6	0.1	0.0	0.0	0.0	0	39	105	1.6
11590	Water chestnuts	0.50 cup	70	35	8.7	0.6	0.0	0.0	0.0	0.0	0	6	82	1.8
11591	Watercress, raw	1.00 cup	34	4	0.4	0.8	0.0	0.0	0.0	0.0	0	14	112	0.4
11478	Zucchini squash, fresh, ck, slice	0.50 cup	90	14	3.5	0.6	0.0	0.0	0.0	0.0	0	3	228	1.3
11477	Zucchini, raw	1.00 cup	130	18	3.8	1.5	0.2	0.0	0.0	0.1	0	4	322	1.6

Diabetes Medical Nutrition Therapy

Nutrient	Food Source	Quantity	Grams per Serving	Cal	Cho (g)	Pro (g)	Fat (g)	SFA (g)	MUFA (g)	PUFA (g)	Chol (mg)	Na (mg)	K (mg)	Total Dietary Fiber (g)
	MEAT & MEAT SUBSTITUTES: VERY LEAN													
05041	Chicken, white meat, no skin	1.00 oz	28	49	0.0	8.7	1.3	0.4	0.4	0.3	24	22	70	0.0
05186	Turkey, white meat, no skin	1.00 oz	28	44	0.0	8.5	0.9	0.3	0.2	0.2	20	18	86	0.0
05310	Cornish hen, no skin	1.00 oz	28	38	0.0	6.6	1.1	0.3	0.4	0.3	30	18	71	0.0
15016	Cod	1.00 oz	28	30	0.0	6.5	0.2	0.0	0.0	0.1	16	22	69	0.0
15029	Flounder	1.00 oz	28	33	0.0	6.8	0.4	0.1	0.1	0.1	19	29	97	0.0
15034	Haddock	1.00 oz	28	32	0.0	6.9	0.3	0.1	0.0	0.1	21	20	163	0.0
15037	Halibut	1.00 oz	28	40	0.0	7.6	0.8	0.1	0.3	0.3	12	20	163	0.0
15219	Trout	1.00 oz	28	54	0.0	7.6	2.4	0.4	1.2	0.6	21	19	132	0.0
15118	Tuna	1.00 oz	28	52	0.0	8.5	1.8	0.5	0.6	0.5	14	14	91	0.0
15121	Tuna, cn, water pack, solids only	1.00 oz	28	33	0.0	7.2	0.3	0.1	0.1	0.1	9	96	67	0.0
15160	Clams, cn, drained solids	1.00 oz	28	42	1.4	7.3	0.6	0.1	0.1	0.2	19	32	179	0.0
15159	Clams, fresh, steamed	1.00 oz	28	42	1.4	7.3	0.6	0.1	0.1	0.2	19	32	179	0.0
15141	Crab, cn, drained solids	1.00 oz	28	28	0.0	5.8	0.4	0.1	0.1	0.2	26	95	106	0.0
15140	Crab, steamed	1.00 oz	28	29	0.0	5.8	0.5	0.1	0.1	0.2	28	80	92	0.0
15148	Lobster, fresh, steamed	1.00 oz	28	28	0.4	5.8	0.2	0.1	0.1	0.1	20	108	104	0.0
2024	Scallops, fresh, steamed	1.00 oz	28	32	0.0	6.6	0.4	0.1	0.1	0.1	15	78	136	0.0
15152	Shrimp, cn, drained solids	1.00 oz	28	34	0.3	6.6	0.6	0.1	0.1	0.2	50	48	60	0.0
15151	Shrimp, fresh, ck in water	1.00 oz	28	28	0.0	6.0	0.3	0.1	0.0	0.2	56	64	104	0.0
15138	Imitation shellfish, from surimi	1.00 oz	28	29	2.9	3.4	0.4	0.1	0.1	0.1	6	238	25	0.0
05154	Duck, wild, breast, raw	1.00 oz	28	35	0.0	5.6	1.2	0.4	0.3	0.3	22	16	76	0.0
05154	Pheasant, no skin, raw	1.00 oz	28	38	0.0	6.7	1.0	0.4	0.3	0.2	19	10	74	0.0
17165	Venison	1.00 oz	28	45	0.0	8.5	0.9	0.4	0.2	0.1	32	15	95	0.0
17157	Buffalo	1.00 oz	28	40	0.0	8.0	0.7	0.3	0.3	0.1	23	16	102	0.0
Assoc	Ostrich	1 oz	28	40	0.0	7.6	0.8	(0.3)	(0.3)	(0.4)	23	21	(110)	0
	Cheeses (<1 g fat/oz)													
Label	Cottage cheese, nonfat	0.25 cup	56	35	2.5	6.5	0.0	0.0	—	—	5	210	948	(0.2)
05015	Cottage cheese, low-fat (2%)	0.25 cup	56	50	2.0	7.7	1.1	0.7	0.3	0.0	5	227	54	0.0
01014	Cottage cheese, dry	0.25 cup	36	31	0.7	6.2	0.2	0.1	0.0	0.0	2	5	12	0.0
Label	Cheese, fat-free	1.00 oz	28	37	3.4	6.1	0.0	0.0	0.0	0.0	0	384	(46)	—
	Processed sandwich meats (<1 g fat/oz)													
13350	Beef, chipped, dried	1.00 oz	28	47	0.0	8.2	1.1	0.5	0.5	0.1	26	948	126	0.0
05287	Turkey ham	1.00 oz	28	36	0.1	5.4	1.4	0.5	0.3	0.4	16	282	92	0.0
01124	Egg whites	2.00 whites	67	34	0.6	7.0	0.0	0.0	0.0	0.0	0	110	96	0.0
Label	Egg substitute	0.25 cup	60	35	1.5	6.5	0.0	0.0	0.0	0.0	0	110	—	0.0
Label	Hot dog, <1 g fat/oz	1.00 oz	28	30	2.5	3.5	0.8	0.3	(0.4)	(0.1)	11	286	(47)	0.0
13324	Kidney, beef, simmered	1.00 oz	28	41	0.3	7.3	1.0	0.3	0.2	0.2	110	38	51	0.0
Label	Sausage, hard, <1 g fat/oz	1.00 oz	28	35	2.5	4.5	0.8	0.3	—	—	12	290	(54)	0.0
	Legumes (see starch group)													

Appendixes

Nutrient	Food Source	Quantity	Grams per Serving	Cal	Cho (g)	Pro (g)	Fat (g)	SFA (g)	MUFA (g)	PUFA (g)	Chol (mg)	Na (mg)	K (mg)	Total Dietary Fiber(g)
	MEAT: LEAN													
13056	Beef, round steak, broiled, lean	1.00 oz	28	55	0.0	8.1	2.3	0.8	1.0	0.1	23	18	118	0.0
13454	Beef, sirloin	1.00 oz	28	54	0.0	8.6	1.9	0.8	0.8	0.1	25	19	114	0.0
13070	Beef, flank steak, broiled, lean	1.00 oz	28	59	0.0	7.7	2.9	1.2	1.2	0.1	19	24	118	0.0
13439	Beef, tenderloin, broiled, lean	1.00 oz	28	67	0.0	7.7	3.7	1.4	1.5	0.1	24	18	114	0.0
13042	Beef, chuck/blade pot roast	1.00 oz	28	62	0.0	9.4	2.4	0.9	1.0	0.1	29	19	82	0.0
13085	Beef, rib roast, lean, roasted	1.00 oz	28	65	0.0	7.8	3.6	1.4	1.5	0.1	23	21	107	0.0
13168	Beef, rump roast, lean, braised	1.00 oz	28	60	0.0	9.0	2.3	0.8	1.0	0.1	27	15	88	0.0
13236	Steak, t-bone, broiled	1.00 oz	28	61	0.0	8.0	3.0	1.2	1.2	0.1	23	19	116	0.0
13232	Steak, porterhouse, broiled	1.00 oz	28	62	0.0	8.0	3.1	1.2	1.2	0.1	23	19	116	0.0
13407	Beef, cubed steak	1.00 oz	28	58	0.0	9.0	2.2	0.7	1.0	0.1	27	15	88	0.0
13434	Beef, ground round	1.00 oz	28	56	0.0	10.2	1.4	0.5	0.6	0.1	26	13	94	0.0
10011	Ham, fresh (pork leg), baked	1.00 oz	28	60	0.0	8.4	2.7	0.9	1.3	0.2	27	18	106	0.0
10185	Ham, cn (fully ck)	1.00 oz	28	48	0.1	6.0	2.4	0.8	1.2	0.3	12	304	100	0.0
10153	Ham, cured, roasted	1.00 oz	28	45	0.0	7.1	1.6	0.5	0.7	0.2	16	378	90	0.0
10182	Ham, boiled lean, sandwich type	1.00 oz	28	46	0.7	5.2	2.4	0.8	1.1	0.3	15	362	84	0.0
10131	Canadian bacon, grilled	1.00 oz	28	53	0.4	6.9	2.4	0.8	1.1	0.2	16	441	111	0.0
10061	Pork tenderloin	1.00 oz	28	47	0.0	8.0	1.4	0.5	0.6	0.1	23	16	125	0.0
10027	Pork loin, roast/chop, roasted	1.00 oz	28	60	0.0	8.2	2.7	1.0	1.2	0.2	23	16	121	0.0
17028	Lamb loin, roast/chop, roasted	1.00 oz	28	57	0.0	7.5	2.8	1.0	1.1	0.2	25	19	76	0.0
17022	Lamb leg, sirloin, roast, lean	1.00 oz	28	58	0.0	8.1	2.6	0.9	1.1	0.2	26	20	95	0.0
17109	Veal loin, chop	1.00 oz	28	50	0.0	7.5	2.0	0.7	0.7	0.2	30	27	97	0.0
17127	Veal, brisket, lean, roasted	1.00 oz	28	47	0.0	7.4	1.7	0.7	0.6	0.1	31	26	101	0.0
05045	Chicken, dark meat, no skin	1.00 oz	28	58	0.0	7.7	2.8	0.8	1.0	0.6	26	26	68	0.0
05188	Turkey, dark meat, no skin	1.00 oz	28	53	0.0	8.1	2.0	0.7	0.5	0.6	24	22	82	0.0
05032	Chicken, light meat with skin, roast	1.00 oz	28	63	0.0	8.2	3.1	0.9	1.2	0.6	24	21	64	0.0
05142	Duck, domestic, no skin, roasted	1.00 oz	28	57	0.0	6.7	3.2	1.2	1.0	0.4	25	19	72	0.0
05149	Goose, no skin, roasted	1.00 oz	28	68	0.0	8.3	3.6	1.3	1.2	0.4	27	22	111	0.0
15042	Herring, smoked	1.00 oz	28	62	0.0	7.0	3.5	0.8	1.5	0.8	23	262	127	0.0
15169	Oysters, medium, ck	6.00 oysters	42	58	3.3	5.9	2.1	0.6	0.3	0.8	44	177	118	0.0
15086	Salmon, fillet broiled/baked	1.00 oz	28	61	0.0	7.7	3.1	0.5	1.5	0.7	25	19	106	0.0
15080	Salmon, cn in water, solids only	1.00 oz	28	40	0.0	6.1	1.6	0.4	0.6	0.4	11	139	86	0.0
15235	Catfish fillet	1.00 oz	28	43	0.0	5.3	2.3	0.5	1.2	0.4	18	23	91	0.0
15088	Sardines, cn in oil, drained	2.00 sardines	24	50	0.0	5.9	2.7	0.4	0.9	1.2	34	121	95	0.0
15119	Tuna, cn in oil, drained	1.00 oz	28	56	0.0	8.3	2.3	0.4	0.8	0.8	5	100	59	0.0
05149	Goose, wild, no skin	1.00 oz	28	(68)	0.0	(8.3)	(3.6)	(1.3)	(1.2)	(0.4)	(27)	(22)	(111)	0.0
17179	Rabbit	1.00 oz	28	58	0.0	8.6	2.4	0.7	0.6	0.5	24	10	85	0.0
01012	Cheese, cottage, 4.5% fat	0.25 cup	52	54	1.4	6.5	2.3	1.5	0.7	0.1	8	213	44	0.0
01032	Cheese, parmesan, grated	2.00 Tbsp	10	46	0.4	4.2	3.0	1.9	0.9	0.1	8	186	10	0.0

277

Diabetes Medical Nutrition Therapy

Nutrient Label	Food Source	Quantity	Grams per Serving	Cal	Cho (g)	Pro (g)	Fat (g)	SFA (g)	MUFA (g)	PUFA (g)	Chol (mg)	Na (mg)	K (mg)	Total Dietary Fiber (g)
	MEAT: LEAN, continued													
	Cheeses (<3 g fat/oz)													
Label	Mozzarella, light	1.00 oz	28	65	0.0	8.0	3.0	2.0	(0.7)	(0.3)	15	180	(23)	0.0
01168	Cheddar/colby cheese, low-fat	1.00 oz	28	49	0.5	6.9	2.0	1.2	0.6	0.1	6	174	19	0.0
Label	Hot dog, low-fat, <3 g fat/oz	1.50 oz (1 dog)	45	50	4.0	6.0	1.5	0.5	—	—	15	450	—	—
05289	Turkey pastrami, <3 g fat/oz	1.00 oz	28	40	0.5	5.2	1.8	0.5	0.6	0.4	15	296	74	0.0
Label	Turkey kielbasa, <3 g fat/oz	1.00 oz	28	45	1.5	4.0	2.5	1.2	(0.6)	(0.5)	16	300	76	0.0
13326	Liver, beef, braised	1.00 oz	28	46	1.0	6.9	1.4	0.5	0.2	0.3	110	20	67	0.0
05028	Liver, chicken, simmered	1.00 oz	28	45	0.3	6.9	1.6	0.5	0.4	0.3	180	15	40	0.0
13322	Heart, beef, simmered	1.00 oz	28	50	0.1	8.2	1.6	0.5	0.4	0.4	55	18	66	0.0
	MEAT: MEDIUM-FAT													
13298	Beef, ground, extra lean, broiled	1.00 oz	28	73	0.0	7.2	4.7	1.8	2.0	0.2	24	20	89	0.0
13305	Beef, ground, lean, broiled	1.00 oz	28	78	0.0	7.0	5.3	2.1	2.3	0.2	25	22	86	0.0
13312	Beef, ground, regular, broiled	1.00 oz	28	82	0.0	6.9	5.9	2.3	2.6	0.2	26	24	83	0.0
B&C	Meat loaf	1.00 oz	28	57	0.9	4.5	3.7	2.5	2.3	0.1	26	186	107	0.0
13347	Beef, corned brisket	1.00 oz	28	72	0.1	5.2	5.4	1.8	2.6	0.2	28	323	41	0.0
13150	Beef, shortribs	1.00 oz	28	83	0.0	8.7	5.1	2.2	2.3	0.2	26	16	89	0.0
13094	Beef, prime rib, roasted	1.00 oz	28	83	0.0	7.8	5.5	2.4	2.4	0.2	23	21	107	0.0
10087	Pork, Boston blade, roasted	1.00 oz	28	66	0.0	6.9	4.1	1.5	1.8	0.4	24	25	122	0.0
10215	Pork cutlet, braised	1.00 oz	28	50	0.0	7.7	1.9	0.7	0.8	0.2	23	13	101	0.0
17033	Lamb rib, roast	1.00 oz	28	67	0.0	7.9	3.7	1.3	1.5	0.3	26	24	89	0.0
17225	Lamb, ground	1.00 oz	28	80	0.4	7.0	5.6	2.3	2.4	0.4	28	23	96	0.0
17100	Veal cutlet, lean, leg	1.00 oz	28	58	0.0	10.5	1.5	0.6	0.5	0.1	38	19	110	0.0
05037	Chicken, dark meat w/skin, roast	1.00 oz	28	72	0.0	7.3	4.5	1.2	1.8	1.0	26	25	62	0.0
05306	Turkey, ground	1.00 oz	28	67	0.0	7.7	3.7	1.0	1.4	0.9	29	30	76	0.0
05008	Chicken, fried, flour coated	1.00 oz	28	76	0.9	8.1	4.2	1.2	1.7	1.0	26	24	66	0.0
15011	Fish, fried, cornmeal coated	1.00 oz	28	65	2.3	5.1	0.8	1.0	1.6	1.0	23	79	96	0.0
	Cheeses <5 g fat/oz													
01019	Cheese, feta	1.00 oz	28	74	1.2	4.0	6.0	4.2	1.3	0.2	25	313	17	0.0
01028	Cheese, mozzarella, part skim milk	1.00 oz	28	72	0.8	6.9	4.5	2.9	1.3	0.1	16	132	24	0.0
01037	Cheese, ricotta, part skim milk	0.25 cup	62	86	3.2	7.1	4.9	3.1	1.4	0.2	19	78	78	0.0
01123	Egg, fresh	1.00 egg	50	74	0.6	6.2	5.0	1.6	1.9	0.7	213	63	60	0.0
Label	Sausage, <5 g fat/oz	1.00 oz	28	45	1.5	4.0	2.5	1.3	(0.7)	(0.5)	15	300	76	0.0
16120	Soy milk	1.00 cup	240	79	4.3	6.6	4.6	0.5	0.8	2.0	0	30	388	—
16114	Tempeh	0.25 cup	42	83	7.1	7.9	3.2	0.5	0.7	1.8	0	2	153	—
16127	Tofu	0.25 cup	116	88	2.2	9.4	5.6	0.9	1.2	3.1	0	8	141	1.4

Appendixes

Nutrient	Food Source	Quantity	Grams per Serving	Cal	Cho (g)	Pro (g)	Fat (g)	SFA (g)	MUFA (g)	PUFA (g)	Chol (mg)	Na (mg)	K (mg)	Total Dietary Fiber(g)
MEAT: HIGH-FAT														
10089	Pork spareribs, braised	1.00 oz	28	113	0.0	8.3	8.6	3.2	3.8	0.8	35	27	91	0.0
10220	Pork, ground	1.00 oz	28	84	0.0	7.3	5.9	2.2	2.6	0.5	27	21	102	0.0
07064	Pork sausage, fresh, patty/link	1.00 oz	28	105	0.3	5.6	8.9	3.1	4.0	1.1	24	369	103	0.0
01042	Cheese, American, processed	1.00 oz	28	106	0.4	6.3	8.9	5.6	2.5	0.3	27	406	46	0.0
01009	Cheese, cheddar	1.00 oz	28	114	0.4	7.1	9.4	6.0	2.7	0.3	30	176	28	0.0
01025	Cheese, monterey jack	1.00 oz	28	106	0.0	6.9	8.6	5.4	2.5	0.3	27	152	23	0.0
01040	Cheese, swiss	1.00 oz	28	107	1.0	8.1	7.8	5.0	2.1	0.3	26	74	31	0.0
Processed sandwich meat <8 g fat/oz														
07008	Bologna, beef & pork	1.00 oz	28	89	0.8	3.3	8.0	3.0	3.8	0.7	16	289	51	0.0
07058	Pimiento loaf	1.00 oz	28	74	1.7	3.3	6.0	2.2	2.7	0.7	10	394	96	0.0
07069	Salami, beef & pork	1.00 oz	28	71	0.6	3.9	5.7	2.3	2.6	0.6	18	302	56	0.0
07013	Bratwurst, pork	1.00 oz	28	85	0.6	4.0	7.3	2.6	3.5	0.8	17	158	60	0.0
07089	Sausage, Italian, pork	1.00 oz	28	92	0.4	5.7	7.3	2.6	3.4	0.9	22	263	87	0.0
07075	Sausage, smoked	1.00 oz	28	96	0.4	3.8	8.6	3.0	4.0	0.9	20	269	54	0.0
07038	Knockwurst	1.00 oz	28	87	0.5	3.4	7.9	2.9	3.6	0.8	16	286	57	0.0
07059	Sausage, Polish	1.00 oz	28	92	0.5	4.0	8.1	2.9	3.8	0.9	20	248	67	0.0
07024	Hot dog, chicken 10/#	1.00 hot dog	45	116	3.1	5.8	8.8	2.5	3.8	1.8	45	617	0	0.0
07025	Hot dog, turkey 10/#	1.00 hot dog	45	102	0.7	6.4	8.0	2.3	3.5	1.6	48	642	80	0.0
10124	Bacon, fried, drained, 20 slices/#	3.00 slice	18	105	0.0	5.4	9.0	3.0	4.2	1.2	15	288	87	0.0
MEAT: HIGH-FAT + 1 FAT														
07023	Hot dog, beef & pork, 10/#	1.00 hot dog	45	144	1.2	5.1	13.1	4.8	6.1	1.2	22	504	75	0.0
16098	Peanut butter, smooth, salted	2.00 Tbsp	32	188	6.6	7.9	16.0	3.1	7.6	4.6	0	153	231	1.9

MONOUNSATURATED FATS

Nutrient	Food Source	Quantity	Grams per Serving	Cal	Cho (g)	Pro (g)	Fat (g)	SFA (g)	MUFA (g)	PUFA (g)	Chol (mg)	Na (mg)	K (mg)	Total Dietary Fiber (g)
09037	Avocado, fresh	0.12 avocado	25	40	1.8	0.5	3.8	0.6	2.4	0.5	0	3	150	1.5
04582	Canola oil	1.00 tsp	5	41	0.0	0.0	4.7	0.3	2.8	1.4	0	0	0	0.0
04053	Olive oil	1.00 tsp	5	40	0.0	0.0	4.5	0.6	3.3	0.4	0	0	0	0.0
04042	Peanut oil	1.00 tsp	5	40	0.0	0.0	4.5	0.8	2.1	1.4	0	0	0	0.0
09194	Olives, ripe, large, pitted	8.00 large	35	40	2.2	0.3	3.7	0.5	2.8	0.3	0	305	3	(1.2)
Label	Olives, green, stuffed, large	10.00 large	(28)	50	2.0	0.0	4.0	0.0	32.3	—	0	660	—	—
12063	Almonds, dry roasted	6.00 whole	8	47	1.9	1.3	4.1	0.4	2.7	0.9	0	1	62	1.1
12085	Cashews, salted	6.00 whole	9	52	2.9	1.4	4.2	0.8	2.5	0.7	0	58	51	0.3
12137	Mixed nuts (<50% peanuts)	6.00 nuts	6	37	1.3	(1.6)	3.3	0.5	1.9	0.8	0	26	35	0.6
16090	Peanuts, dry roast, no salt, all types	10.00 nuts	9	44	1.9	2.1	4.5	0.6	2.2	1.4	0	1	59	0.7
12143	Pecans	4.00 halves	7	46	1.6	0.6	4.5	0.4	2.8	1.1	0	0	26	0.5
16098	Peanut butter, smooth, salted	2.00 tsp	11	63	2.2	2.6	5.3	1.0	2.5	1.5	0	51	77	0.9
12023	Sesame seeds	1.00 Tbsp	9	52	2.1	1.6	4.5	0.6	1.7	2.0	0	1	42	1.1
12166	Tahini paste	2.00 tsp	10	59	2.1	1.7	5.4	0.8	2.0	2.3	0	11	41	0.9

POLYUNSATURATED FATS

Nutrient	Food Source	Quantity	Grams per Serving	Cal	Cho (g)	Pro (g)	Fat (g)	SFA (g)	MUFA (g)	PUFA (g)	Chol (mg)	Na (mg)	K (mg)	Total Dietary Fiber (g)
04132	Margarine, stick, >80% veg oil	1.00 tsp	5	34	0.0	0.0	3.8	0.7	1.7	1.2	0	44	2	0.0
Label	Margarine, tub, >75% veg oil	1.00 tsp	(5)	30	0.0	0.0	3.7	0.7	0.3	1.3	0	33	—	0.0
Label	Margarine, squeeze, >70% veg oil	1.00 tsp	4	30	0.0	0.0	3.3	0.5	0.8	1.7	0	37	—	0.0
Label	Margarine, red-fat, 30–50% veg oil	1.00 Tbsp	14	50	0.0	0.0	6.0	1.0	1.5	1.5	0	60	4	0.0
Label	Margarine, reduced-calorie	1.00 Tbsp	14	50	0.0	0.0	5.6	1.0	2.8	1.8	0	90	2	0.0
04025	Mayonnaise	1.00 tsp	5	33	0.0	0.0	3.7	0.5	1.0	1.9	3	26	1	0.0
Avg	Mayonnaise, light/reduced-fat	1.00 Tbsp	15	40	3.0	0.0	3.0	(0.7)	(1.3)	(2.6)	6	120	40	0.4
12155	Walnuts, English	4.00 halves	8	51	1.5	1.1	4.9	0.5	1.1	3.1	0	1	40	0.4
04518	Oil, corn	1.00 tsp	5	44	0.0	0.0	5.0	0.6	1.2	2.9	0	0	0	0.0
04510	Oil, safflower (over 70% linoleic)	1.00 tsp	5	44	0.0	0.0	5.0	0.5	0.6	3.7	0	0	0	0.0
04044	Oil, soybean (glycine max)	1.00 tsp	5	44	0.0	0.0	5.0	0.7	1.2	2.9	0	0	0	0.0
Avg	Salad dressing, reg	1.00 Tbsp	15	64	1.9	—	6.1	—	—	—	—	150	—	—
Avg	Salad dressing, lite/red-cal/red-fat	2.00 Tbsp	30	80	5.0	0.0	6.3	1.0	—	—	—	307	—	0.0
04018	Miracle Whip salad dress, reg	2.00 tsp	10	39	2.4	0.1	3.3	0.5	0.9	1.8	3	71	1	0.0
Label	Miracle Whip salad dress, red-fat	1.00 Tbsp	14	45	2.0	0.0	4.0	1.0	1.0	2.0	5	95	0	0.0
12016	Pumpkin seeds, roasted	1.00 Tbsp	14	70	1.8	4.5	5.7	1.0	1.8	2.6	0	3	110	0.8
12037	Sunflower seeds, dry roasted	1.00 Tbsp	8	47	1.9	1.5	4.0	0.4	0.8	2.6	0	0	68	0.7

Appendixes

Nutrient	Food Source	Quantity	Grams per Serving	Cal	Cho (g)	Pro (g)	Fat (g)	SFA (g)	MUFA (g)	PUFA (g)	Chol (mg)	Na (mg)	K (mg)	Total Dietary Fiber(g)
	SATURATED FATS													
10124	Bacon, fried, drained	1.00 slice	6	35	0.0	1.8	3.0	1.0	1.4	0.4	5	96	29	0.0
01018	Bacon grease	1.00 tsp	4	36	0.0	0.0	4.0	1.6	1.8	0.4	4	(64)	0	0.0
04136	Butter, stick	1.00 tsp	5	36	0.0	0.0	4.1	2.5	1.2	0.1	11	41	1	0.0
Label	Butter, whipped	2.00 tsp	6	40	0.0	0.0	4.7	3.3	—	—	13	50	—	0.0
Label	Butter, reduced-fat	1.00 Tbsp	14	50	0.0	0.0	6.0	4.0	—	—	20	70	—	0.0
10099	Chitterlings, boiled	2.00 Tbsp	14	42	0.0	1.4	4.0	1.4	1.4	1.0	20	6	1	0.0
12109	Coconut, shredded, dried, swtnd	2.00 Tbsp	11	52	5.2	0.4	3.5	3.1	0.2	0.0	0	28	35	2.6
01049	Cream, half and half	2.00 Tbsp	30	39	1.3	0.9	3.5	2.2	1.0	0.1	11	12	39	0.0
01017	Cream cheese, regular	1.00 Tbsp	14	49	0.4	1.1	4.9	3.1	1.4	0.2	15	41	17	0.0
Label	Cream cheese, reduced-fat	2.00 Tbsp	28	60	2.0	3.0	5.0	3.0	1.4	0.2	15	160	34	0.0
10165	Salt pork, raw, cured	0.25 oz	7	52	0.0	0.4	5.6	2.1	2.7	0.7	6	100	5	0.0
04031	Shortening	1.00 tsp	4	35	0.0	0.0	4.0	1.0	1.8	1.0	0	0	0	0.0
10108	Lard	1.00 tsp	4	36	0.0	0.0	4.0	1.6	1.5	0.4	4	0	0	0.0
01056	Sour cream, regular	2.00 Tbsp	24	52	1.0	0.8	5.0	3.1	1.5	0.2	10	12	34	0.0
Label	Sour cream, reduced-fat	3.00 Tbsp	(45)	45	2.0	1.0	3.5	2.5	0.9	0.1	15	20	58	0.0
	FREE FOODS: LOW-FAT OR FAT-FREE FOODS													
Label	Cream cheese, fat-free	1.00 Tbsp	12	15	1.0	2.5	0.0	0.0	0.0	0.0	2	80	—	0.0
Label	Creamer, nondairy, liquid, regular	1.00 Tbsp	15	18	1.5	0.0	1.0	0.2	0.8	0.0	0	5	29	0.0
01069	Creamer, nondairy, powder, regular	1.00 tsp	4	22	2.2	0.2	1.4	1.3	0.0	0.0	0	7	33	0.0
Label	Mayonnaise, fat-free	1.00 Tbsp	15	10	2.0	(0.2)	0.0	0.0	0.0	0.0	0	105	(5)	0.0
Label	Mayonnaise, light/low-fat/red-fat	1.00 tsp	5	5	1.0	0.0	1.0	(0.1)	(0.3)	(0.5)	(2)	40	(2)	0.0
Label	Margarine, fat-free/nonfat	4.00 Tbsp	48	20	0.0	0.0	0.0	0.0	0.0	0.0	0	360	—	0.0
Label	Margarine, low-fat/light	1.00 tsp	5	17	0.0	0.0	1.9	0.3	0.7	0.6	0	30	2	0.0
Label	Miracle Whip, nonfat dressing	1.00 Tbsp	15	15	3.0	0.0	0.0	0.0	0.0	0.0	0	105	—	0.0
Label	Miracle Whip, light	1.00 tsp	5	19	1.2	0.0	1.7	0.2	0.4	0.9	1	36	1	0.0
Label	Nonstick cooking spray	1.00 spray (⅓ of 10" pan)	0	2	0.0	0.0	0.2	0.0	0.0	0.0	0	0	0	0.0
Avg	Salad dressing, fat-free	1.00 Tbsp	16	20	4.5	0.0	0.0	0.0	0.0	0.0	0	145	(13)	0.0
Label	Salad dressing, Italian, fat-free	2.00 Tbsp	31	15	3.2	0.2	0.2	0.0	0.0	0.0	0	290	5	0.0
06164	Salsa	0.25 cup	64	14	3.2	0.8	0.2	0.0	0.0	0.0	0	168	120	0.8
Label	Sour cream, light	1.00 Tbsp	16	18	2.0	0.5	1.0	0.8	0.2	0.0	5	15	(21)	0.0
Avg	Sour cream, fat-free	1.00 Tbsp	16	15	2.5	0.5	0.0	0.1	0.0	0.0	0	20	(23)	0.0
Avg	Whipped topping	2.00 Tbsp	8	24	2.0	0.0	1.5	1.0	0.0	0.0	0	2	—	0.0
Avg	Whipped topping, light	2.00 Tbsp	8	19	2.0	0.0	1.0	0.5	0.0	0.0	0	2	—	0.0

281

Diabetes Medical Nutrition Therapy

Nutrient	Food Source	Quantity		Grams per Serving	Cal	Cho (g)	Pro (g)	Fat (g)	SFA (g)	MUFA (g)	PUFA (g)	Chol (mg)	Na (mg)	K (mg)	Total Dietary Fiber (g)
FREE FOODS: LOW-SUGAR OR SUGAR-FREE FOODS															
Label	Candy, hard, sugar-free	1.00	candy	5	20	4.7	0.0	0.0	0.0	0.0	0.0	0	0	—	0.0
19176	Gelatin dessert, sugar-free	0.50	cup	117	8	0.8	1.3	0.0	0.0	0.0	0.0	0	56	0	0.0
19177	Gelatin, unflavored	1.00	envelope	7	23	0.0	6.0	0.0	0.0	0.0	0.0	0	14	1	0.0
Label	Jam/jelly, low-sugar/light	2.00	tsp	11	15	3.5	0.0	0.0	0.0	0.0	0.0	0	4	(8)	0.0
Label	Syrup, sugar-free	2.00	Tbsp	30	18	4.5	0.0	0.0	0.0	0.0	0.0	0	53	—	0.0
FREE FOODS: DRINKS															
06413	Broth type	1.00	cup	242	28	0.5	3.8	1.0	0.4	0.4	0.2	1	779	70	—
06081	Bouillon or broth, granular/cubes	1.00	tsp	2	5	0.6	0.4	0.1	0.0	0.1	0.0	0	576	9	0.0
Label	Bouillon/broth, low-sodium	1.00	tsp	6	13	1.5	0.9	0.3	0.1	0.1	0.1	1	5	24	0.0
14384	Carbonated or mineral water	1.00	cup	237	0	0.0	0.0	0.0	0.0	0.0	0.0	0	3	0	0.0
19165	Cocoa powder, unsweetened	1.00	Tbsp	5	11	2.7	1.0	0.7	0.4	0.2	0.4	0	0	76	1.5
14209	Coffee, brewed	0.75	cup	177	4	0.8	0.1	0.0	0.0	0.0	0.0	0	4	96	0.0
14121	Club soda	12.00	oz	355	0	0.0	0.0	0.0	0.0	0.0	0.0	0	75	7	0.0
14416	Diet soft drinks, sugar-free	12.00	oz	355	2	0.3	0.2	0.0	0.0	0.0	0.0	0	21	0	0.0
14289	Drink mixes, sugar-free	1.00	cup	2	7	1.7	0.1	0.0	0.0	0.0	0.0	0	0	0	0.0
14355	Tea, brewed	0.75	cup	178	2	0.4	0.0	0.0	0.0	0.0	0.0	0	5	66	0.0
Label	Tonic water, sugar-free	1.00	cup	240	0	0.0	0.0	0.0	0.0	0.0	0.0	0	35	—	0.0
FREE FOODS: CONDIMENTS															
11935	Catsup, tomato	1.00	Tbsp	15	16	4.1	0.2	0.1	0.0	0.0	0.0	0	178	72	0.2
1136	Horseradish	1.00	Tbsp	15	6	1.4	0.2	0.0	0.0	0.0	0.0	0	14	44	1.2
09153	Lemon juice	1.00	Tbsp	15	3	1.0	0.1	0.0	0.0	0.0	0.0	0	3	15	0.1
09160	Lime juice	1.00	Tbsp	15	4	1.4	0.1	0.0	0.0	0.0	0.0	0	0	17	0.1
1371	Mustard, prepared	1.00	tsp	5	4	0.3	0.2	0.2	0.0	0.0	0.0	0	63	7	0.0
11937	Pickles, dill	1.50	large	98	18	4.0	0.6	0.2	0.0	0.0	0.2	0	1256	114	1.2
16125	Soy sauce	1.00	Tbsp	18	7	1.4	0.4	0.0	0.0	0.0	0.0	0	1024	27	0.0
16125	Soy sauce, lite	1.00	Tbsp	18	7	1.4	0.4	0.0	0.0	0.0	0.0	0	605	27	0.1
B&C	Taco sauce	1.00	Tbsp	14	7	2.0	0.2	0.0	0.0	0.0	0.0	0	102	36	—
2406	Vinegar, cider	0.25	cup	60	8	3.6	0.0	0.0	0.0	0.0	0.0	0	1	60	0.0

Nutrient	Food Source	Quantity	Grams per Serving	Cal	Cho (g)	Pro (g)	Fat (g)	SFA (g)	MUFA (g)	PUFA (g)	Chol (mg)	Na (mg)	K (mg)	Total Dietary Fiber (g)
	FREE FOODS: SEASONINGS													
11215	Garlic	1.00 clove	4	1	0.2	0.0	0.0	0.0	0.0	0.0	0	0	12	0.1
11943	Pimiento, cn, s+l	1.00 Tbsp	12	3	0.6	0.1	0.0	0.0	0.0	0.0	0	0	19	0.1
06169	Tabasco sauce	1.00 tsp	5	1	0.0	0.1	0.0	0.0	0.0	0.0	0	30	6	0.0
B&C	Worcestershire sauce	1.00 tsp	5	4	0.9	0.1	0.0	0.0	0.0	0.0	0	49	40	0.0
	COMBINATION FOODS, FROZEN ENTREES, SOUPS													
B&C	Tuna noodle casserole	1.00 cup	255	259	33.5	13.4	7.9	(1.6)	(2.9)	(2.9)	(42)	1043	198	(1.8)
B&C	Lasagna	1.00 cup	227	302	27.2	22.2	11.8	(3.5)	(3.9)	(0.7)	34	885	363	(1.8)
B&C	Spaghetti tom sauce/meatballs	1.00 cup	250	258	28.5	12.3	10.3	2.2	(4.0)	(0.6)	(39)	1220	245	(2.9)
21042	Chili with beans	1.00 cup	253	256	21.9	24.6	8.3	3.4	3.4	0.5	134	1007	691	(7.1)
B&C	Macaroni and cheese	1.00 cup	240	228	25.7	9.4	9.6	4.2	(4.4)	(0.9)	(20)	730	139	(1.5)
B&C	Chow mein, beef (no ndles/rice)	2.00 cups	453	160	13.3	16.0	2.7	1.1	(1.0)	0.0	43	2373	400	5.3
B&C	Pizza, cheese, thin crust (10")	0.25 (≈ 5 oz)	126	317	27.8	14.2	16.6	7.0	3.0	1.0	20	770	268	(2.2)
B&C	Pizza, meat, thin crust (10")	0.25 (≈ 5 oz)	135	368	29.2	15.0	21.3	7.0	7.0	2.0	15	1000	284	2.4
B&C	Pot pie, individual (dbl crust)	1.00 (7 oz)	198	450	34.9	13.3	28.2	—	—	—	34	778	199	—
	Frozen entrees													
Label	Salisbury steak, gravy, mshd pot	1.00 (11 oz)	314	500	26.0	23.0	34.0	—	—	—	80	600	—	—
Label	Turkey, gravy, mshd pot, dressing, veg	1.00 (11 oz)	314	390	35.0	18.0	20.0	—	—	—	40	1110	—	—
Avg	Entree, <300 kcal	1.00 (≈ 8 oz)	243	220	29.3	12.0	6.3	1.5	1.8	1.5	35	483	70	3.0
	Soups													
06402	Bean	1.00 cup	247	116	19.8	5.6	1.5	0.4	0.5	0.5	0	1198	273	(4.4)
06443	Cream of mshrm, w/water	1.00 cup	244	129	9.3	2.3	9.0	2.4	1.7	4.2	2	1032	100	0.5
06410	Cream of celery, w/water	1.00 cup	244	90	8.8	1.7	5.6	1.4	1.3	2.5	15	949	122	0.7
06451	Split pea, made with water	0.50 cup	127	95	14.0	5.2	2.2	0.9	0.9	0.3	4	504	400	5.1
06559	Tomato, made with water	1.00 cup	244	85	16.6	2.0	1.9	0.4	0.4	1.0	0	871	264	0.5
06471	Vegetable beef, w/water	1.00 cup	244	78	10.2	5.6	1.9	0.9	0.8	0.1	5	956	173	0.5
06409	Beef noodle, w/water	1.00 cup	244	83	9.0	4.8	3.1	1.1	1.2	0.5	5	952	100	0.7
06419	Chicken noodle, w/water	1.00 cup	241	75	9.4	4.0	2.5	0.7	1.1	0.6	7	1106	55	0.7

FAST FOODS

Nutrient	Food Source	Quantity	Grams per Serving	Cal	Cho (g)	Pro (g)	Fat (g)	SFA (g)	MUFA (g)	PUFA (g)	Chol (mg)	Na (mg)	K (mg)	Total Dietary Fiber (g)
21006	Burritos with beef	2.00 burritos	220	523	58.5	26.6	20.8	10.5	7.4	0.9	65	1492	739	(2.2)
21037	Chicken nuggets, plain	6.00 nuggets	102	290	15.5	16.9	17.7	5.6	8.7	2.3	61	543	251	0.4
21036	Chicken, breaded & fried (side breast & wing)	1.00 each	163	494	19.5	35.7	29.5	7.8	12.2	6.8	149	975	566	(0.6)
21105	Fish sandwich & tartar sauce	1.00 sandwich	158	431	41.0	16.9	22.8	5.2	7.7	8.3	55	615	340	(1.4)
21138	French fries, 1–2" long strips	20–25 strips	76	235	29.3	3.0	12.2	3.8	6.0	1.9	0	124	541	(1.5)
21107	Hamburger, single patty, plain	1.00 burger	90	275	30.5	12.3	11.8	4.1	5.5	0.9	36	387	145	(1.2)
21112	Hamburger, large	1.00 burger	137	425	31.7	22.6	22.9	8.4	9.9	2.1	71	474	268	(1.2)
21118	Hot dog with bun	1.00 hot dog	98	242	18.0	10.4	14.5	5.1	6.9	1.7	44	671	143	(1.0)
21028	Soft-serve cone	1.00 regular	142	226	33.2	5.4	8.4	4.9	2.5	0.5	38	126	233	(0.5)
Pizza Hut	Individual pan pizza	1.00 pizza	327	722	70.0	33.0	34.0	12.0	(13.9)	(5.8)	66	1760	(739)	6.0
21124	Submarine sandwich (6")	1.00 sub	228	456	51.0	21.8	18.6	6.8	8.2	2.3	35	1650	394	(2.0)
21082	Taco, hard shell, small (6 oz)	1.00 taco	171	369	26.7	20.7	20.6	11.4	6.6	1.0	56	802	474	(0.7)
Taco Bell	Taco, soft shell (3 oz)	1.00 taco	99	220	19.0	12.0	11.0	(6.3)	(3.5)	(0.3)	30	464	374	(1.1)

Index

A
Acarbose, 36-37
   hypoglycemia as rare in clients using, 75-76
Acceptable daily intake (ADI) of nonnutritive sweeteners, 23
Acesulfame K use by diabetics, 23
ADA diet as not endorsed by American Diabetes Association, 25
Adolescents
   blood glucose goals for, 63-64
   continuous assessment of, 64
   nutrition assessment of, 61-63
   optimal diabetes management in, 61-64
   role of diabetes medical nutrition therapy in growth and development of, 61
African Americans, nephropathy incidence in, 81
Aging as risk factor in development of type II diabetes, 11
Alcohol
   beverages made with, nutritional composition of, 84-85
   as cause of hypoglycemia and hyperglycemia, 83-84
   composition of beverages made with, 86
   effects on triglycerides of, 84
   interactions of drugs and, 85
   moderation in use of, 131
   oral glucose-lowering medication used concurrently with, 84
   in recipes, 175
   recommendations for persons with diabetes regarding, 24, 86
   sugar, calculations for, 175
Alpha-glucosidase inhibitors, 36-37
   combination therapy with, 37
   time activity of, 36
American Association of Diabetes Educators, 248
American Diabetes Association
   address of, 248
   Carbohydrate Counting published by American Dietetic Association and, 179
   education goals of, 105-6
   exchange lists developed by, 167
   fiber intake recommendations by, 23
   First Step in Diabetes Meal Planning published by American Dietetic Association and, 137
   Healthy Food Choices published by American Dietetic Association and, 139, 175
   historic perspective of distribution of total calories from past recommendations of, 19-20
   Month of Meals developed by, 162
   1994 Diabetes Nutrition Recommendations of, 4, 17, 19, 25
   Single-Topic Diabetes Resources published by American Dietetic Association and, 148
American Dietetic Association
   Carbohydrate Counting published by American Diabetes Association and, 179
   Diabetes Care and Education Practice Group of, 248
   endorsement of 1994 Nutrition Recommendations of American Diabetes Association of, 4
   exchange lists developed by, 167
   First Step in Diabetes Meal Planning published by American Diabetes Association and, 137
   Healthy Food Choices published by American Diabetes Association and, 139, 175
   Single-Topic Diabetes Resources published by American Diabetes Association and, 148
Arrhythmia as risk factor of exercise for clients with cardiovascular disease, 31
Aspartame use by diabetics, 23

B
Beta blockers, 45
Beverages
   alcohol in, 84-85
   low in calories, 89
Biguanides, 35-36
   combination therapy with, 37
   reaction to using alcohol with certain, 84
   time activity of, 36
Binding defect of insulin receptors, 11
Blood glucose control, exercise by clients with type II diabetes as improving, 29, 30
Blood glucose levels
   goals for, 63-64, 65, 204
   in HHNS, 77
   identifying patterns in, 181
   individualized target, 51
   notifying physician about, 91
   nutrient-related factors affecting, 187-88
   in pregnancy, normalizing, 64-65
   recording, 181, 196
   snacks to help prevent fluctuations in, 87
   strategies for, 182
Blood glucose monitoring, 4. *See also* Self-monitoring of blood glucose (SMBG) records
   to avoid hypoglycemia, 88
   client education for, 204, 208, 218, 220, 225, 226, 230-31, 236
   for client with gastrointestinal neuropathy, 81
   to determine effect of alcohol on person with diabetes, 24
   in diabetes medical nutrition therapy, 43
   equipment and supplies for, 51
   insulin adjustments facilitated by, 53
   with morning sickness, 66
   for pregnant client with GDM, 67
   for pregnant client with preexisting diabetes, 67
   sample daily record for, 44
Blood glucose records
   for children or adolescents with diabetes, 64
   sample blank form for, 243
Blood glucose response to exercise, 32
Blood glucose tests
   daily, 42
   frequency of, for pregnant clients, 67
Body mass index (BMI), 100, 252-53

C
Caloric modification for weight control in type II diabetes, 18
Calorie counting, 193-95
   advantages and disadvantages of, 194-95
   clinical setting for, 194
   exchange list use compared to, 193
   historical background of, 193
   intended population for use of, 194
   length of time to teach approach of, 194
   method of using, 194
   summary of, 247
Calories
   in alcohol, 84
   "banked," 87
   calculating, 172
   calculating child's or adolescent's needs for, 61-62
   daily requirements for, estimating, 195, 255
   overrestriction in children of, 61
   setting levels of, 163
   snacks and beverages low in, table of, 89
   wasted through glycosuria, 186
Carbohydrate choice method to determine carbohydrate-to-insulin ratio, 182-83, 184-86
Carbohydrate Counting (American Dietetic Association and American Diabetes Association), 179-91
   advantages and disadvantages of, 186-87, 189-90
   case studies using, 228, 234-37
   clinical setting for, 189

285

historical background of, 180
intended population for use of, 188
length of time to teach approach of, 189
levels of, 179–90
method of using, 180–88
ordering information for, 191
summary of, 247
Carbohydrate gram method to determine carbohydrate-to-insulin ratio, 182–84, 186
Carbohydrate quiz, 180
Carbohydrate-counting approach to meal planning, 173, 179–91
for clients who work shifts, travel, or have erratic schedules, 186–87
Level 1 of, 180–82, 188–90
Level 2 of, 181–90
Level 3 of, 188–90
Carbohydrate-to-insulin ratios (carbohydrate counting), 51, 56, 173, 184–86
developing, 182–83
matching insulin to carbohydrate using, 180
practice worksheet for figuring, 242
Carbohydrates
adjusted depending on blood glucose monitoring results, 46
in alcohol, 84
calories from, 20
intake of, figuring, 180
nutrition recommendations for, 21, 26
sources of, for treating hypoglycemia, 89–90
Cardiovascular disease in young people with diabetes, 64
Case study
of Jackie (Case Study 7), 231–44
of Joey (Case Study 5), 223–28
of John (Case Study 3), 215–17
of Marion (Case Study 4), 217–22
of Mattie (Case Study 2), 206–14
of nutrition assessment, 111–13
of Sarah (Case Study 1), 201–205
of Sheri (Case Study 6), 228–31
Cerebrovascular disease as macrovascular complication of diabetes, 78
Children
blood glucose goals for, 63–64
continuous assessment of, 64
diagnosis of diabetes in, 13
nutrition assessment of, 61–63
optimal diabetes management in, 61–64
recommended energy intake for, 255
reduced IQ scores in, 67
role of diabetes medical nutrition therapy in growth and development of, 61
role of parents and caregivers in diabetes management of, 63
school versus weekend routine for, 63
Chlorpropamide, reaction from concurrent use of alcohol and, 84
Chromium deficiency, 25
Client empowerment approach, 95–97
Complete Book of Food Counts, 237
Complications of diabetes, 75–82
acute, 75–78
chronic, 78–81
Congestive heart failure, vitamin/mineral supplement evaluation for clients with, 25
Continuous subcutaneous insulin infusion (CSII). *See* Insulin pumps
Council on Nutritional Science and Metabolism, *Month of Meals* developed by, 162

Counterregulatory hormones, decreased effects of, 29
Counting approach to meal planning, 155
resources for, 156
Coxsackie virus, 11

D

Daily fat allowance, calculating, 195–96
Daily Food Guide Pyramid, 26
Dawn phenomenon, 40, 46
Delay of meals, 86–87
Delayed glycemic peak, 80–81
Desirable body weight (DBW) defined, 254
Diabetes. *See also* individual types
classification of, 9–10
complications of, 75–82
diagnosis of, 13
impact and incidence of, 9
interrelation of malnutrition and, 70
laboratory values for, 251
management of, 1–92
nutrition services as vital in treatment of, 3
pathophysiology of, 10–12
promoting self-management of, 5
resources for, 147–52
Diabetes Care and Education Practice Group, Scope of Practice for Qualified Professionals in Diabetes Care and Education of, 4–7
roles and responsibilities in, table of, 6
Diabetes Care and Education Practice Group of American Dietetic Association, 248
Diabetes Care Made Easy: A Simple Step-by-Step Guide for Controlling Your Diabetes, 142
Diabetes care team
discussion of carbohydrate counting between inpatient client and, 189
experience with IIT of, 51
members of, 4, 5–7, 51
target blood glucose goals set by client and, 43
Diabetes Control and Complications Trial (DCCT), 15–17
affirmation of importance of meal planning by, 16
carbohydrate-counting approach used in, 180
demonstration of effectiveness of IIT in, 51
nutrition intervention in, 15–17
participant subgroups of, 15
relationship between control of glucose levels and development of complications confirmed by, 63
results of, 4, 16
severe hypoglycemia incidence noted in, 88
Diabetes education advisory committee, 5
Diabetes educators, 5
as counselors, 106–7
goals negotiated between clients and, 106, 107
information on nutrition assessment for, 100, 105
Diabetes Knowledge Checklist blank form, 259
Diabetes medical nutrition therapy
defined, 3
four-pronged approach to, 61, 99, 151, 246
goals of, 17, 43, 105–6
individualizing, 4
introduction to, 3–8
in management of diabetes, 15–28
milestone events in, 3–4
overview of, 141
philosophy of care for, 95–97
practice guidelines for, 4, 7, 108
process of, 99–123
purpose of, 99

reinforcing, 109
time frames for, 110
weight loss in, 79
Diabetes Nutrition Education Goals, 106
Diabetes nutrition education resources, 245–49
Diabetes Self-Care Daily Record, 43–44
blank form for, 257
sample completed, 241
Diabetes Self-Care Record, 103
sample completed, 239–40
Diabetic ketoacidosis (DKA), 78, 91
Dietary Guidelines for Americans (USDA-HHS), 26, 131–32, 134–35, 137
advantages and disadvantages of, 132
historical background of, 131
for inpatient and ambulatory care settings, 132
intended population for use of, 132
length of time to teach approach of, 132
methods for using, 131–32
ordering information for, 135
summary of, 247
Dietetic technician, registered (DTR)
as provider of diabetes medical nutrition therapy, 5
roles of, 6
Dyslipidemia with insulin resistance, 79

E

Eating behavior diary, sample completed, 120
Eating habits
"beginning" changes in, 127
promoting change in clients', 99
Eating out, meal planning for, 86–87
Economic information about client, 103–4
Education plan, case study for, 112–13
Educational interventions, 107
Elderly, vitamin/mineral supplement evaluation for, 25. *See also* Older adults
End-stage renal disease (ESRD), 81
Enteral nutrition support for older adults, 71
Epstein-Barr virus, 11
Evaluation, 107–10
defined, 107
outcome and impact, 108
practice, 108
process, 108
types of, 108–9
Exchange list approach to meal planning, 155
calorie counting compared to, 193
resources for, 156
Exchange Lists for Meal Planning, 139, 162, 167–75
advantages and disadvantages of, 173, 175
carbohydrate choice method based on, 184
case study using, 226–27
clinical setting for, 173
database of nutrient sources for, 265–84
hints for calculating exchange lists meal plans for, 172
historical background of, 167–69
intended population for use of, 171, 173
length of time to teach approach of, 173
method of using, 169–71, 174–75
1995 updates to, 168–69
ordering information for, 178
summary of, 247
Exchanges, 167–78
Exercise, 51
benefits of, 30
client education for, 204, 208, 217, 220, 225, 226, 230–31, 234

Index

guidelines for, 32–33
in management of diabetes, 29–33
metabolic effects of, 29
recommendations for, 32
relationship of food, insulin, and, 18
risks of, 30, 31
Exercise schedule, case study for, 111
Exercise specialists as diabetes educators, 5, 51

F

Facilitating Lifestyle Change: A Resource Manual, 99, 102, 103–4, 106, 108
   case studies using, 111–13, 204, 207, 225
   summary of, 247
Family history as risk factor in development of type II diabetes, 11
Fast-food restaurants, nutrient information pamphlets in, 196
Fat
   "banked," 87
   calculations for meal plans of, 172, 174
   entrees prepared with minimal, 87
   laboratory values for, 251
   nutrition recommendations for, 20–21
Fat counting, 195–97
   advantages and disadvantages of, 196–97
   clinical setting for, 196
   historical background of, 195
   intended population for use of, 196
   length of time to teach approach of, 196
   method of using, 195–96
   summary of, 247
Fat intake as affecting blood glucose levels, 187
Fiber, nutrition recommendations for, 23
Fiber intake as affecting blood glucose levels, 188
First Step in Diabetes Meal Planning (American Dietetic Association and American Diabetes Association), 137–39, 151
   advantages and disadvantages of, 139
   case studies using, 204
   clinical setting for, 139
   historical background of, 137–38
   intended population for use of, 138
   length of time to teach approach of, 139
   method of using, 138
   ordering information for, 145
   summary of, 247
Follow-up in diabetes medical nutrition therapy
   defined, 109
   time frame for, 110
Food and blood glucose records, 181, 183
Food and Physical Activity Record, 108
   Sarah's (Case Study 1) sample completed, 205
Food Guide Pyramid (USDA and Food Marketing Institute), 133, 134–35
   for diabetes. *See First Step in Diabetes Meal Planning*
   historical background of, 134
   intended population for use of, 135
   methods for using, 134–35
   ordering information for, 135
   summary of, 247
Food history, 62–63
Food intake trends, 102
Food jags, 62
Food label calculations, guidelines for, 174–75
Food labs, hands-on, 180
Food Marketing Institute and US Department of Agriculture, *Food Guide Pyramid* developed by, 134

Food Record Form, 102–3
   blank, 256
   to implement calorie counting, 194
   sample completed, 116
Food, relationship of insulin, exercise, and, 17, 18
Foods low in calories, 89
Fructose in meal plans for people with diabetes, 23

G

Gestational diabetes mellitus (GDM), 9
   blood glucose goals in pregnancy for clients with, 65
   congenital anomalies in infants of mothers with, 58, 65
   development of type II diabetes following, 10
   diagnosis of, 13
   monitoring for. *See* Blood glucose monitoring
   pathophysiology of, 12
   risk factors for, 12
   risk of macrosomia in, 58
   screening for, 66
Glucose, hepatic, 29
Glucose level in blood in diabetes, 9, 13
   laboratory values for, 251
   nutrition behaviors that improve control of, 16–17
   sucrose and, studies of, 21–22
Glucose tolerance test, 13
Glucose toxicity, 11–12
Glycemic control
   caloric restriction as associated with improved, 193
   with fat counting approach, 196
   value of, 4
   weight loss for improving, 19
Glycosuria, wasting calories through, 186
Goal setting in diabetes self-management training, 105–6
   blank form for, 260
   defined, 105
   negotiation in, 106
Guide to Good Eating (NDC), 132–35
   advantages and disadvantages of, 134
   case study using, 208
   food groups and leader nutrients of, 132–33
   historical background of, 133
   for inpatient and ambulatory care settings, 134
   intended population for use of, 133
   length of time to teach approach of, 134
   methods for using, 133
   ordering information for, 135
   summary of, 247

H

Health care institutions
   meal-planning options of, 26
   translation of American Diabetes Association's 1994 Nutrition Recommendations for, 25–26
Healthy Eating (International Diabetes Center), 142–44
   advantages and disadvantages of, 144
   clinical setting for, 143
   historical background of, 142
   intended population for use of, 143
   length of time to teach approach of, 144
   method of using, 143
   ordering information for, 145

Healthy Food Choices (American Dietetic Association and American Diabetes Association)
   advantages and disadvantages of, 142, 177
   case study using, 225
   clinical setting for, 142, 177
   guidelines section of, 139–42
   historical background of, 139, 175–76
   intended population for use of, 141, 177
   length of time to teach approach of, 142, 177
   method of using, 139–41, 177
   ordering information for, 145, 178
   poster section of, 175–78
   summary of, 247
Histocompatibility locus antigens (HLAs)
   in children, 10
   function of, 11
Human placental lactogen (HPL) as insulin antagonist, 12
Hyperglycemia
   as acute complication of diabetes, 75
   alcohol as cause of, 83–84
   causes, symptoms, and treatment of, 77
   chronic, 79, 81
   defined, 76
   medications that may increase, 70
   microvascular chronic complications related to, 78
   persistent, 77
Hyperglycemia in type I diabetes after exercise with inadequate insulin, 29, 31
Hyperglycemia in type II diabetes, 11
   preventing postmeal, 19
   sulfonylureas to control, 35
Hyperglycemia, rebound, 46
Hyperglycemic hyperosmolar nonketotic syndrome (HHNS), 77
Hyperinsulinemia, benefits of exercise for clients with, 30
Hyperinsulinemia, chronic, 11–12
Hyperlipidemia, 30
Hypertension
   association between types I and II diabetes and, 24
   benefits of exercise for clients at risk for, 30
   retinal and renal complications worsened by, 78
Hypoglycemia
   as acute complication of diabetes, 75–76
   in afternoon, 46
   alcohol as cause of, 83
   before lunch, 46
   carbohydrate sources for treating, 90
   causes, symptoms, and treatment of, 76, 89–90
   correction of, resulting from oral glucose-lowering medications, 37
   defined, 75
   in first trimester of pregnancy, 65–66
   increased risk of, with IIT, 56n., 57–59, 186
   meal planning for avoiding, 88–91
   medications that may increase, 70
   at night, 46, 186
   overtreatment of, 89, 186
   reducing risk of, 63
   as risk of exercise, 31
   self-management training for, 90–91, 128, 186
   severe, 40
Hypotension, postural, 79

287

I

Impaired glucose tolerance (IGT), 9
   diagnosis of, 13
   management of, 10
   pathophysiology of, 12
   risks for clients with, 10
   treatment goals for, 10
Impotence, erectile, 79
In-depth nutrition intervention, 153–78
   advancing to stage of, 155–56
   defined, 155
   introduction to, 155–56
   resources for, 156
Individualized menus, 157–61
   advantages and disadvantages of, 160
   clinical setting for, 159
   historical background of, 158
   intended population for use of, 159
   length of time to teach approach of, 160
   method of using, 158–61
   summary of, 247
Infant
   anomalies caused by mother's diabetes in, 58, 65
   nutrition history for, 62
   recommended energy intake for, 255
Insulin
   low levels of, in type II diabetes, 9
   in pregnancy, need for, 12, 66
   relationship between food and, 17, 18
   role of, in diabetes mellitus, 9
   short course of, 38
   sources of, 38
   total daily requirements for, estimating, 56
Insulin adjustment, 53–56
   individualized formula for, 54–55
   for more or fewer carbohydrate choices, 185
   with morning sickness, 66
   prospective compensatory or anticipatory, 54, 56
   retrospective method of, 54–55
   sample algorithms/records for, 53–55, 57
Insulin delivery systems, advances in, 51. *See also* Insulin pumps
Insulin injections
   multiple daily (MDI), 51–52, 58, 179
   into non-exercising area to minimize effects of exercise on absorption, 33
   in type I diabetes, 9, 37, 51
   in type II diabetes, 10, 38
Insulin pens, 52
Insulin pumps, 41–42
   Regular insulin used in, 38
   subcutaneous insulin infusion (CSII) using, 51, 52–53, 58, 179
Insulin regimens, 39–41
   idealized periods of insulin effect in, 41, 52
   individualized, 39, 40
   multiple-component, 51
   one through four, 40–41
   sample multiple daily, 41, 52
   selecting, 51–53
Insulin release, impaired, 11
Insulin resistance
   dyslipidemia seen with, 79
   medications to lower, 36
   in older adults, 68
   in type II diabetes, 11–12, 35, 38
Insulin sensitivity, 30
   caloric restriction as associated with improved, 193
   during first trimester of pregnancy, 66
   insulin dose adjusted after physical activity according to, 88

Insulin therapy
   factors in deciding to initiate, 38
   intensive, 51–60, 67, 86, 179, 186–87
Insulin types
   intermediate-acting (NPH or Lente insulin), 38–39, 40, 46, 51–52, 56
   long-acting (Ultralente), 38–39, 40, 46, 51–52, 56
   rapid-acting (insulin analog–Lispro), 38–39, 40, 51–52
   short-acting (Regular insulin), 38–39, 40, 46, 51–52, 87
Insulin users, alcohol use guidelines for, 24
Insulinase, 12
Intensive insulin therapy (IIT), 51–60
   advantages of, 58
   candidates for, 56–58
   carbohydrate counting and, 179
   for clients who work shifts, travel, or have erratic schedules, 186–87
   disadvantages of, 58–59, 186
   elements of, 51
   expense of, 57
   flexibility in timing of meals in, 86
   goals of, 51
   in treating pregnant client with preexisting diabetes, 67
   time requirements for teaching, 58
International Diabetes Center, diabetes nutrition guidelines published by, 142
Intervention, 106–7. *See also* individual types
Ischemic heart disease as macrovascular complication of diabetes, 78, 79
Islet cells, antigens to, 11

J

Jet injectors, 52

K

Ketoacidosis. *See also* Diabetic ketoacidosis (DKA)
   circumstances for development of, in people with type II diabetes, 9
   development of, in people with type I diabetes, 9
Ketone monitoring records, 68
Ketones, testing urine, 91
Ketonuria, 67

L

Lactating women, vitamin/mineral supplement evaluation for, 25
Life stages in management of diabetes, 61–73
Lifestyle Change forms, 108, 112–13
   sample completed, 114–19, 122. *See also* Food and Physical Activity Record
Lifestyle change goals, 105
Lifestyle Change Plan, sample completed, 121
Lifestyle Questionnaire, 102
   sample completed, 114–19, 209–14
Lipid. *See* Fat

M

Macroalbuminuria, 81
Magnesium depletion, 25
Malabsorptive disorder, vitamin/mineral supplement evaluation for clients with, 25
Malnutrition, interrelation of diabetes and, 70
Management of diabetes, 1–92
   by child, 63
   complications in, 75–82
   diabetes medical nutrition therapy for, 15–28

   for different life stages, 61–73
   exercise for, 29–33
   intensive insulin therapy for, 51–60
   medications for, 35–42
   self-monitoring of blood glucose for, 43–49
   in type I diabetes, 9
   in type II diabetes, 10
Mannitol, uses and energy value of, 23
Meal plan
   alcohol substituted for fat in, 83
   calculating exchange lists in, hints for, 172
   carbohydrate goals in, 180
   for child or adolescent with diabetes, 62, 64
   collaborating to develop, 96
   evaluating effectiveness of, 43
   individualized, 43, 99, 169–71
   nutrition history for developing or revising child's, 62–63
   for older adult residents in LTC settings, 70–71
   for pregnant client with diabetes, adjustments in, 66
   renal, 172
   resources for, 142
Meal planning, 51, 83–92
   alcohol use in, 83–86
   approach to, 132, 155
   client education for, 204, 216–17, 220, 225, 226–28, 230–31, 234, 235, 237
   delay of meals in, 86
   eating out in, 86–87
   Exchange Lists for Meal Planning used for, 168–71
   hypoglycemia in, 88–91
   selecting approaches for, based on type of diabetes, 248
   sick-day management in, 91
   snacking in, 87–88
   summary of approaches for, 246–47
   timing of meals in, 128
   tools for, 138
Meal-planning form, 181–82
Meats, calculating fat content of, 172
Medical nutrition therapy. *See also* Diabetes medical nutrition therapy
   case study of diabetes treatment regimen using, 201
   defined, 3
Medications affecting blood glucose, 70
Medications in management of diabetes, 35–42. *See also* Insulin
   oral glucose-lowering, 35–37
Mental health professionals as diabetes educators, 5, 51
Menus, 157–65
   as approach to meal planning, 155
   individualized, 157–61
   odd-day and even-day, 159
   resources for, 156
   sample preprinted, 160–61
Metformin, 35–36
   hypoglycemia as rare in clients using, 75, 76
   reaction from concurrent use of alcohol and, 84
Mexican Americans, nephropathy incidence in, 81
Microalbuminuria, 81
Micronutrients, nutrition recommendations for, 24–25
Mixers for beverages, carbohydrates and calories from, 84–85
Monitoring practice of client, 103
Monounsaturated fats (MUFAs), calories from, 20

Month of Meals (American Diabetes
    Association), 161–64
    advantages and disadvantages of, 164
    clinical setting for, 164
    historical background of, 162
    intended population for use of, 162–64
    length of time to teach approach of, 164
    method of using, 162–64
    ordering information for, 165
    summary of, 247
Morning sickness, blood glucose control
    during, 66
Myocardial infarction
    as risk factor of exercise for clients with
        cardiovascular disease, 31
    vitamin/mineral supplement evaluation
        for clients with, 25

N

National Cholesterol Education Program
    (NCEP), children's treatment
    guidelines of, 64
National Dairy Council, adaptation of *Guide
    to Good Eating* by, 133
National Research Council RDAs, 255
Native Americans, nephropathy incidence in,
    81
Nephropathy as microvascular complication
    of diabetes, 78, 81
Neuropathy
    autonomic, 79
    gastrointestinal, 79–81
    as microvascular complication of diabetes,
        78
    peripheral, 79
Non-insulin users, alcohol use guidelines for,
    24
Nonnutritive sweeteners, 23
Normoglycemia, achieving, 51
NPH injections
    initiating insulin therapy with, 38–39
    in regimen two insulin regimen, 40
Nutrition assessment, 99–105, 169
    case studies involving, 111, 202–3, 206–7,
        215–16, 218–19, 224, 229–31, 233–34
    collection of data for, 104–5
    components of, 100–104
    defined, 99–100
    initial, 102, 110
    preliminary data collected before, 100–101
    resources for, 140–41
Nutrition care plan
    for child or adolescent, 61
    individualizing, 245
Nutrition change goals, case study for, 112
Nutrition education for diabetes, 93–123
    for parents and caregivers of children with
        diabetes, 63
    resources for, 129, 132, 138–39, 139–45,
        147–52
    time frame for, 128
Nutrition guidelines
    basic, 127, 131–35
    for diabetes, 127, 137–45
Nutrition history for child or adolescent
    case study for, 224
    food history/preferences for, 62–63
    24-hour recalls and food records for, 62
Nutrition history for client with diabetes, 100
    for basic food guideline uses, 131, 133,
        134
    blank form for, 256
    case studies for, 111, 202–3, 207, 216,
        218–19, 229–31, 233
    for exchange lists uses, 169–70

information in, 101
    sample completed form for, 115, 258
Nutrition intervention, 15–17, 125–52
    case studies of, 203–4, 206, 216–17, 219,
        225
    components of, 107
    in-depth, 153–78
    determining priorities for, 189
    documenting effectiveness of, 245
    introduction to basic, 127–29
    for older adults with diabetes, 71
    resources for, 107
    time frame for, 110
Nutrition practice guidelines for types I and II
    diabetes, 7, 26
Nutrition prescription in diabetes medical
    nutrition therapy, 4
    as based on nutrition assessment and
        individual treatment goals, 25
    for inpatients, 127
    physician-determined, 25
Nutritional supplements
    for clients with gastrointestinal
        neuropathy, 80
    for older adults, 71
Nutritive sweeteners, 22–23

O

Obesity in person with type II diabetes, 11
    association of hypertension and, 24
    calorie-counting approach as appropriate
        for treating, 194
    decreased cardiovascular risk factor with
        exercise for, 30
Older adults, 68–72
    HHNS in, 77
    incidence of protein-energy malnutrition
        in, 70
    incidence of type II diabetes in, 68
    meal plans in LTC settings for, 70–71
    nutrition intervention for, 71
    special problems of, 69–70
Oral glucose-lowering medications, 51
    reactions to concurrent use of alcohol and
        certain, 84
    response of older adults to, 69
Outcome measures, client, 109

P

Pancreatic beta cells
    defective insulin-secretion response of,
        in type II diabetes, 11
    in emergence of type I diabetes, 11
Parenteral nutrition support for older adults, 71
Peripheral neuropathy, 31
Peripheral vascular disease as macrovascular
    complication of diabetes, 78
Pharmacists as diabetes educators, 5
Philosophy as guiding nutrition education
    programs, 95–97
Physical Activity History, 103
    sample completed form for, 118
Physicians
    in diabetes care team, 5, 51
    as diabetes educators, 5
Podiatrists as diabetes educators, 5
Polydipsia, 13
Polyols, 23
Polyphagia, 13
Polyunsaturated fats (PUFAs), calories from, 20
Polyuria, 13
    prior to development of HHNS, 77
Practice guidelines for diabetes medical
    nutrition therapy, 4

Preconception counseling for women with
    preexisting diabetes, 65
Preconception planning, 65
Prednisone, 45
Pregnancy
    metabolic changes during first trimester
        of, 65–66
    metabolic changes during second and
        third trimesters of, 66
Pregnant women. *See also* Gestational
    diabetes
    development of gestational diabetes
        mellitus in, 12
    diagnosis of diabetes in, 13
    role of diabetes medical nutrition therapy
        in, 61
    SMBG for, 43
    tight blood glucose control for, 58
    vitamin/mineral supplement evaluation
        for, 25
Protein
    nutrition recommendations for, 20
    snacking recommendations for, 88
Protein intake as affecting blood glucose
    levels, 187–88
Protein source, effect of, on progression of
    renal disease, 20
Protein-energy malnutrition (PEM) in older
    adults, 70
Psychosocial information about client, 103–4

R

RD/certified diabetes educator (CDE)
    as provider of diabetes medical nutrition
        therapy, 5
    roles of, 6
Reasonable body weight, goal of, 254
Recipe exchanges, guidelines for, 174–75
Registered dietitians
    in diabetes care team, 4, 5–7, 51
    as diabetes educators, 5
    as nutrition experts, 245
    as providers of diabetes medical nutrition
        therapy, 5
    roles of, 6, 25, 96
Registered nurses
    in diabetes care team, 5, 51
    as diabetes educators, 5
Rehydration, 91
Restaurant Companion, The, 237
Restaurant dining, meal planning for, 86–87
Retinal ischemia, 79
Retinopathy, 15
    as microvascular complication of diabetes, 78
    preventing, 79
    worsening of, as risk factor of exercise, 31

S

Saccharin use by diabetics, 23
Sedentary lifestyle as risk factor in
    development of type II diabetes, 11
Self-management of diabetes
    adjustments to training plan for, 246
    client training for, 51, 186
    clinical setting for introduction of, 58
    dietitian as leading nutritional aspect of, 5
    plan for, fine-tuning, 180–81
    promoting, 5
Self-monitoring of blood glucose (SMBG)
    flexibility for client of using, 88
    frequency of, 43–45, 51, 53, 57
    as important for deciding when to
        exercise, 32
    in Level 1 carbohydrate counting, 180
    in management of diabetes, 43–49

289

in monitoring effectiveness of meal plan, 169
in prevention of DKA, 78
in prevention of hypoglycemia after alcohol consumption, 83
in prevention of hypoglycemia with intensive insulin therapy, 186
in prevention or correction of ketosis in pregnant client, 67
problem patterns found in, common, 46
purpose of, 43
records from, evaluating, 3
Self-monitoring of blood glucose (SMBG) records
case study for type I diabetes using, 48–49
case study for type II diabetes using, 47–48
reviewing, 45–46
sample form for, 44
Sexual dysfunction, 79
Sick-day management for clients with diabetes, 91, 128
Simplified exchange system, 139–42
Simplified form for assessment of food intake, 258
Single-Topic Diabetes Resources, 147–52
advantages and disadvantages of, 151–52
case studies using, 204, 207, 225–26, 230–31
clinical setting for, 151
historical background of, 148
homework assignments for, 149
intended population for use of, 150–51
length of time to teach approach of, 151
method of using, 148–50
ordering information for, 152
professional guide for, 149–50
sample completed handouts for, 261–64
summary of, 247
tips for use of, 150
Smoking as worsening complications of diabetes, 78
Snacking for clients with diabetes, 87–89, 128
Social workers as diabetes educators, 5
Sodium
diet moderate in, 131
nutrition recommendations for, 24
Somogyi effect, 40, 46
Sorbitol, uses and energy value of, 23
Standardized meal patterns, advantages and disadvantages of, 25–26
Starvation ketosis, preventing, 66
modification of meal plan for, 67
Stress history, sample completed form for, 119
Stress-management skills in self-management of diabetes, 51
Sucrose
nutrition recommendations for, 21–22
nutritive sweeteners compared to, 22
unnecessary restriction in some meal-planning options of, 26
Sulfonylureas, 35
combination therapy with, 37
hypoglycemia in clients taking, 75
reaction to using alcohol with certain, 84
time activity of, 36
Summary Record, Lifestyle Change, 108
sample completed, 222
Sweeteners. *See also* Sucrose
nonnutritive, 23
nutritive, 22–23
Syringes, low-dose, 52

T

Thiazolidinediones, 36
Toddler, food records for, 62. *See also* Infant
Triglycerides, effects of alcohol on, 84
Troglitazone
hypoglycemia as not occurring in clients using, 76
to reduce insulin resistance, 36
Type I diabetes
association between hypertension and, 24
benefits of exercise for clients with, 30
complications of, 16
DKA in clients with, 78
goals of medical nutrition therapy for, 18, 61
IIT for clients with, 56
insulin deficiency in, 9
laboratory values of lipid and glucose for, 251
lipid levels in children with, 64
metabolic response to exercise in clients with, 29
nutrition practice guidelines for, 7, 26
onset of, 9, 11
pathophysiology of, 10–11
pregnancy in clients with, 66
recommendations for exercise for clients with, 32
SMBG for, 43–45
weight gain with IIT in clients with, 186
Type II diabetes
association between hypertension and, 24
benefits of exercise for clients with, 30
calorie-counting approach for obese clients with, 194
complications of, 16, 79
developed postpartum in clients with GDM, 10
goals of medical nutrition therapy for, 18–19, 128
laboratory values of lipid and glucose for, 251
loss of vision in clients with, 79
management of, 9–10
metabolic response to exercise in clients with, 29–30
nephropathy in clients with, 81
nutrition practice guidelines for, 7, 26
in older adults, 68
onset of, 9
pregnancy in clients with, 66
recommendations for exercise for clients with, 32
risk factors for development of, 11
SMBG for, 44–45
snacking discouraged for clients with, 88
weight loss in clients with, 18–19, 128, 186

U

Ultrafine needles, 52
US Department of Agriculture
and Department of Health and Human Services, *Dietary Guidelines for Americans* by, 131
and Food Marketing Institute, *Food Guide Pyramid* by, 134
US Department of Health and Human Services and US Department of Agriculture, *Dietary Guidelines for Americans* by, 131
US Department of Public Health, exchange lists developed by, 167
US Food and Drug Administration, sorbitol food labeling required by, 23

V

Vegetables in carbohydrate group for meal plans, 172
Vegetarians
exchange list values for meal planning for, 172
vitamin/mineral supplement evaluation for, 25
Very-low-calorie diets (VLCDs), 19
Viruses in emergence of type I diabetes, 11
Vision, loss of, 79
Vitamin/mineral supplements, recommendations for, 24–25
Vitrectomy, 79

W

Weight gain
in children and adolescents with diabetes, excessive, 61
as disadvantage of IIT, 59, 186
in pregnancy in clients with diabetes, 68
Weight history
information for, 103
sample completed form for, 117
Weight loss
in diagnosing diabetes, 13
in diabetes medical nutrition therapy, 79
focus of fat counting approach on, 197
as goal of medical nutrition therapy for type II diabetes, 18–19, 128, 186
study of calorie counting–lifestyle change approach to, 193
Weight ranges for men and women, table of healthy, 254
Wheeler, Madelyn L., 265

X

Xylitol, uses and energy value of, 23